D1245850

HUMOR

THE LIGHTER PATH TO RESILIENCE AND HEALTH

Paul McGhee, PhD

authorHOUSE®

AuthorHouse™
1663 Liberty Drive
Bloomington, IN 47403
www.authorhouse.com
Phone: 1-800-839-8640

First published by AuthorHouse 1/19/2010

ISBN: 978-1-4490-6069-5 (sc)
ISBN: 978-1-4490-6070-1 (e)

Printed in the United States of America
Bloomington, Indiana

This book is printed on acid-free paper.

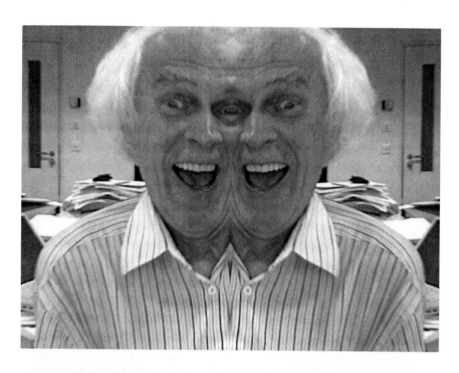

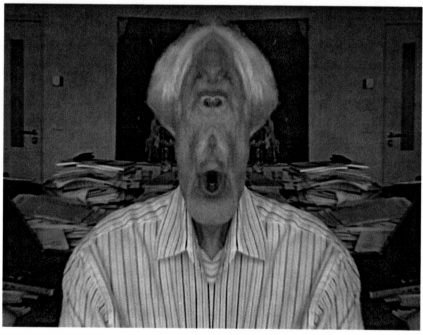

THE AUTHOR

ABOUT THE AUTHOR

Paul McGhee has a PhD in Psychology and is internationally known for his own research on humor, having published many scientific articles and 11 books on humor. He spent 20 years conducting basic research on humor and laughter and is generally viewed as a pioneer in the field.

He now works full time as a professional speaker and is President of The Laughter Remedy, in Wilmington, Delaware. He is at the cutting edge of the current movement to put humor to work in healthcare settings and corporations. He shows physicians, nurses and other healthcare professionals how to use humor to 1) cope with the growing pace of change and uncertainty in the healthcare system and 2) build the resilience needed to remain productive and provide quality care and service in the midst of growing job stress. In corporate settings, he shows how humor provides the emotional resilience needed to meet the challenges provided increasing work demands.

Dr. McGhee is internationally recognized as an authority on the physical and mental health benefits associated with humor. He has provided humor programs in 12 countries. His work has been featured in the *Scientific American: Mind, the New York Times, USA Today, The Learning Channel, PBS,* Dutch, Swiss and German television, and German, French, Swiss, Norwegian, Japanese and Italian magazines and newspapers.

His hands-on humor skills training program is the only program of its kind. It shows how to develop the basic skills required to use humor to become more effective in your work and cope with job stress. The program has been shown to be effective in four countries.

For additional information Dr. McGhee's keynotes, as well as both a discussion of research on the health and coping benefits of humor and guidelines for improving your own humor skills, see his web site at www.LaughterRemedy.com.

Contents

PREFACE

"After God created the world, He made man and woman. Then, to keep the whole thing from collapsing, He invented humor."

(Guillermo Mordillo)

THIS BOOK IS AN UPDATE of the first half of my 1999 book, *Health, Healing and the Amuse System: Humor as Survival Training.* The first half of that book included chapters on humor and physical health, using humor to cope with stress and humor in the workplace. The second half presented my hands-on Humor Skills Training Program. That book has now been split into two new books for several reasons. One is that an enormous amount of new research has been conducted which either directly examines the link between humor and physical health or has clear implications for the impact of humor on health. Another is that in the year 2000, studies using new neuroimaging technologies began to study how the brain is engaged in the comprehension and enjoyment of humor. I felt that it was important to include this exciting new information in the same volume as the new work relating humor to health and resilience.

Finally, an entire new field, called Positive Psychology, was created in 1999. As noted in the Introduction, humor is considered a key "character strength" within this new field, but researchers who call themselves positive psychologists have shown little interest in humor. And yet, some of the findings from new this field are of direct relevance to our understanding of humor. I felt that it was essential to include this work in any discussion of the physical and emotional benefits associated with humor. Similarly, a great deal of research on humor has direct relevance to key concerns of Positive Psychology. Most positive psychologists seem to be unaware of this research, so the present book is, in part, designed to acquaint them with humor research that is directly related to their own interests.

Including a detailed discussion of all of these areas, while retaining the presentation of the 8-Step Humor Skills Training Program included in the previous book, would have doubled the size of the earlier volume. So it simply made more sense to break the previous book into two separate books. The chapter on Humor in the Workplace, included in *Health, Healing and the Amuse System*, was omitted here partly for space reasons and partly to create a sharper focus in this book on humor's impact on health and personal/emotional resilience. The 8-Step Program for learning to use humor to cope with stress is published as a separate book (with the new title, *Humor as Survival Training for a Stressed-Out World*) with Author House, and will be available in the Spring of 2010.

Who is this Book Written for?

As with *Health, Healing and the Amuse System*, I have tried to write this book in a manner that is interesting to both the general reader and those who either conduct research on humor or have a general background in some area of psychology. It is also written for nurses, physicians, social workers, therapists and counselors, and anyone else who works in a broad range of allied fields concerned with promoting good physical and mental health. I have specifically geared much of the book toward the rapidly growing numbers of people interested in applications of Positive Psychology. Many who are already working in this new field are unaware of the direct relevance of the evidence presented here for their own interest in supporting the development of character strengths and resilience. Finally, the book is designed to be suitable as a textbook for university courses focusing specifically on the health and coping benefits associated with humor.

If you have no background in any health-related field, some of the material included here may seem overly-detailed and difficult to follow. In anticipation of this, I have included at the beginning of each chapter a "preliminary summary" which is designed to provide a general understanding of the contents of the chapter before getting into the details. If you find yourself getting bogged down in the details at any point, go back to the summary again to get a good sense of the "big picture" before going back to the details.

Skill-Building Exercises

Each chapter contains a series of boxes entitled, "Build Your Humor Skills." Each box contains two or three jokes with a key part of the punch line missing. A clue is provided to get you thinking in the right direction without giving the answer. These verbal humor exercises are designed to demonstrate one way to build your skill at playing with language. As with all aspects of humor, strengthening your verbal sense of humor is a matter of developing the habit of playing with language in different ways.

My book, "*Small Medium at Large*" (also published by Author House), provides several hundred jokes and stories using this technique, enabling you to cultivate the habit of coming up with your own spontaneous verbal humor. Developing this skill when you're not under stress enables you to have access to it as a coping tool when you are under stress. I have published a similar book for 7- to 12-year-old children, *Stumble Bees and Pelephones*; that book is designed to build children's verbal humor skills at the point where they are very excited about learning and telling riddles, knock-knock jokes, etc. (See my website, www.LaughterRemedy.com, for more information on this book.)

Professional Organizations Devoted to Improving Your Understanding of Humor

There are many organizations devoted to humor in one way or another. Two of these are especially important to improving your understanding of humor. One is for either the general lay person who has an active interest in the benefits of humor or any person working in a health-related field. It is called the Association for Applied and Therapeutic Humor (see www.aath.org for information about the organization and their annual conferences). As the name suggests, AATH is committed to providing information on practical applications of humor. As their website says, "Our mission is to serve the community of professionals who study, practice & promote healthy humor & laughter."

For those interested in basic research on humor and laughter, the annual meetings of the International Society for Humor Studies (Google this name to get to their website) may be of greater interest. This is an inter-disciplinary scholarly organization which has been dedicated for the past 30+ years to the advancement of humor research. It publishes a quarterly journal for researchers called *Humor: International Journal of Humor Research.*

Special Thanks

I would like to extend a special thank you to Frank Appletree Rodden and Barbara Wild (University of Tuebingen, Germany) and Andrea Samson (University of Fribourg, Switzerland) for their comments on earlier versions of Chapter 3, Humor and the Brain.

Introduction

Humor and Positive Psychology

During the 1990s, a group of psychologists became increasingly dissatisfied with the decades-long emphasis on negative emotion, stress and mental illness within psychology. They determined to change this, and the end result was the creation of a new field of research devoted to the study of such topics as character strengths, resilience, happiness, life satisfaction, and psychological and physical well-being, among others. This new field was called Positive Psychology, and is sometimes referred to as the study of what makes life worth living . . . the "good life."[1] One underlying goal of this new field has been to achieve enough understanding of these positive qualities to help people "evolve toward their highest potential." Abraham Maslow long ago discussed this notion as becoming a "self-actualizing" person.[2] Positive psychologists have more recently referred to it as "human flourishing."

From its inception, Positive Psychology has consistently moved along two parallel lines. One involves basic research on the nature and determinants of happiness, resilience, life satisfaction and other positive aspects of life. The other has a clear applied focus. Even as the basic research remains in its infancy, rapidly growing numbers of practitioners around the world now eagerly work to help both individuals and organizations build a more positive focus into their life and business. Because of this strong applied focus, one of the newest thrusts of research in the field now focuses on the impact of specific positive interventions.

Widespread interventions are already occurring on an individual basis through people who are generally referred to as "coaches."[3] In contrast to therapists, who typically work with individuals struggling with serious emotional conflicts or mental disorders, personal (or life) coaches work with healthy and high-functioning individuals to help them thrive or flourish.

Many companies are also now addressing the issue of character strengths (or lack thereof) within their organization—sometimes as a result of the questionable conduct of CEOs and other business leaders in recent years.[4] Character strengths presumably generally lead people to "do the right thing," and businesses increasingly realize that they need to hire people who can be expected to do the right thing precisely because they possess such strengths. Because of the growing belief in the importance of such character strengths, positive interventions aimed at improving morale, communication and productivity have become much more common in recent years.[5]

The explosion of interest in Positive Psychology is not restricted to the United States; it is occurring world-wide.[6] And it has already led to the development of several Masters Degree programs specifically devoted to applications in this field. The first of these was the Master of Applied Positive Psychology (or MAPP) program at the University of Pennsylvania. The University of Pennsylvania website notes that this degree program is ". . . for psychologists, educators, life coaches and other professionals interested in the application of a psychology that focuses on positive emotions, strengths-based character and healthy institutions. The program trains students in the history, theory and research methods of Positive Psychology and helps them to apply the concepts and techniques in their professional settings."

The burgeoning body of research in this exciting new field will not be reviewed here. Many recently-published reviews are already available. These include *The Science of Subjective Well-Being* (2008), by Michael Eid and Randy Larsen, *Happiness: Unlocking the Mysteries of Psychological Wealth* (2008), by Ed Diener and Robert Biswas-Diener, the *Oxford Handbook of Positive Psychology* (2009), by Shane Lopez and C. R. Snyder, and *The Collected Works of Ed Diener* (2009), among others. The goal of this introduction is to call attention to the surprising lack of interest in humor—an acknowledged character strength—among Positive Psychology researchers.

Throughout the first decade of intense research within Positive Psychology, the topic of humor has been consistently neglected—in spite of the fact that (as this book shows) many well-established humor research findings clearly relate to many key concerns of the field. This book is designed to help overcome that neglect.

The Core Character Strengths and Virtues

One of the key starting points of Positive Psychology was the identification and study of enduring positive human traits. This led to the identification of 24 core strengths of character.[7] Each strength is seen as part of one of six basic virtues. The virtue of wisdom and knowledge is composed of five character strengths: these include creativity, curiosity, open-mindedness, perspective (wisdom) and love of learning and. Four strengths compose the virtue of courage, including bravery (valor), persistence, integrity and vitality. The virtue called humanity is composed of the strengths love, kindness (nurturance, compassion), and social/emotional intelligence. Justice is a virtue defined by strengths of citizenship (social responsibility, teamwork), fairness and leadership. The virtue of temperance includes strengths of forgiveness/mercy, humility/modesty, prudence and self-regulation. Finally the virtue of *transcendence* includes strengths related to the appreciation of beauty and excellence, gratitude, hope/optimism, *humor/playfulness* and spirituality.

Lack of Interest in Humor within Positive Psychology

As of 2010, the core character strength of humor has received little attention from Positive Psychology researchers—in spite of evidence that a sample of nearly 1100 young American adults reported humor to be (on average) their third greatest strength (behind only kindness and love.[8] Major books by acknowledged leaders in the field do not include the word humor in the subject index—let alone devote a chapter to it. This includes *A Psychology of Human Strengths* (edited by Aspinwall & Staudinger in 2003), *Happiness: Unlocking the Mysteries of Psychological Wealth* (by Diener & Biswas-Diener in 2008) and the *Oxford Handbook of Positive Psychology* (edited by Lopez and Snyder in 2009), among others. In some cases, the word is included in the subject index, and a few paragraphs—less than one page—give a token nod to its importance (e.g., *The Science of Subjective Well-Being* by Eid & Larsen in 2008).

This consistent failure of leaders in Positive Psychology to give any attention to humor has long puzzled me. When the field was created a little over a decade ago, I assumed that interest would quickly emerge because of humor's obvious and well-established link to the some of the main concerns of Positive Psychology. Since a full decade has passed, and humor as a character strength has still not appeared on the radar screen of the field, the question is why? Among the 64 chapters in the latest (2009) *Oxford Handbook of Positive Psychology*, none of the 131 contributors to the volume saw any basis for including humor or laughter in their discussion of the field. The most obvious place for inclusion would be the numerous chapters in Part 10 of the book focusing on "Specific Coping Approaches." (It should be noted that a chapter on humor was included in the first edition of the *Handbook*, but then excluded in the revised edition.)

My own conversations with several leaders in the field have led me to the conclusion that many positive psychologists (researchers and applied practitioners) are unaware of the widespread research on humor and laughter; others are simply interested in other things. Hopefully, this book will begin to inform those who are interested in the topic, but unaware of the research, and generate interest among those who have had no interest in humor in the past.

One interesting exception to this pattern of neglect in books on Positive Psychology was the inclusion of a chapter on laughter in the recent (2007) *Oxford Handbook of Methods in Positive Psychology* (edited by Ong and van Dulmen). The two writers of this chapter emphasize that Positive Psychology has failed to consider the importance of laughter to the field.[9] They correctly note that "The neglect of laughter is unfortunate because the topic of laughter has much to offer the study of positive psychology." Interestingly, at no point do they mention the idea that humor, similarly, has much to offer the field of Positive Psychology, in spite of their admission that considerably more research has been completed on humor than on laughter. This appears to simply reflect the authors' special interest in laughter, as opposed to humor.

These authors emphasize, however (and I agree), that since the benefits offered by laughter may be independent of (and different from) those associated with humor, the two must be independently measured. This distinction has been consistently neglected during the resurgence of humor research over the past 25 years. Among the many studies of humor completed, some researchers talk about their data by discussing humor, while others focus on laughter. There is an obvious confounding here, since the humor and laughter occur together. In virtually all humor research, no effort has been made to sort out whether the findings of interest are due to the emotional and mental experience of humor or the physical act of laughter that follows—even when data on both laughter and some kind of humor judgment are obtained.

It should be noted from the outset that the present book focuses on the importance of humor *and* laughter for Positive Psychology. However, for virtually all of the findings discussed here, the relative contribution of humor vs. laughter is not known and not discussed. It seems likely that both make a contribution to varying degrees. Thus, when a statement is made about humor, it should be assumed that the effect or benefit attributed to humor is actually in response to some unknown combined influence of humor and laughter. This avoids the cumbersome habit of repeating "humor/laughter" or "humor and laughter" throughout the book. In a few exceptions to this rule, specific separate influences of the two are discussed.

At the 1st International Positive Psychology Association World Congress held in Philadelphia in June of 2009, there were 15 invited presentations, 15 symposia (including 60 different presentations), nine workshops and 265 poster presentations. Only two poster sessions—one of which was my own—(and no other presentations) included the word humor in the presentation title. This is consistent with the failure to consider the topic in books claiming to cover the entire field of Positive Psychology.

On the other hand, among the conference attendees who stopped by my poster (entitled "Can a sense of humor be trained? Evidence from the 8-Step Program.") in order to discuss the findings, the great majority emphasized that this topic was an important piece that was clearly missing within Positive Psychology. Current and former

MAPP students wondered why it was not given greater attention in their courses. I spent five hours (without leaving my poster, except for a 3-minute bathroom break) speaking to a non-stop stream of conference attendees who wanted to learn more about humor's importance and whether you really could train people to improve their humor skills to the point that they might be used to cope with life stress and improve the quality of one's life. (As already noted, intervention approaches which have lasting effects in strengthening key character strengths are currently of great interest in Positive Psychology.)

This expression of interest was not restricted to Americans. Attendees from many different countries wanted to learn more about the benefits of humor and how to help people get those benefits into their lives. Among those who stopped by my poster were people from Germany, Belgium, Israel, Japan, Russia, England, Australia, the Azores, Netherlands, and New Zealand, among numerous others. Representatives of two countries specifically expressed interest in translating the Humor Skills Training Program for use in their own country. This poster experience and many conversations throughout the conference suggested to me that the interest in humor among non-researchers (especially those engaged in applications of Positive Psychology) is very strong.

In part, then, this book is designed to update those already interested in (or working in) the field of Positive Psychology on the ways in which humor and laughter contribute to positive emotion, resilience, mental and physical health and well-being, and life-satisfaction. Practitioners clearly are yearning for more information on this topic; hopefully, Positive Psychology researchers will follow their lead and begin to address the role of humor in Positive Psychology, as well.

Importance of Positive Emotion in Daily Life

The single most important theme within Positive Psychology is the importance of positive emotion in one's daily life. Quite simply, people who have more positive emotion in their lives are happier and more satisfied with their lives.[10] Greater amounts of positive emotion are also associated with greater success in coping with adversity,[11] greater trust in others,[12] more successful relationships,[13] greater success at work,[14] and even a longer life.[15]

Of course, much of this research is correlational in nature and does not demonstrate that positive emotion has caused these positive outcomes. It could also be that the positive emotion experienced is the result of accumulated successful outcomes in these areas. The most convincing case for positive emotion being the cause of such outcomes would be a demonstration of their occurrence in response to interventions which increase positive emotion. Some research along these lines has been completed, and there is growing evidence that interventions which boost one's daily dose of positive emotion do build key psychological, mental and social resources.[16]

When measures are taken at two different times (a prospective study), more frequent positive affect at time predicts (at a later time) greater happiness,[17] psychological growth,[18] and resilience in the face of adversity.[19] It similarly predicts several general mechanisms associated with better physical health, including lower blood levels of cortisol, reduced inflammatory response to stress[20] and reduced pain the next day.[21] It also predicts increased resistance to the common cold,[22] reduced incidence of stroke among the elderly[23] and even greater longevity.[24]

A meta-analysis was completed of 70 prospective studies linking psychological well-being to subsequent mortality. Half of these studies were on initially healthy individuals, while the other half focused on people with some illness. Those showing high initial positive psychological well-being had lower subsequent mortality rates, both among initially healthy individuals and people already dealing with some disease. This finding held even when controlling for the level of negative affect experienced. So ". . . the protective effects of positive psychological well-being were independent of negative affect."[25]

As will be seen throughout this book, similar findings have been obtained in connection with humor and laughter—with the exception of a longer life.

The Broaden-and-Build Theory of Positive Emotion

The obvious question that arises in the midst of the large (and rapidly growing) mass of data pointing to the importance of positive emotion is why it generates such tremendous benefits in promoting happiness, life satisfaction and a general sense of well-being. What is it about positive emotion that promotes resilience? The most promising explanation offered to this point was put forth by Barbara Fredrickson and is called the Broaden-and-Build theory of positive emotion.[26] The Broaden-and-Build theory proposes that positive emotions serve to build many different kinds of lasting personal resources—intellectual, social and emotional. It suggests that positive emotion produces various kinds of approach behaviors which lead to increased exploration and interaction with the environment. These exploratory behaviors lead to increased cognitive, social and emotional resources, which, in turn, result in more flexible and more successful adaptation or coping, along with better health and personal flourishing. Greater flexibility is possible because of the lack of any immediate outside threat which serves to put constraints on behavior. And it is this broadened set of personal resources which allows one to bounce back from adversity.

In support of her notion of "broadening," Fredrickson and a colleague[27] note that positive emotion leads to increased attention to peripheral objects,[28] more flexible[29] and more creative[30] thinking, increased receptiveness to new information,[31] more careful consideration of different problems,[32] greater trust,[33] and greater bonding with others.[34]

This is very reminiscent of the long-established benefits offered by play—a key source of positive affect. When animals are playing in the wild, they are cultivating skills and acquiring information that is crucial to their survival as adults.[35] During play activities (e.g., play fighting), they develop key skills that their life may depend on some day. Similarly, play among human children has long been recognized as a crucial means of learning and building skills that are important for successfully adapting to their world. I have argued for the past 30 years[36] that humor is actually a form of mental play—play with ideas. Just as physical play helps animals develop skills that are crucial for their survival later on, the mental play that is at the core of humor plays an important role in our psychological survival. It does this by boosting emotional resilience in the midst of stress.

Chapter 3 presents evidence that humor activates known dopamine-based pleasure centers in the brain. This may be one of the mechanisms by which play and humor support children's (and adults') learning. Consistent with this notion, one pair of researchers has argued that positive emotion leads to the release of dopamine, and that this is the basis for the intellectual gains (including creative problem solving) associated with positive emotion.[37]

There is evidence that positive emotion initiates a reciprocal relationship with coping in which the experience of positive emotion enhances coping, which—in turn—leads to greater positive affect.[38] This generates what the researchers called an "upward spiral of emotional well-being." It is important to note that this upward spiral only occurred for positive forms of coping, not negative ones. This upward spiral of mutual influence may well be one of the key mechanisms via which positive emotion boosts resilience.

Resilience

A second major theme within Positive Psychology is the notion of resilience. Resilience can be viewed as the ability to cope with the adversity in one's life and "bounce back" from the negative emotions that accompany that adversity.[39] Those who demonstrate this capacity on an ongoing basis are considered to have trait resilience; it is an enduring part of their personality.

An enormous amount of research over the past 50 years has been devoted to the negative impact of stress and trauma on people. However, it has always been clear that many people exposed to major life trauma somehow have the emotional strength and resilience to pull through it all with minimal lasting impact on their mental health. This was noted long ago by Victor Frankl in the Nazi death camps during WWII.[40] In fact, some individuals actually thrive in the midst of difficult life circumstances.[41]

People with high trait resilience have been shown to adapt more successfully to stressful life events, whether they are of a traumatic nature or not.[42] They also show more complete emotional recovery when an anticipated negative event does not actually occur.[43]

Positive Emotion is the Key to Building Resilience

Fredrickson and her colleagues argue that resilient individuals find ways to generate positive emotion for themselves when they encounter stress.[44] A growing body of evidence suggests that it is this higher level of positive emotion that accounts for the enhanced ability of resilient individuals to prevent depression and bounce back from stressful events[45]. . . and flourish generally.[46] This resilience-boosting influence of positive emotion is quite distinct from the processes that regulate negative emotion in the midst of stress.[47] And interventions which serve to increase positive emotions boost one's resilience.[48]

While we generally think of only negative emotion being present in times of stress, both positive and negative emotions have been found to occur in some people when stress is chronically present. When the same stress is present day after day, positive emotions provide a "respite" and help replenish depleted personal/emotional resources.[49] This has been found in connection with a wide range of conditions, including caregiving partners of men with AIDS[50] and patients with spinal cord injuries[51] or chronic illness.[52]

One way to build positive emotion into your daily life whenever you need or want it, of course, is to simply build more humor into your life, by either immersing yourself in the humor of others (via TV, DVDs, going to comedy movies, etc.) or finding more humor in your own everyday life. It is no surprise, then, that people with high levels of trait resilience often use humor as a coping strategy.[53] Even children with high trait resilience initiate more humor when under stress than children with low trait resilience.[54] Increased use or appreciation of humor has also been found to be associated with increased resilience among cancer patients,[55] surgical patients[56] and even combat veterans (from the Vietnam War).[57] Fortunately, it has now been shown (as discussed in Chapter 1) that it is possible strengthen humor skills among adults, so that they can be used to cope with life stress.

The Importance of Experiencing More Positive than Negative Emotion

Recent epidemiological research has indicated that roughly the same percentage of the U.S. population that meet established criteria for mental illness (about 20%) can be considered to be flourishing in terms of mental health.[58] That means that about 60% (most of us) lie somewhere in the middle. Since I abandoned my own research career in the field of humor (to become a professional speaker), I have seen countless numbers of these middle-of-the-roaders putting in their time at their increasingly stressful jobs (which they don't enjoy), dealing with relationships that are neither wonderful nor distressing and just going through the motions of life generally. I don't see a lot of joy, enthusiasm or excitement in these lives. Many in this middle group are stressed out at work and are missing a lot of days at work due to illness, burnout, etc. When they are at work, their job performance is down. The cost to the economy of this general "languishing" on the job, and in life generally, has been estimated to be in the billions of dollars every year.[59] Clearly, it is crucial—even at the economic level—to provide people with tools that boost mental health and coping . . . and help people flourish.[60]

An important early insight into this issue was the recognition 25 years ago that positive and negative affect are basically independent of each other.[61] More recently, it has been recognized that a key determinant of happiness and life satisfaction is the ratio of positive to negative affect experienced in a typical day.[62] Ed Diener and his colleagues determined early on that the frequency of positive emotional states in comparison to negative ones over a person's life strongly predicts global life satisfaction.[63]

A higher ratio of positive to negative emotional states predicts overall subjective well-being.[64] Among individuals in treatment for depression, those who show optimal recovery from depression have positivity ratios that jump from lower than 1:1 to higher than 4:1.[65] Partners in happy, stable marriages have positivity ratios of about 5:1, while those heading for divorce have ratios below 1:1.[66]

Fredrickson's research on individuals who are flourishing also suggests that the thing that distinguishes them is that they have higher ratios of positive to negative affect in their daily life than people who are not flourishing.[67] The threshold for achieving this resilient state of flourishing mental health appears to be about three positive emotional experiences to every negative one experienced. Of course, some emotions are more intense and lasting than others; but this pattern—on average—characterizes resilient people with flourishing mental health. This issue is further discussed below.

Given the importance of a 3:1 ratio of positive to negative emotions for emotional well-being, it is crucial to have effective tools for assuring that positive emotions are built into your daily life when you need them. There are many ways of doing this, including counting your blessings, prayer, meditation and finding positive meaning within negative events.[68] While there are no data on the impact of humor upon this ratio, the findings discussed in Chapter 1 make a strong case for humor's effectiveness in keeping the positive side of the ratio at an elevated level.

When you're having a bad day, the ratio of positive to negative progressively shifts toward negativity. Once the ball starts rolling in a negative direction, it is hard for most of us to change course. The negative emotion of the moment generates negative thoughts about what might happen next (e.g., "I'll get fired if I can't get this project done by the deadline"). *Some kind of well-practiced habit is needed to jump-start a good positive feeling in the midst of the negative things happening at the moment.*

Humor is one quick and effective means of generating a positive emotion, but most of us find that our sense of humor abandons us right when we need it the most—when we are angry, tense, anxious or depressed. That's why it is important to cultivate basic humor skills like playing with language and finding a light side of things happening at the moment when you're in a good mood . . . so you'll have access to this habit when you're in a bad mood. For those who don't want to make this effort, you can always try carrying around your favorite book of cartoons (The *Far Side* works for me), since mere exposure to humor also generates a more positive mood.[69]

There is also some evidence that laughter alone may be sufficient to elevate a positive mood—even when there's nothing particularly funny to laugh at.[70] Laughter Clubs around the world now invite people to do "laugh for no reason" exercises with this idea in mind.

Stronger and More Lasting Impact of Negative Emotion. There is mounting evidence that negative events have a stronger and more lasting emotional impact than positive ones;[71] that is, we carry the resulting negative emotion around with us for a longer period of time. This is not surprising, since negative emotion often signaled a genuine threat to survival early in our evolution. While we now rarely experience a threat to our physical survival, the same biological systems that initially prepared us for "fight or flight" remain active when we experience a threat to our psychological survival—when we are chronically angry or anxious. In extreme cases, we "stew in our emotional juices" day after day when things are going badly.

Given this greater impact of negative emotion, it is not surprising that a 3:1 ratio of positive to negative emotions is essential for human flourishing. This means that we need extra sources of positivity in our lives when things start heading south. It is also essential to have effective tools for "letting go" of negative emotions when they are no longer adaptive. Humor and laughter provide an ideal tool for achieving both of these goals. As discussed in Chapter 1, they are very effective in letting go of negative emotion (especially frustration, upset and anger), while adding frequent small doses of positive emotion throughout the day.

More Rapid Adaptation to Positive Events. The flip side of the greater persistence of negative emotion is the fact that we habituate to positive events more rapidly than to negative ones.[72] As a result of this, some individuals appear to consciously look for ways to generate and maintain a positive mood during their daily life. "Counting your blessings" is one way to do this,[73] and purposefully committing acts of kindness is another.[74] I have seen several bumper stickers on cars suggesting that people commit random acts of kindness. One familiar act along these lines is to pay the toll of the car behind you—even though you have no idea who that may be. Such acts have been shown to boost the positive mood of the person committing the acts.[75] And, of course, we all know people who use music or their spiritual faith to boost their spirits and stay positive.[76]

The active use of your sense of humor is simply one additional tool you can use to elevate your mood when you need or want to.

Positive Emotion and Life Satisfaction/Happiness

We all encounter stress in our lives, but it is less likely to have a negative impact if we are happy in general.[77] One's happiness and emotional well-being at any given time reflects the overall balance of positive and negative emotions felt at the moment. On some days, our mood persists in the same positive or negative direction throughout the day. On others, it fluctuates back and forth as mood-changing events thrust themselves into our lives. One's emotional state at any given moment is certainly important for happiness and life satisfaction, but the extent to which a given positive or negative state is present day after day is much more important. This is viewed as an emotional "trait"—a stable part of one's self over time.

Some of us have personality traits (like extraversion) that predispose us to experience positive affect (and happiness) more often, while others have personality traits (like neuroticism) which predispose us to more negative affect (and unhappiness).[78] Other personality traits, like optimism, self-esteem, hardiness and a desire for control have also been found to be strong predictors of happiness.[79] Such stable temperaments/dispositions have long been assumed to have a strong genetic component. It was recently reported that as much as 50% of the variability in people's general happiness level can be accounted for by genetic factors.[80] Of course, this also means that 50% of people's happiness level can be changed. The use of positive emotion to manage one's daily mood can play a major role in assuring that this modifiable half of daily happiness is biased in the direction of greater happiness.

My own view of such "heritability" studies is that while genetic factors may well account for 50% of the variance in people's happiness levels in any given sample of people, this does not mean that the 50% finding cannot be changed by purposefully providing effective interventions which have a lasting impact on one's daily diet of positive emotion. If you were to take the same subjects that generated the 50% happiness heritability score and (assuming that you have a large enough sample) expose half of them to an intervention which had a lasting impact of their (increased) daily experience of positive emotion from that point onwards, and compare them with those who did not receive this intervention, I would be startled if the intervention failed to reduce the heritability estimate.

In the case of life satisfaction, which involves a more conscious reflection about (and evaluation of) the developments in one's life to this point, a key question that arises within both Positive Psychology generally, and humor research specifically, is whether it is increased positive emotion or reduced negative emotion that is most important in sustaining high levels of life satisfaction. In a study of over 8,000 people from 46 countries, when all the countries were combined, "the experience of positive emotions was more strongly related to life satisfaction than the absence of negative emotions."[81]

Consistent with this finding, when individuals' emotional states were monitored daily for a month, the level of positive emotion experienced predicted subsequent increases in resilience. Equally important was the finding that *"Changes in resilience mediated the relation between positive emotions and increased life satisfaction, suggesting that happy people become more satisfied not simply because they feel better but because they develop resources for living well."*[82] (Italics are McGhee's.) So this study suggests that it is not just the sum of good and bad feelings that combine to determine one's level of life satisfaction. Rather, it is the boost in resilience associated with positive emotion that accounts for increased life satisfaction. (It is also worth noting that positive emotion predicted the resilience/life satisfaction boost even when the amount of negative emotion experienced was considered.)

One key focus of this book is the impact of humor on resilience. While some of the research specifically links humor to resilience, most of the data discussed focus on humor's effectiveness in helping individuals cope with life stress. Good coping skills are assumed here to be crucial to achieving high levels of resilience, since they help reduce the negative emotion that goes with stress, substituting positive emotion in its place. As we shall see, humor is very effective in simultaneously reducing negative emotion and increasing positive emotion. Thus, even when the term resilience is not used (especially in Chapter 1), it remains the author's underlying assumption that evidence of increased coping skills are tantamount to increased levels of personal/emotional resilience.

As just noted, resilience-linked boosts in positive emotion are central to the achievement of increased life satisfaction. It will be shown in Chapter 1 that humor is a reliable tool for boosting positive emotion and mood. There is also evidence (discussed in Chapter 1) that my humor skills training program boosts humor skills, and that they are sustained three months after completion of the training.[83] This training program is presented in my book, *Humor as Survival Training for a Stressed-Out World*.[84]

CHAPTER 1

HUMOR AND RESILIENCE

"If it weren't for the brief respite we give the world with our foolishness, the world would see mass suicide in numbers that compare favorably with the death rate of the lemmings."

(Groucho Marx)

"If I had no sense of humor, I should long ago have committed suicide."

(Mohandas K. Gandhi)

IF YOU RANDOMLY SELECT 100 people on the street and ask them if it's important to have a good sense of humor, most will say yes without hesitation. They would recognize that humor helps get through the tough times ("If I didn't laugh, I'd cry!"). But what appears to be an obviously important set of skills for getting through our daily life has not always been considered important enough for researchers to study in a "serious" fashion. As noted in Chapter 2, it was not until the 1980s that psychologists and others began to systematically look at the ways in which humor contributes to both physical and emotional health and well being.

Imagine for a moment that you are an alien from another planet (perhaps you are a logic-oriented Vulcan, like Spock in the old television series, *Star Trek*). You arrive on Earth and observe a most bizarre behavior in humans. They see or say something incongruous or otherwise unusual/unexpected and then go through a puzzling sequence of behaviors. Major facial muscles contract and pull upward and to the side (producing what they call a "smile"), their mouth opens up and their diaphragm and stomach muscles start a series of contractions which produce a strange repetitive sound—a kind of "ha-ha-ha-ha-ha" that sometimes goes on and on to the point where they have trouble standing up. Their body seems to be out of control with involuntary spasms. Sometimes they hold their sides when they've been doing this for several minutes. Surely, it must be very painful . . . and yet they look so happy. But many of them do have tears coming out of their eyes, so they must be very sad when they do this.

You continue to watch more closely, and you notice that they seem to be gasping for air. This odd breathing pattern causes them to push out as much air as possible from their lungs before taking a deep breath and starting the whole process all over again. You discover that their heart is also racing and their blood pressure jumps much higher. Their faces are pinker because of the increased blood flow to their cheeks. Many of them slump over in their chairs; or if they're standing up, it looks like they're about to fall over. In fact, you notice that the young humans really do fall down on the floor while they're doing this . . . they can't stand up! Some are rolling on the floor. Again, it all looks so painful, and yet they look so happy.

When the humans explain that this is called laughter, and that they can't help themselves, you become all the more concerned about its impact on their well being. They finally explain why they're laughing and you become all the more puzzled. They laugh at things that are just absurd and make no sense. As an alien who does not have the strong drive to play (physically or mentally) as part of your biological heritage, you never manage to understand either humor or laughter, no matter how often humans explain it. And you would never be convinced that this strange behavior might be good for you or help you cope with stressful times.

Even if you are someone who has always been pretty serious in your adult life, you are certain to have more insight into the importance of humor than this alien. Chances are, however, that—because of this seriousness—you've never had any direct personal experience with how humor and laughter can ease life's burdens on the tough days. This chapter shows how your sense of humor contributes to personal resilience, focusing mainly on how it provides you with a crucial skill to help cope with the mounting stress we all find in our lives these days. As Groucho Marx suggested more that half a century ago, a

2

good sense of humor helps keep your sanity in the worst of conditions. It is a natural stress remedy that you want to take full advantage of.

As I was writing this chapter in February of 2009, the insight within the Groucho Marx and Gandhi quotes became tragically poignant. The news media had just reported that the number of suicides by military personnel returning from Iraq had risen dramatically (24 in January of 2009 among those already back in the United States). Throughout 2007 and 2008, I remember hearing endless reports about the high level of post-traumatic-stress-syndrome among returning soldiers. Spouses of returning soldiers reported relationship difficulties, noting that their spouse was just not the same person who had gone to Iraq a couple of years earlier.

In September of 2009, an article by a writer for *Military Times* reported that 106,726 American veterans of the wars in Afghanistan and Iraq had been diagnosed with mental health issues after leaving the service (data were from a Department of Veterans Affairs study). Within this figure, 22% had been diagnosed with post-traumatic stress disorder. (The article notes that this figure is probably higher, since it does not include troops still on active duty or those who have sought help outside the VA system.) But major efforts were finally underway to provide better mental health support to our returning troops by 2009. As we shall see later in this chapter, humor has long had an important role to play in military conflicts, where one's life is continually at risk.

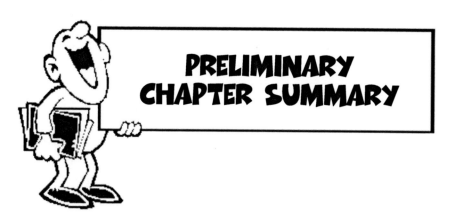

PRELIMINARY CHAPTER SUMMARY

For the past two decades, the stress level in most people's lives has continued to mount—especially because of rising job demands, but also because of rising healthcare costs, the threat of terrorism, gasoline prices, personal health problems, and finally the economic crisis of 2008-2010 on top of everything else that had us feeling we were approaching our stress limits. There is ample evidence that stress is taking a heavy toll on the nation's health—both physically and mentally/emotionally. The negative emotion accompanying stress, and the underlying physiological changes associated with it, plays a key role in generating a broad range of health problems. The ability to manage this negative emotion effectively is crucial to sustaining good physical and mental health. Humor is shown here to be a powerful tool in managing one's emotions.

In the midst of this tsunami of stress sweeping over ever-increasing numbers of people, it is more important than ever to cultivate basic skills that boost our personal and emotional resilience. As already noted in the Introduction, your sense of humor plays a key role in resilience; it helps you bend without breaking on your worst days— and cope better in meeting the challenges posed by the stress in your life. As noted below, it is a powerful ally in any effort to bounce back from adversity.

A broad range of research has documented the effectiveness of humor as a tool for coping with life stress. This includes experimental studies in which people are purposefully put in stressful situations, as well as studies of people who score higher on sense of humor tests. In both cases, humor is associated with reduced levels of anger, anxiety, depression and sadness. Consistent with these findings, exposure to humor reduces the level of stress hormones circulating in the blood. Just as importantly, humor boosts the level of positive emotion experienced at the same time that it reduces negative emotion. In fact, *this boost in positive emotion appears to be one of the key mechanisms through which humor increases emotional resilience.*

Humor also strengthens a general sense of psychological well being and is associated with a heightened sense of self-esteem. A good sense of humor is seen as a desirable quality in dating couples, and a great deal of evidence points to its importance in sustaining a healthy marriage.

While most of the research on humor and stress supports the positive outcomes just described, some studies have not demonstrated humor's effectiveness as a coping tool. One reason for this appears to be that measures of sense of humor have—until very recently—failed to distinguish between positive and negative forms of humor. (Failure to make this distinction may also help explain some of the inconsistent findings relating sense of humor to physical health.) New measures that do make this distinction have shown positive forms of humor to be associated with higher levels of optimism, hope, happiness, self-esteem and interpersonal competence—and lower levels of depression and anxiety. These qualities, along with humor's ability to pull you out of a negative state and substitute a positive one in its place, play an important role in accounting for the coping power of humor.

Negative and maladaptive forms of humor are associated with poorer self-esteem and interpersonal competence and higher levels of depression and anxiety. These findings make it clear that *simply having a well-developed sense of humor is not enough to obtain the mental health and resilience-boosting benefits humor offers, since a well-developed negative sense of humor can actually interfere with good psychological health and effectiveness in social interaction.*

There is a great deal of evidence from real-life, high-stress situations that supports the experimental research documenting humor's capacity to boost resilience. This includes findings for cancer patients, doctors and nurses (and other hospital staff), mental health professionals, victims of natural disasters, emergency personnel who respond to crises and disasters, military personnel during a war, POWs and others who must deal with a personal life crisis. These real-life findings add strength to the evidence from more artificial laboratory experiments showing the importance of humor as a coping tool.

Serious studies of the mental and physical health benefits associated with humor and laughter began a couple of decades before the creation of the new field of Positive Psychology at the beginning of the present century. However, Positive Psychology has supported key findings already obtained for humor, even though many in the field of Positive Psychology appear to be unaware of these findings. For example, Positive Psychology has shown that positive emotion in general facilitates effective coping with both acute and chronic stress and is associated with better psychological health. It is also the key to boosting resilience. This makes a strong case for the notion that it is the positive emotion that results from humor and laughter that is primarily responsible for much of their coping and resilience-boosting power. (Chapter 3 shows that humor activates known reward or pleasure centers in the brain, which helps account for the positive emotion resulting from humor.)

Several different mechanisms—in addition to the generation of positive emotion—combine to account for humor's amazing ability to help cope with life stress. One of the most important of these is the muscle relaxation (and easing of psychological tension that goes with it) that results from humor and laughter (muscle relaxation is the #1 goal of all stress management techniques). Humor also reduces the cardiovascular reactivity (increased heart rate and blood pressure) that accompanies stress, as well as the level of stress hormones circulating in the blood. It provides a means of managing your daily mood or emotional state, giving you a sense of control over at least your emotions—even when you can't control the specific circumstances causing your anger, anxiety, etc. The notion of control is a key concept in stress; your stress level mounts quickly when you feel powerless to control any stress-causing circumstance.

The ability to manage your emotions is a key component of emotional intelligence. You can consciously use humor to pull yourself out of a negative mood (whether from anger, anxiety or non-clinical depression) and substitute a more positive, upbeat frame of mind in its place. While in this more positive frame of mind, it is easier to take active steps to deal with the situation causing you stress. Equally important, humor appears to help you make a more accurate appraisal of stressful events. (This is a difficult thing to do for most people when they are angry, anxious or depressed.) Also, the ability to use humor to generate or sustain a more positive mood helps keep everyday problems and stressors in perspective. (We've all heard the phrase, "Don't sweat the small stuff.")

Finally, you will be heartened to know that it's not too late for you to learn to improve your own humor coping skills. A common assumption held by adults is that "you're either born with a good sense of humor or you're not; I wasn't, and there's nothing I can do about it." We all have a sense of humor as our biological heritage. As children, we are designed to play with our ideas. While many adults lose this quality as they go through adulthood, it's not too late to get it back. Numerous studies have now shown that adults can improve the basic foundation skills (like playing with language, finding humor in everyday life and laughing at yourself) required to use humor to cope.

In the book, *One Flew over the Cuckoo's Nest*, McMurphy (played by Jack Nicholson in the film) says, "When you lose your sense of humor, you lose your footing." Another character says about McMurphy, "He knows you have to laugh at the things that hurt you, just to keep yourself in balance, just to keep the world from running you plumb crazy." This is great wisdom from someone who lives in a psychiatric institution. Your sense of humor is one of the most potent tools you have to cope with those days when life seems determined to deal you enough stress to make you crazy. In the midst of the global economic crisis confronting us all as this book is published, most of us are finding more and more days like this showing up in our lives.

President Abraham Lincoln once read something to his advisors which he found very funny, but they didn't laugh. He said, "Why don't you laugh? With the fearful strain that is upon me night and day, if I did not laugh I should die, and you need this medicine as much as I do." When the president has a good sense of humor, we all benefit. It eases our tensions about the country's problems. As Robert Orben, a former director of the White House Speech Writing Department, once said, "A sense of humor implies a confident person . . . If you can joke about a tough situation, you're saying, 'Yes, it's serious, but I'm in control.'" President Reagan eased the anxiety of an entire country after he was shot. While being taken to the hospital, he looked into the TV cameras and spoke to his wife saying, "Honey, I forgot to duck." Before his surgery, he joked with his surgeons, saying, "I hope you guys are all republicans." With memories of the assassinations of President Kennedy, Robert Kennedy and Martin Luther King two decades earlier still fresh in our minds, stress levels across the country were noticeably relieved following Reagan's joking remarks.

Like tea bags, people never discover how strong they are until they get into hot water. In this chapter you will see how your sense of humor helps provide the strength you need to survive and cope well in the hottest of water.

Your Sense of Humor
The Secret Ingredient for Making Lemonade

We've all heard the expression, "When life deals you lemons, make lemonade." What no one told you, however, is that the secret ingredient in this recipe is your sense of humor. It can take a sour event in your life and make it sweet(er). By learning to find a light side of the situation, you can transform the hand you've been dealt. So don't let the fact that you're feeling miserable keep you from getting some fun and joy out of life.

We will see below that humor has the power to weaken negative emotions and even transform a negative mood into a positive one. In the process, it substitutes a frame of mind that is more conducive to finding solutions to the problem that generated this negative emotion in the first place. It eases your momentary level of tension and upset and gives you a greater sense of control over your lemons. And for everyday problems, it helps keep them in perspective in terms of life's big picture. As you get better at making good comic lemonade in the midst of adversity, you'll find yourself serving it to others—comfortably and naturally—giving them the same benefits of humor that you enjoy yourself.

"Life is full of misery, loneliness, and unhappiness, and it's all over much too quickly."   (Woody Allen)

"It is because they can be frivolous at times that the majority of people do not hang themselves."   (Voltaire)

Hopefully, you're not ready to hang yourself because of the stress in your life. But if you're like most people, your daily stress has gone up in recent years—especially on your job. The mushrooming growth of the stress management industry provides ample evidence of the increasing stress in our lives. We have seen a proliferation of stress management techniques, such as progressive relaxation, deep breathing, meditation, biofeedback, yoga, and more.

Amazingly, many of us have completely neglected one of the most effective stress reducers available to us—our sense of humor. This natural stress remedy is one of the most important tools you have for maintaining a more relaxed and joyful life—yes, even a happy life—a life that always has room for fun, even in the midst of stress from jobs (or loss of your job), relationships, health, the threat of terrorism—from life, in the 21st century.

> **Donovan the bartender is walking to his pub one day when a perfect stranger walks up and gives him a punch in the face, trying to start a fight. He says, "That'll teach you O'Brien!" To which Donovan roars with laughter, after recovering from the shock.**
>
> **"Why are you laughing?" asks the stranger. "Do you want me to hit you again?"**
>
> **"No, please," comes the reply, "It's just that the joke's on you . . . I'm not O'Brien."**

The problem, of course, is that your sense of humor probably abandons you right when you need it the most—during your most stressful days. This is why I've written a companion book to this book. It is called *Humor as Survival Training for a Stressed-Out World.* It shows how to develop the basic foundation habits and skills you need to use humor to cope with life stress. Learning to adopt these humorous habits on the good days—when you're in a good mood—strengthens them to the point that you're capable of a light response even in the stress of the moment. (This Humor Skills Program is discussed at the end of this chapter.) You may even achieve the coolness of the New York hot dog vendor who had a guy aim a gun at him in a robbery attempt. The vendor came up with the following line: "Now what do I need a gun for on a job like this? Try selling it to that cop over there." The gunman panicked and ran off—even though there was no cop.

We've All Had Days Like This

It's Monday morning, and you have an important meeting to attend, so you absolutely have to be there on time. Imagine that the following sequence of events happens to you. We've all had days like this, so think about how you react when it happens to you.

Since it's crucial that you not be late, you give yourself two hours to get there—twice the time you really need. You head out the door, but can't find your keys. You don't panic, because you've allowed for this. After looking everywhere twice, you start to feel anxious. But just then, your son finds them on his way out to school—in the front door! You grab them and smugly congratulate yourself on having decided to start early. You get to your car and find that a freezing rain has fallen during the night, covering everything with a layer of ice. Not only do you have to scrape the ice off the windshield, you can't even open the door; it's frozen shut. After making your feelings about this situation known to everyone in the neighborhood, it finally occurs to you to go back inside and get a screw driver. You return to the car and force the door open as you lift the handle. You're in!

After one block, you glance at the gas gauge. Less than one eighth of a tank! You'll never get there without stopping for gas. You pull into the first gas station your see. You quickly fill the tank, but the credit card machine doesn't accept your card. As you run in to pay, you find two other people waiting to do the same. None of the credit card machines on the pumps are working! One guy has his card rejected . . . and has to use a different card.

Finally, your turn comes. As the attendant is about to slide your credit card, the phone rings. It's her boss. She feels obliged to give him her full attention and just holds your card. You grab the card from her and throw $40 down and walk out. Your jaw is clenched as you head for the door.

You pull back on the road just in time to catch a red light. A school bus then turns in front of you as you wait at the light. There's so much traffic that you can't pass. The bus makes 11 stops before you get around it. You've also managed to hit every light red! But you're almost to the interstate and you know you're home free from there.

"When you're down in the mouth, remember Jonah. He came out ok." (Thomas Edison)

As you approach the entry ramp to the freeway, the lights start flashing and the gate comes down in front of the one set of railroad tracks you have to cross—the ones you've crossed every day for a year without ever seeing a train! Two minutes later, the end of the train is in sight. Then it comes to an agonizing halt . . . and starts backing up! Does this sound familiar so far?

You finally get across the tracks and onto the freeway, and you're cruising at 60 mph. You come over a little hill and are stunned by a string of red lights—break lights—as far down the road as you can see. It's an accident. Traffic is backed up over a mile.

You realize now that you're running out of time. You notice that the other lane is moving faster, so you force your way into that lane as the driver you cut in front of compliments you on your maneuver. Within seconds, that lane slows down and the cars from the lane you just left zip by. You're determined to prove that you made the right decision, so you stay put, as traffic from the original lane continues to pass you. Just before you reach the site of the accident, a tow truck pulls the damaged car off the road and traffic speeds up again.

You've got 15 minutes until your meeting begins. As you exit the freeway, you run into construction; two lanes have been funneled into one. So you take an alternate route, where traffic is moving freely. You hear sirens in the distance. They are getting closer, but your path is finally clear. No problem! Five minutes to go, but you're a mile away from your destination.

The sirens are getting very loud now. Suddenly, from out of nowhere, two fire engines careen around the corner and stop at the intersection in front of you. Another one emerges behind you and blocks your only escape. You look up and realize that the fire is in the building you just happen to be in front of at that moment. Three cars are trapped between the fire trucks, and yours is one of them.

Every one of these incidents has occurred in my life at one time or another, although not all on the same trip. I came close, though, the day I got surrounded by fire engines in New York City, after every traffic problem imaginable made me late for my meeting. (It didn't help that I made a wrong turn that forced me onto the Brooklyn Bridge. I had to cross over to Brooklyn, find a way to turn around, and then return to Manhattan.) At some point, you've had your own version of this episode. How did you react?

My own reaction was to burst out laughing when the fire trucks surrounded me. I couldn't believe it. The gathering crowd looked at me oddly, thinking I was laughing at the fire. But all the tension and upset that had built up in the previous hour and a half just exploded in the form of a good belly laugh. After the laughter, I stopped worrying about the fact that I was late and focused my attention on the problems this would cause and how I would deal with them.

I broke through the blockade and arrived 10 minutes late. I later realized that the fire trucks actually helped me; they reversed the bad mood I would have been in when I arrived at the meeting. The belly laugh and resulting positive mood didn't get me there any faster, but instead of arriving tense, upset, and unable to concentrate, I walked in relatively relaxed and able to focus on the tasks at hand.

The real power of humor and laughter shows up when you learn to use it under stress. It keeps the problem in perspective, dissipates negative emotions (anger, anxiety, or depression) that burgeon up within you when things go wrong, and puts you in a more positive frame of mind that is much better equipped to handle the situation.

The Mounting Stress of Everyday Life

One of the most striking features of American life (as well as life in most other countries) as we enter the second decade of the 21st century is the constantly escalating level of daily stress in the lives of people from all sectors of society. The staggering cost of healthcare alone was pushing many families to their economic limits even before the economic meltdown of 2008-2009. Those who are lucky enough to still have a job are commonly forced into spending greater time and energy on the job. The familiar phrase, "doing more with less," probably now applies to most of the jobs in the country. By the end of 2009, many who had lost their jobs in the previous year longed for the "good old days" when their constant concern was job stress—not lack of a job.

Increasingly, couples are finding it more difficult to sustain the quality of family relationships they want. The quality of our air, water, and other aspects of our environment is steadily breaking down. Global warming is creating new sources of environmental stress, including (in some years) more frequent and more intense hurricanes. Political divisiveness in the U. S. A. has been increasing for the past decade. We have the threat of biological and other forms of terrorism hanging over our heads. With all of these sources of stress confronting us at the same time, it is crucial that we somehow become more resilient in our daily lives.

Impact of Stress on Health

So what is all this stress doing to our health? A tremendous amount of research has documented the impact of distressing negative emotions on physical health. As early as the mid-1980s, the American Academy of Family Physicians estimated that 60% of the problems that people go to their doctors about are either caused or worsened by stress.[1] Other estimates put this figure as high as 80%. Stress has been found to contribute to a broad range of diseases, including cancer, cardiovascular disease, osteoporosis, arthritis, and type 2 diabetes.

But what is it about stress that makes us more vulnerable to disease? The most important part of the answer to this question clearly lies in the negative emotion that accompanies stress. We all have our own way of reacting emotionally to stress. Some of us get angry, while others get depressed, tense, or anxious. Often, it's a combination of these emotions that take over when we're under stress. Whatever your own typical responseis, if you're stressed-out and immersed in negative emotion day after day, this makes you more susceptible to disease.

Chronic anger, for example, has long been known to be closely linked to heart disease.[2] (We long ago learned about the health risk associated with the classic Type A personality, characterized

13

by hostile or angry feelings and a strong drive to succeed.) In fact, men high in hostility and anger have more than twice the risk of death from cardiovascular problems in comparison with low hostility men.[3] Anxiety has also been linked to heart disease, as well as to gastrointestinal disorders.[4]

By far the greatest evidence documenting a damaging health effect resulting from chronic negative emotion has been found for depression. *Depression contributes to heart disease, osteoporosis, and a general suppression of the immune system.*[5] An excellent example of this research is a recent study in which measured levels of depression at one time were used to predict occurrence of heart attacks over the next 13 years. Those who had major depression at time one were found to have 4.5 times the risk of heart attacks than people who had no history of depression.[6] Depression, of course, is a common response to many serious illnesses, and we now know that it can increase the risk of death from a broad range of health problems. *Depressed mood is an independent risk factor for death among hospital inpatients—regardless of their illness.*[7] This is an especially important finding; it makes it very clear how crucial it is for families and hospitals alike to find effective ways to elevate patients' spirits when they are seriously ill. This is one reason (as noted in Chapter 2) why a growing number of hospitals are making some form of "therapeutic humor" program available to patients during their hospital stay.

So the negative emotion that accompanies stress is the key to understanding the effect of stress on health. This suggests that *learning to both prevent stress from occurring and manage your emotional state more effectively in the midst of stress (through a combination of reducing the level of negative emotion experienced and increasing positive emotion) is the key to controlling the potential harmful health effects of stress.*

The question of just how negative emotion worsens health, of course, must still be answered. We do know at this point that one way in which stress and chronic negative emotion do this is by *reducing our resistance to disease.* This is often a result of suppression of the immune system[8], although emotions have also been found to directly influence health "through alterations in the functioning of the central nervous system, immune, endocrine, and cardiovascular systems."[9] A great deal of attention has also been given to increased inflammation in response to stress; this has been linked to cardiovascular disease, osteoporosis, arthritis, type two diabetes and certain cancers. One reviewer of research in this area recently concluded that "There is excellent evidence that depression and anxiety enhance the production of proinflammatory cytokines, including IL-6."[10] In addition to the inflammatory effect in the body, these cytokines can also suppress the immune system.

BUILD YOUR HUMOR SKILLS

[Turn the page for answers. Work on both jokes before checking answers.]

1. The day after his return from the hospital, John says to his wife, "I have to say, I really am feeling better since the operation. But for the life of me, I can't figure out how I got this bump on my head. "Oh," says his wife, "Well, they _____ in the middle of your operation.

Clue: What do they use to "put you out" during major surgery?

2. A 75-year-old man came home from a round of golf and his wife asked him how it went. "Well, I hit it pretty well, but my eyes have gotten so bad I couldn't see where the ball went." So his wife suggests talking his brother along. The man says, "Nah, he's eight years older than me, and he doesn't even play golf anymore." But his wife points out that he's got perfect eyesight. So the next day he tees off with his brother watching. The ball disappears down the middle of the fairway. So he asks his brother, "Did you see it?" "Yup." "Well, where is it?" His brother says, "I _____."

Clue: His eyes are great, but his mind is not.

Depression-induced elevated levels of cortisol also weaken the immune system. And it is not only the release of cortisol in extreme cases of clinical depression that pose a health risk. Frequent minor cortisol increases resulting from typical daily stressors can also contribute to the onset or worsening of disease.[11] This research on the effect of emotions on health is discussed in detail in Chapter 2.

We all have stress in our lives. How you react to it is the key, and certain personalities or coping styles promote disease, while others support resistance to disease. There is a growing conviction among both researchers and practitioners that the *ability to "unwind" after a stressor—i.e., to "let go" of the stressful event and return to one's neuroendocrine baseline—is the key to minimizing the damaging effects of these hormone-related processes upon one's health.* This is where the wellness-promoting power of humor comes in. At the physiological level, humor and other sources of positive emotion can play a key role in undoing the damaging effects of negative emotion by substituting a positive "frame of body" that is incompatible with the physical state associated with negative emotion—at the same time that it substitutes a positive frame of mind that reduces the simultaneous presence of negative feelings.[12]

Humor is just one tool which helps achieve this goal. As another expert in the rapidly growing field of mind/body medicine recently put it, "*A potent resilience factor for health outcomes may be the induction and maintenance of positive emotion* through personality and coping styles . . . The pathways through which positive emotions impact health outcomes are not well known at this point, but likely occur through endocrine and immune mechanisms, as well as indirectly through health behaviors."[13] (Italics are McGhee's.)

The Growing Need for Emotional Resilience

Prior to the keynotes I do for hospitals and corporations, I have a series of telephone conversations with people who are representative of the group I'll be speaking to. The one thing that I almost always see—with rare exceptions—is that people are feeling pushed harder than ever before in both their personal and work lives. I can see that stress is taking their toll on the quality of their lives. More than ever before, we all need effective sources of emotional resilience that help us cope and remain happy. The main thrust of this chapter is that humor provides a much more powerful means of sustaining resilience on a daily basis than you ever imagined. Hardiness and emotional intelligence have similarly been emphasized as sources of emotional resilience, so we will briefly discuss these, as well.

ANSWERS TO JOKES

1. ran out of ether (or other general anesthetic)   2. forgot

---

Hardiness

A good sense of humor is just one quality which helps you deal effectively with stress. Stress–resistant (resilient) people also have other qualities which have been described as making people more "hardy." 1) They view change as a challenge, rather than a threat— even when it's unwanted change. It's seen as an opportunity for personal growth. 2) They feel a greater sense of control, believing that they are in charge—even when things don't go the way they want them to. They also see themselves as having greater control over their emotions. They know they can change their feelings by taking active steps to deal with the problem. Poor copers tend to feel like victims, believing that life is not fair, and wondering, "Why should this happen to me?" This leads to feelings of helplessness, depression and anxiety. 3) They maintain a more optimistic outlook in life. They feel that things will turn out for the best—not in a naive Pollyanna sense, but because of confidence in their own abilities.[14] These qualities enable stress–resistant people to maintain their effectiveness in potentially stressful situations.

"Tragedy and comedy are but two aspects of what is real, and whether we see the tragic or the humorous is a matter of perspective." (Dr. Arnold Beisser)

Numerous studies have now shown that a good sense of humor is closely linked to these three defining features of hardiness. We'll just discuss a couple of examples here. Among college students, exams are the biggest ongoing stressor, since they define success or failure in school. Students who scored higher on a measure of using humor to cope with stress were more likely than those scoring lower on the measure to appraise upcoming exams as a challenge—not a threat.[15] Similarly, high sense of humor individuals were more likely to view a difficult experimental task as a challenge rather than a source of stress.[16]

Later sections of this chapter demonstrate humor's effectiveness as a tool for boosting feelings of control in a bad situation (partly because of its ability to manage your emotions) and sustaining a positive, optimistic attitude. It substitutes a frame of mind which enables you to both view the current problem as a challenge and find innovative solutions to the problem. It helps keep things in perspective, allowing you to take greater control over both the problem and your emotional reactions to it.

Do you smoke after sex?
I don't know, I never looked.

Resilience has been defined by some as the ability to sustain flexibility in one's behavior as the demands of the situation change, as well as the ability to quickly and efficiently bounce back from highly stressful experiences.[17] Recent evidence suggests that *highly resilient individuals actually experience some degree of positive emotion in the midst of stressful situations, and that it is this positive emotion that helps them bounce back from negative emotional experiences.*[18] (See the discussion of positive emotion below for a detailed discussion of this.)

Barbara Fredrickson and her colleagues, who have done some exciting research on positive emotion during the past decade, were able to demonstrate the role of positive emotion in coping with the September 11 attacks in New York City and Washington, D. C. She had already obtained measures of trait resilience on a group of individuals prior to the attacks. High-resilience individuals reported greater experience of such positive emotions as gratitude, love and interest in the midst of their negative emotions (e.g., fear, sadness and anger) following the attacks than did low-resilience subjects. The high-resilience subjects also showed more psychological growth after the crisis (as indicated by a sense of tranquility and subjective well-being, along with greater optimism about the future) than lows.

Statistical analyses showed that *it was the positive emotion experienced after the attacks that was responsible for the post-attack psychological growth that occurred.*[19] This real-life demonstration of the importance of positive emotion for resilience and well-being is an important addition to laboratory studies (discussed below) showing the same effect for humor. It also suggests that *any skills (such as humor) that you develop which increase your ability to create positive emotion for yourself in the midst of stressful events may boost your ability to become a stronger, more resilient person in the midst of adversity.*

Emotional/Psychological Restoration

Another source of emotional resilience is the opportunity to replenish yourself in some way—to "recharge your batteries." And psychologists have begun looking at things we can do every day to restore ourselves emotionally to face the challenges ahead. *This emotional replenishing is now recognized as playing an important role in our psychological well being.*

The need for regular psychological restoration should come as no surprise, since we have long been aware of a similar need at the physiological level.

"Restoration refers to the fact that physiological systems (such as the nervous system and its constituent neurons) need time to restore their ability to react. A neuron that has fired cannot fire again until refraction is accomplished. After refraction, neurons can respond fully and rapidly. Similar effects are seen with skeletal muscle and its ability to respond and grow. During physical training, muscle hypertrophy occurs in which repeated injury to muscle fibers results in overcompensation of protein synthesis during rest. After resting, muscle fibers are able to respond with similar or increased strength. *Similar processes appear to govern behavior and well-being. Restoration is also a useful method for buffering, reducing, and coping with the harmful effects of stress on the body.*[20] (Italics are McGhee's.)

Everyone who has a job and a family is acutely aware of the need for restoration in everyday life. As job stress mounts and time with family drops, and as the pace of life continues to accelerate, growing numbers of people feel physically and emotionally drained. A sense of urgency in learning to manage this stress has emerged in recent years as the evidence mounts showing that chronic stress increases vulnerability to such diseases as heart disease,[21] cancer,[22] autoimmune disorders,[23] diabetes,[24] infectious illness[25] and more.

We now know that, along with vacations and days off from work, exercise, good social support or interaction, better sleep, and increased time in natural environments all have psychological restorative power. Anything capable of substituting a positive daily mood for the tense and pressured mood many now consider normal contributes to psychological restoration. As shown in this chapter, *your sense of humor provides a built-in tool for psychological restoration.* The key to reaping the many benefits of humor described here is getting yourself to the point where your sense of humor does not abandon you during your own high-stress moments.

Emotional Intelligence

There has been tremendous interest in the notion of emotional intelligence (EI) in the past decade and a half. Intelligence has long been viewed as a quality of the rational side of ourselves—our mind—and it is only in the past couple of decades that researchers have brought the notion of intelligence to the realm of emotions. This new development is a result of evidence that the cognitive and emotional systems of the brain are far more integrated than previously thought.[26] Corporations now spend a great deal of money in efforts to boost their managers' EI in the belief that this will sharply improve job performance and quality of service. A growing number of educators are also convinced that improving children's EI will improve performance in school.

The experts in this area, however, have been unable to agree upon a definition of EI. According to Jack Mayer and Peter Salovey, two leading researchers studying this topic, EI consists of four components: 1) the perception and identification/appraisal of emotions, 2) emotional facilitation of thought, 3) emotional understanding, and 4) *the management of emotions—in oneself and others. This 4th component is considered by them to be the highest level of EI.*[27]

Daniel Goleman, author of two popular books on EI, has argued that EI includes five distinct skill areas: 1) knowing one's emotions, 2) *managing emotions (including the ability to soothe oneself and shake off rampant irritability, anxiety or gloom)*, 3) motivating oneself, 4) recognizing emotions in others, and 5) handling relationships (including skill in managing others' emotions and interacting smoothly with others).[28] Another leading expert on EI defines it in terms of non-cognitive *skills that influence one's ability to cope with the stress of everyday life.* These include both intrapersonal and interpersonal skills, general mood and adaptability and stress management skills.

Peter Salovey argued that EI plays a key role in psychological or emotional resilience.[29] Amazingly, neither he nor other researchers (or popularizers) of EI have given any attention to the role of humor skills in EI. It will become obvious, however, as you read this chapter that humor makes a significant contribution to EI, regardless of whose definition you adopt (especially in those areas italicized in the two preceding paragraphs). You will see that *humor 1) helps manage one's own emotions, as well as the emotions of others—a skill considered to be a cornerstone of EI, 2) helps sustain a frame of mind conducive to creative thinking and effective problem solving (especially in the midst of stress), 3) helps sustain satisfying and effective personal relationships, and 4) helps cope with life stress.*

Having a better understanding of emotions is also associated with a larger repertoire of possible strategies to regulate one's emotion.[30] Humor is clearly a good example of one strategy. You can consciously and purposefully use humor to manage both your emotional experience and physiological changes occurring in the body.[31] In fact, one study has shown that 34% of people consciously use humor to pull themselves out of a negative mood or sustain a positive mood.[32] Among resilient people, humor is likely to be simply one means (among others) of sustaining a positive mood in the midst of negative life events.

Does Stress Happen to You? Or Do You Create it?

If you've ever attended a stress management seminar, you've probably heard the idea that "you create your own stress." This initially makes no sense at all to most people. After all, you didn't create the tornado that wiped out your house, the extra work you inherited when your colleague was laid off, the increase in your health insurance payments or the economic woes of 2009. The victims of the devastating tsunami of 2004 and hurricane Katrina in 2005 did not create these events. But you do create the level of stress such events generate—depending on how you interpret and react to them.

If you've ever been in a situation where several people have had identical stressors (e.g., cancer, loss of a job, or impossible job demands), you've probably noticed that they handle it in very different ways. Some get so angry, anxious, or depressed that their relationships collapse, they lose their effectiveness on their job, and their life falls apart in general. Others have the same initial upset, but quickly face up to the reality of the situation and get on to coping with it.

> *"Perhaps I know why it is man alone who laughs; he alone suffers so deeply that he had to invent laughter."* (Friedrich Wilhelm Nietzsche)

One way we create stress is by constantly worrying about things that might happen. Unforeseen and unwanted events will always occur in our lives. You want to take reasonable precautions against these, but must also learn to accept the fact that you can't control everything. Once you've done what you can to prevent unwanted events in your life, the next step is learning to manage them effectively when they do occur. As we shall see, learning to lighten up in the midst of your problems helps you do exactly that.

Humor Overcomes the Law of Psychological Gravity

I coined the phrase "The Law of Psychological Gravity" a few years ago. This law says that people become heavier when they're under stress. When you have one terrible day after another, you can feel yourself start to drag. You become emotionally heavy. For some, this heaviness takes the form of anger. For others, it shows up as anxiety, depression, or general sadness. Regardless of how it shows in you personally, it weighs you down on your job and in your relationships; and it robs you of your ability to experience real satisfaction (and be effective) in both. But your sense of humor overcomes this law by preventing the weight build-up (or reducing it if it has already occurred) and improving your effectiveness on the job and in life generally.

I witnessed the anti-gravity power of humor while visiting my parents some years ago. My father was in his mid-80s and had a number of health problems and physical limitations. As he often said, "My day is full of misery; you just don't know what it's like. My job is to put in my 24 hours and get through the day." I heard him say many times, "I just ain't no good any more." He said it was hard for him to keep his spirits up, because he had nothing to hope for. He knew that things were never going to get better; they could only get worse.

But a funny thing happened when the in-home-care lady who had been helping my mother was replaced. The new care provider had a good sense of humor and often engaged my father in playful banter and good-natured ribbing. The impact on his mood was immediately apparent. You can imagine how wonderful it was to see a playful grin come across his face when the new woman began talking about how the two of them had "a thing" going, and that she hoped my mother wouldn't be too jealous.

He even started telling jokes and funny stories. He asked me one day, "Did you hear about the guy who bowled 301?" "301? That's impossible!" I said. He couldn't keep from grinning as he added, "Well, did you ever see anyone who bowled three hundred and lost?" (The ambiguity here only works orally.) Since he rarely told jokes, I saw this new joking style as a direct effect of the new aide's ability to bring out his own playfulness. I discovered later that he had recently heard Archie Bunker tell this joke on an *All in the Family* rerun. While I don't ever recall him being a joke-teller during his middle-adult years, this care provider clearly had the impact of making him more interested in sharing humor with others.

On the same trip, I had some animal noses and a silly-looking "Smile on a Stick" sitting around the house. On Christmas day, I took some photographs of him and my mother wearing these and making silly faces. From that point on, whenever friends or relatives would come over, he would grab the Smile on a Stick and suddenly turn toward the guest, holding it under his nose with his eyebrows sharply raised (as shown below). Or he would hand them the animal-nose photos and wait for their reaction. These simple little props brought many moments of joy to his difficult, dreary days. This is just one of the ways in which humor adds to the quality of life. It may or may not add years to your life, but it will certainly add life to your years.

Bounce-Back-Ability

Your sense of humor gives you what I have long called "bounce-back-ability"—a quality noted in the Introduction to be part of the definition of resilience. By this point in your life, you've probably developed some good coping skills, so that minor problems generally only get you down momentarily. You're able to bounce back quickly and do whatever is required to deal with them. But some days are tougher than others, and on those days it takes every bit of energy you can muster to bounce back and cope. You can do it, but it takes a committed effort on your part, and it leaves you emotionally drained.

And then there are other days—you know the ones I mean—where your problems just seem to overwhelm you, maybe because they all happen at once. No matter what you do, you just can't bounce back and make lemonade from all the lemons thrown your way. Your resistance is weakened, and you become a victim of the Law of Psychological Gravity.

This is precisely where your sense of humor can help. It helps you bounce back in situations where you'd otherwise succumb. Just as the elasticity of a ball enables it to absorb the energy created by gravity and produce the force necessary to bounce back up against the pull of gravity, *your sense of humor gives you the emotional elasticity you need to overcome psychological gravity and bounce back in a more positive direction.*

You will feel the force of gravity pulling you down as you first start trying to use your sense of humor in the midst of stress. It will seem unnatural as you ask yourself, "OK, what's funny about this situation?" Because you know there's absolutely nothing funny about it! This soon will pass, however, as you learn to distinguish between the seriousness of the situation and the little things that still could be funny to someone who has the habit of noticing them.

"I have seen what a laugh can do. It can transform almost unbearable tears into something bearable, even hopeful."

(Bob Hope)

Finding something to laugh at during hard times does not mean you're failing to take the situation seriously. You will learn that having a good laugh actually helps you handle the problem stressing you out—if you're determined to deal with it effectively to begin with. Meetings in corporations often begin with a joke or funny story, because this generates a (positive) frame of mind that makes the meeting flow better, and more gets accomplished. The same thing happens when you manage to have a good laugh in the midst of a personal conflict. It helps you bounce back and deal with the conflict more effectively.

Humor as Verbal Aikido

Aikido is a martial art in which you use an attacker's own force to disarm him and defend yourself. Instead of countering his force by striking back, you add to it or deflect it in a slightly different direction. If someone rushes toward you, you use his own energy to thrust him aside.

Joel Goodman noted some years ago that humor can be used as a kind of verbal aikido. In the midst of a conflict, a humorous remark can disarm a verbal attack in a way that establishes a more positive—even playful—atmosphere for resolving the conflict; and it doesn't put the other person down. It removes the bitterness and leaves both parties in a better position to deal with the problem at hand.

Despite the high cost of living . . . it's still very popular.

For example, Robert F. Kennedy was asked in the early 1960s why he felt qualified to become attorney general for the United States. His answer was, "If a person wants to become attorney general, that person should first go to a good law school, study hard, get good marks, establish a reputation, and most important of all—have a brother who is president of the United States." The remark totally defused the implicit suggestion that it was inappropriate for a brother of the president to receive the post.

A few years ago, many public schools in New York City were late in opening for classes because of a scandal in which schools which had presumably been tested for asbestos were found not to have been tested. In the midst of tension-filled meetings between parents and school authorities, one group of parents congregated around a school wearing T-shirts which said, "We're doing asbestos we can." They provided a welcome release of the tension and upset felt by both sides.

A group of bus drivers got tired of people in cars behind them honking their horns all day long. So they got the bus company to put a big sign on the back of the busses saying, "Honk if you love life!" Drivers stopped honking as soon as the signs went up.

Evidence that Humor Builds Resilience and Helps You Cope

Freud pointed out nearly a century ago that humor offers a healthy means of coping with life stress. George Vaillant, in his book *Adaptation to Life*, reported that humor was a very effective coping mechanism used by many people under stress. Gail Sheehy, author of *Pathfinders*, similarly found humor to be an effective was to overcome crises and find one's own path. These books were based on in–depth interviews with people about their lives.

Rigorous research has similarly documented the coping power of humor. That research is divided into three general categories below. We will first discuss the findings of experimental studies in which stress was created in some kind of controlled laboratory setting. This is the only kind of study that allows you to demonstrate that humor really is the *cause* of reduced stress or an improved emotional state. Studies relating measures of sense of humor to stress reduction or a change in emotional state will then be reviewed. If we can first demonstrate that humor is capable of causing a reduction in stress or negative emotion and an increase in positive emotion (or psychological well-being), we can feel a bit more comfortable in interpreting correlational studies linking sense of humor to measures of stress or psychological well-being. It should be remembered, however, that this second group of studies doesn't prove anything about causality.

If a study shows a positive relationship between sense of humor scores and psychological well-being, it can always be argued that a person has a better sense of humor because of a more positive psychological state, and not vice versa. Chances are that both of these directions of influence are operating in the real world. We simply have a stronger foundation for talking about humor causing the observed relationship if we've already established it through good experimental research.

The third general category of findings relating to humor and stress involves the use of humor in a broad range of high-stress life circumstances or work environments. These are real world situations in which people have learned that using humor is crucial to coping in very emotionally demanding situations.

Experimental Research

Experimental studies of the coping power of humor have used various techniques to generate stress in a laboratory setting. The stress-inducing procedures used are tested in advance to assure that they are, in fact, generating stress. The goal is to arouse feelings of anger, anxiety, sadness, depression, etc., and then measure humor's power to alleviate those feelings and reduce the perception of stress. Funny cartoons or videos are then presented to these angry, anxious or depressed subjects, and the impact of humor on these feelings (or the level of stress experienced) is compared to the effect of non-humorous materials. People are randomly assigned to humor or non-humor groups, so the effect of humor on stress or negative emotion can be precisely determined.

Using this approach, humor has been shown in many studies to reduce feelings of anger or aggression,[33] anxiety,[34] and depression.[35] In the case of anxiety, progressive relaxation (in which you focus attention on specific muscle systems, going from head to toe, or vice versa, relaxing one set of muscles after another) is one technique often used to help anxiety-prone individuals manage their anxiety. When watching a comedy video was compared to this progressive relaxation procedure, humor was just as effective as the 20-minute relaxation procedure in reducing anxiety.[36] The great advantage of shared humor and a good belly laugh, of course, is that it's quicker and a lot more fun. And, let's face it, in the middle of most people's typical bad day, it's not possible to sit down and meditate or do 10 minutes of progressive relaxation. Although humor and laughter are obviously inappropriate in many settings, it's certainly much easier to find an appropriate place to share a funny anecdote and *laugh yourself loose* than to do a progressive relaxation exercise.

"Human life is basically a comedy. Even its tragedies often seem comic to the spectator, and not infrequently they actually have comic

touches to the victim. Happiness probably consists largely in the capacity to detect and relish them."

(H. L. Mencken)

Sometimes any form of distraction can take your mind off whatever is making you anxious and provide a bit of relief from the constant tension that goes along with anxiety. So it's not surprising that some research has shown non-humorous videos to be just as effective as humorous ones in reducing anxiety. In one example of this kind of outcome, subjects first watched a movie segment known to cause stress and then viewed either a humorous or non-humorous videotape. Several stress-related measures were taken both before and after each of the two video segments. Both the humorous and non-humorous videos were effective in reducing anxiety generated by the film, presumably because of their shared ability to distract subjects from the previously-seen stressful content. However, only the humorous video also increased positive emotion.[37]

This increase in positive emotion occurred even though no attempt was made to match the funny video seen to participants' own humor preferences. When exposed to one's favorite comedians or forms of humor, this effect should be all the stronger. *It is this combination of increased positive emotion and reduced stress-linked negative emotion that makes humor such a powerful and desirable stress management tool.* This emotional shift leaves the previously distressed person in a much better position to take steps to eliminate the source of stress—if s/he is inclined to do so.

If you consider yourself to be among the humor-impaired in life, it's comforting to know that you can get some of the stress-reducing benefits of humor from a passive humor experience. That is, you don't have to have a great sense of humor yourself, and you don't have to actively initiate humor to reduce your anger, anxiety or depression. Simply sitting down and watching your favorite sit com will often do the trick.

No experimental studies have compared this kind of passive exposure to humor to a more active effort to producing humor to determine which is a more effective means of coping with stress. And only a few studies have asked subjects to actively produce their own humor in a laboratory situation where stress was experimentally induced. My own conclusion, in considering all the available data, is that the coping benefits of humor increase when you generate your own humor in a stressful situation.

In one study, individuals were asked to generate either a humorous or serious accompanying monologue to a silent film that was stress-inducing.[38] Compared to people who produced a serious narrative, those who made up a funny commentary were less tense and showed less negative emotion to the film. But sometimes writing a non-humorous narrative is just as effective in reducing such stress, so humor may not be unique in its ability to do this.[39]

A doctor calls his patient and says, "The check you gave me for my bill came back." The patient replied: "So did my arthritis!"

One of the difficulties with studies done in laboratory settings, of course, is that even though evidence is obtained that participating subjects do feel more angry, anxious or depressed as a result of the stress-inducing intervention, this is quite different from the kinds of stress experienced in everyday life in the real world. So although it is crucial to establish in good experimental studies that humor is capable of reducing the negative emotions resulting from stress—and increasing positive ones—the argument for humor's stress-reducing power becomes much stronger if it can be shown that people who regularly use humor to cope in everyday life experience this same stress-reduction effect. This research will be discussed following the discussion of stress hormones.

Stress Hormones. If humor and laughter do have a significant impact in reducing stress, this should be evident in direct physical changes going on in the body, as well as in reduced feelings of anger, anxiety, or depression experienced by stressed research subjects. This kind of evidence has now been obtained. In the case of the immune system, for example, we have known for decades that stress (especially the chronic variety) weakens the immune system. The evidence (discussed in Chapter 2) mounts each year showing that humor and laughter (as well as other sources of positive emotion) strengthen the immune system. Humor and laughter also reduce blood pressure (in the long run)—an important finding, since chronic stress is generally associated with increased blood pressure. The most important direct physical evidence of the stress-reducing power of humor, however, would be a demonstration that humor reduces the level of stress hormones circulating in the blood.

Most studies of the relationship between stress hormones and the experience of stress have focused on cortisol. Cortisol levels increase not only when stress is experienced, but even when it is anticipated.[40] Since humor is effective in both reducing the stress experienced and shifting attention away from the source of stress, it should be an effective means of reducing circulating cortisol levels. As demonstrated in Chapter 2, this is, indeed, the case.

There is further evidence that positive affect in general (i.e., from other sources, as well as from humor) is associated with lower cortisol levels. One group of researchers who found this cortisol-reducing effect of positive emotion noted that "The impact of daily stressors on cortisol secretion was no longer significant after statistically controlling for the relationship between daily stressors and affect as well as between affect and cortisol."[41] While this sentence is hard for a non-researcher to understand, its implications are crucial to our understanding of how humor reduces stress. It means that *your emotional state of the moment is the key in determining the amount of cortisol released in a stressful situation.* This led the researchers conducting this study to suggest that *the affect experienced in the midst of stressful situations "may mediate the relationship between stress and cortisol."* (Italics are McGhee's)

If you develop tools (one of which is humor) that minimize the negative emotion experienced when under stress, and boost joyful positive emotions at the same time, the result should be a reduction in cortisol (and other stress hormones) circulating in the body. *The effect of stress on cortisol (and your health, when stress is chronic), then, depends on your emotional state in the midst of the stressful situation. If you have poor coping skills, the negative emotion that typically accompanies stress persists, along with elevated cortisol levels in the body.* Again, then, good coping skills are the key.

Studies of People Who Have a Good Sense of Humor

The second major approach to assessing humor's coping power involves correlating measures of sense of humor with the level of stress or negative emotion experienced. If watching a comedy video in a research laboratory, or exposure to some other form of "outside" humor, helps reduce feelings of anger, anxiety or depression, or otherwise helps cope with stress, then people who find or produce a lot of humor in everyday life should receive this stress-reducing benefit every day. It has already been noted (in the Introduction) that people with high levels of trait resilience more often use humor as a coping strategy.

Three different types of research have been conducted using sense of humor measures to study the relationship between humor and stress. The strongest approach uses an experimental procedure to induce stress. The expectation is that subjects with a stronger sense of humor will experience the event as being less stressful than those with a weaker sense of humor. A variation of this approach (noted earlier) requires subjects to actively produce humor in some way following a procedure designed to generate stress.

The second approach is to assess the number and level of stressful events going on in people's lives and determine the relationship between their sense of humor and measures of negative emotion occurring at different stress levels. The expected finding here is that if humor does reduce the level of stress experienced in the midst of negative life events, then negative emotion should increase among low sense of humor individuals as life stress increases. This relationship should not be present, however, among high sense of humor individuals. Sense of humor would serve as a "buffer" to protect them from the usual negative emotional impact of negative life events.

The third (and weakest) approach is to simply correlate scores on a sense of humor test with a measure of stress, anger, anxiety, or depression. In this case, there is no consideration of the level of stress participating subjects are under. The expected finding here is that people with a better sense of humor will score lower on these measures of stress. That is, if they really are actively using their sense of humor, this should produce the same lowering of stress and negative emotion that experimental studies have demonstrated.

Experimentally-Induced Stress. Some researchers have asked subjects to produce humor in a lab setting. For example, exposure to a stressful film caused less mood disturbance (less negative emotion) among individuals who actively produced humor while watching the film than among those who did not produce a humorous narrative to accompany the film.[42] This effect was strongest among those who did not habitually produce humor in everyday life. This is consistent with the idea that *people who do not normally initiate humor on their own can benefit (in terms of stress reduction) from any form of help that gets them engaged in humor*—whether it be watching a funny video or responding to a request to generate humor.

In another important study, subjects were led to believe that they would receive an electric shock a bit later in the experiment.[43] This is a clear anxiety-generating situation, since no one enjoys electric shocks (although it was a mild shock). Watching a funny video prior to the anticipated shock reduced anxiety levels at several points prior to the expected time of the shock (the shock was still some time away at all of these points). This occurred for both high and low sense of humor subjects.

In this case, then, having a good sense of humor offered no particular advantage in managing anxiety at the early stages of the study—when the anticipated shock was still some time away. But as the anticipated time of the shock became immanent, those with a stronger sense of humor showed less anxiety than their low sense of humor counterparts. This suggests that *a good sense of humor may well serve to protect us against elevated stress right when we need it the most.* The problem for most of us, of course, is that this is precisely when our sense of humor usually abandons us.

Stress in Current Real-Life Situations. Many studies have now shown that people who score higher on a sense of humor measure—especially measures that directly assess the extent to which you use humor as a coping tool in everyday life—experience less negative emotion during the stressful event than those who score lower on the tests. These findings again suggest that *a good sense of* *humor serves as a kind of buffer, helping to protect against stress.* In the earliest (now classic) study like this, Rod Martin and Herb Lefcourt, at the University of Western Ontario in Canada, found that among individuals who did not often use humor as a coping tool, levels of anger, anxiety, depression, and fatigue all increased as the amount of stress in their life increased. This is the general outcome we expect when people are faced with stress. These negative emotions did not increase with escalating stress, however, among people who frequently used humor to cope.[44]

This finding was subsequently replicated using five different ways of measuring sense of humor, several of which measured sense of humor in a general sense, rather than focusing specifically on the use of humor to cope. So *there is something about having a better sense of humor that helps keep people from suffering the depression, anxiety and anger that most of us experience when our stress goes up.* This supports the notion that a good sense of humor is a key component of a "hardy" personality, as discussed above. The ability to keep from being overcome with negative emotion when under stress is a crucial component of personal and emotional resilience.

BUILD YOUR HUMOR SKILLS

[Turn the page for answers. Work on both jokes before checking answers.]

1. "Mental health hotline. If you are obsessive-compulsive, press _____."
Clue: The key symptom of an obsessive-compulsive person.

2. "Mental health hotline. If you are codependent, _____."
Clue: Codependent people have difficulty doing things on their own.

Similar findings have been obtained for depression,[45] anxiety,[46] perceived stressfulness of an exam,[47] and negative emotion in general.[48] I spent 18 years teaching college students before becoming a professional speaker. Since I was aware of the power of humor to reduce text anxiety, I often suggested at exam time that students should share a few jokes or other funny incidents with each other before the exam to loosen themselves up and eliminate the tension that kept them from using the information they knew they had mastered before the exam. Most students—especially those who generally tightened up under exam pressure—told me afterwards that this was good advice.

Other studies have looked at the relationship between sense of humor and negative emotion or stress among people dealing with specific diseases or other stressful circumstances. For example, more frequent use of humor to cope was associated with lower depression and anxiety among older patients suffering from chronic obstructive pulmonary disease,[49] less distress among breast cancer patients,[50] fewer depressive symptoms among both chronic arthritis patients[51] and older widows who recently lost their spouse,[52] better adaptation among the elderly to being moved to a new residential care facility (relocation is a major stressor for most elderly people),[53] and reduced stress during dental surgery.[54]

> *"Don't wait to laugh until you're completely happy."*
>
> (Anonymous)

An especially interesting study investigated the extent to which different factors boosted the level of resilience shown by individuals being treated with drugs for post-traumatic stress disorder. Those with higher scores on a sense of humor scale showed significantly better levels of response to the drug treatment.[55] The implications for military personnel suffering from PTSD upon returning from the war in Iraq (as discussed at the beginning of this chapter) are clear.

Studies Not Considering Current Level of Life Stress. People who more often use humor to cope have been shown to have lower levels of depression[56] and anxiety,[57] worry about things less often,[58] experience less job stress and burnout[59] and experience less stress in life generally.[60] The problem with this kind of research, as we've already noted, is that there is no way to determine which is the cause and which is the effect. People who are less stressed, depressed, or anxious in everyday life may use humor to cope with problems more often because they are in a better frame of mind to do so from the beginning. Or the opposite may also be true; they may be less stressed, depressed, and anxious precisely because they use humor to cope. There is no way of knowing what is responsible for the negative relationship between humor and stress in this kind of study. But these findings are consistent with experimental studies which have demonstrated humor's power to cause a reduction in stress and negative emotion.

Positive Emotion When Under Stress. A section on positive emotion in the midst of stress may make no sense to you, since real stress is anything but positive. But if the ability to find a light side of things in the midst of stress really does help keep you from being overcome with negative emotion, this leaves the door open to remaining more positive during your bad days. Two studies have shown that this is exactly what happens. As expected, individuals who don't laugh very often or very heartily showed less positive emotion as the number of negative events in their life increased; those who laugh more often and more heartily were able to sustain a more positive emotional state even as the number of negative events increased.[61] This finding fits very nicely with the evidence already discussed showing that *a good sense of humor helps you keep from being swallowed up by the anger, anxiety or depression that often goes along with being under stress*. While we're not in as positive a state as we would be if the situation causing us stress had never presented itself, we're still able to sustain some degree of positivity.

ANSWERS TO JOKES

1. 3 repeatedly   2. please ask someone to press 2 for you

Studies in laboratory settings have produced similar findings. For example, watching a comedy video simultaneously reduced anxiety and increases positive affect.[62] Also, people who more often use humor to cope with life stress were better able to resist falling into a negative mood after watching a sad cartoon video.[63]

While a good sense of humor does sustain a more upbeat and positive mood, frequent laughter during the day doesn't necessarily do so. This may seem puzzling, since we laugh in response to something we find funny. But this laughter-humor connection is not as obvious as you might think. Some people have acquired laughter as a general style of interacting with others. They do laugh when something is funny, but also laugh when there is no humor. I have observed many people who laugh one or more times virtually every minute when they are engaged in a typical everyday conversation with someone. This laughing conversational style may have evolved as a way of easing their own social tension, or for some other reason. You probably know such a person yourself. In many cases, this laughing conversational style seems to simply serve as a way to connect or bond with others.

When the laughter that individuals showed over a three-day period was monitored, more frequent laughter during the day was not significantly related to the extent of either their positive or negative emotional state in the evening or the next morning.[64] This suggests that *the experience of humor may be more important that the act of laughing for sustaining a positive mood.* The same study, however, found that when you consider the level of stress experienced during the day, laughter does become important in sustaining positive (at least among males) and reducing negative emotion (for both genders). That is, as daily stressors increased among people who laughed infrequently during the day, the extent of positive emotion was reduced while negative emotion increased. This did not happen among more frequent laughers. *So laughter does help sustain a positive mood and avoid a negative one when you're under stress—which is when you need this benefit the most!* When you're not under stress, being a good laugher does not appear to have a significant impact on your ongoing emotional state.

In everyday life, most laughter occurs while interacting with other people; it is not in response to jokes or other forms of humor per se.[65] As already noted, some of us have developed laughter as a style of interaction with others, while others laugh only when we find something funny. If you find yourself in the former category, then simply keeping this quality in the midst of stress will give you the mood-enhancing effects described above. If you tend to laugh only when you find something funny, you'll want to make a special effort to strengthen your humor skills so that they become part of your personal style when you're under stress. Since your sense of humor now probably abandons you when you're under stress, it is essential to build the habit of playing with language, finding humor in everyday life and poking fun at yourself on the good days so that you'll have access to these habits on the bad days.

Psychological Well-Being. Another way to look at the relationship between humor and stress or mental health is in terms of general psychological well-being. Since people with a better-developed sense of humor do experience lower levels of negative emotion in the midst of everyday life stress, this should boost their perception of the quality of their own life. Consistent with this view, higher scores on measures of psychological well-being or perceived quality of life have been obtained for those showing higher sense of humor scores among a broad range of groups of people, including physically healthy men,[66] older adults,[67] older adults suffering from chronic obstructive pulmonary disease,[68] and men with HIV.[69]

One aspect of psychological well-being is one's self-concept or sense of self-esteem. Numerous studies have shown that people who initiate humor more often or score higher on measures of sense of humor tend to have a healthier and more positive self-concept and higher self-esteem[70] and less discrepancy between the way they actually view themselves and the way they would ideally like to be.[71] This relationship has also been found for people coping with arthritis—a chronic source of health-related stress.[72]

Did you hear about the Buddhist who refused Novocain during a root canal? He wanted to transcend dental medication.

Two studies have focused exclusively on negative self-esteem, showing that university students who less frequently used humor as a coping strategy showed greater negative self-esteem and had a more negative body image, as well.[73] Finally, among high school students, using humor as a coping strategy (along with other problem-focused coping strategies) was again associated with high self-esteem. Students with low self esteem did not often use humor to cope; the strategies they did use centered around avoiding dealing with the problem.[74]

People who use humor to cope with life stress also tend to show greater confidence in their interactions with others and to enjoy social interactions more than those who less frequently use humor to cope. So the quality of their social life is higher.

Humor and Marriage. It comes as no surprise that most people attach a great deal of importance to a sense of humor in both choosing a mate and remaining happy once married.[75] In the case of dating relationships, both male and female college students put "displaying a good sense of humor" at the top of the list were asked to rate a large

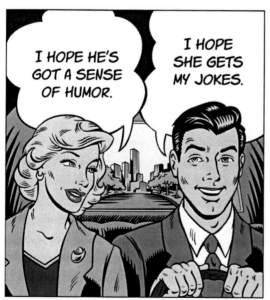

set of behaviors in terms of how important they were in attracting the opposite sex,.[76] Among students who were already dating, couples with greater similarity in the things they found funny expressed higher levels of liking, loving and desire to marry their partner.[77] Even complete strangers are viewed as more attractive if they laugh at your attempts at humor. This is the case even when the other person's attitudes are seen as very dissimilar to your own.[78]

As a side note, it is worth remembering that this bonding through humor and laughter is not restricted to romantic links between people. You may recall from your own experience that if you were ever at a party where you knew no one and felt very ill at ease in the situation, once you shared a laugh with someone the barriers began to come down—first with the person you laughed with, and then others. Laughter helps you feel connected with others. The famous piano-player comedian (from the 1950s-1970s) Victor Borge captured this notion with his statement that "Laughter is the shortest distance between two people." This was demonstrated in a laboratory setting by asking pairs of same-sex strangers to work together to complete either a humorous or non-humorous task. Those who shared humor while working on their task later reported greater feelings of closeness to their partner than those whose task contained no humor.[79]

"Among those whom I like, I can find no common denominator; but among those I love, I can: all of them make me laugh."

(W. H. Auden)

Once a couple marries, satisfaction with the marriage makes a stronger contribution to general life satisfaction than anything else—including one's work and career.[80] A good marriage fills our fundamental human need for intimacy. The emotional and social support provided by marriage plays an important role in helping partners cope with all kinds of stress in their lives.[81] At the same time, however, the coping skills of every married couple are often put to the test throughout their relationship. Every marriage or other long–term intimate relationship eventually encounters some stress or strain. While marital problems may seem minor in comparison to the stressors discussed elsewhere in this chapter, marital stress has a tremendous impact on our lives. And the high divorce rate attests to the extent of relationship stress in the country. *If humor is an effective tool for handling conflict, couples who value humor and have a good sense of humor should have healthier, happier—and longer—marriages. They should be drawn closer together and have a stronger foundation for battling marital stress when it arises.* Even reminiscing about past incidents of shared laughter may strengthen the marriage. Among young couples (college students—some married and some unmarried), those who reminisced about past events involving shared laughter reported higher relationship satisfaction than those who did not reminisce about such events.[82]

Among older couples (who have been married several decades), both husbands and wives generally believe that a good sense of humor is important for the long–term success of a marriage.[83] For couples married at least 45 years, laughing often with their partner was one of the top three stated reasons for the success of their marriage. Within these long-term satisfying marriages, nearly 80% said that they laughed together once a day or more. Similarly, enjoying and creating humor within the relationship boosts marital satisfaction among both husbands and wives.[84] As we age, it is very common for one or both spouses to have to put up with pain (e.g., due to arthritis). Among couples where either one or both partners are experiencing chronic pain, increased use of humor between the couple is associated with higher marital satisfaction.[85]

> *"Laughter is the shortest distance between two people."*
>
> (Victor Borge)

> *"The couple that plays together stays together."*
>
> (Paul McGhee)

The belief that you share similarities in what you and your spouse find funny also contributes to marital satisfaction after you're married.[86] A lack of appreciation of the humor of one's partner tends to be a sign of marital discord—a relationship that is no longer healthy. When husbands or wives indicate that they don't appreciate their spouse's sense of humor, this is often an indication of problems within the relationship.[87]

In one study, a distinction was made between positive and negative uses of humor within the relationship. Positive use was defined as humor which draws the couple toward intimacy and helps manage conflict. Negative use was defined as hostile humor or humor which increased distance between partners. Not surprisingly, couples showing positive forms of humor showed better marital adjustment than those using negative humor.[88]

There is some evidence that women are better than men at using humor to reduce relationship conflicts. In a study of young married couples (married an average of eight years), wives' use of humor to soften conflict situations was associated with increased happiness and marital satisfaction. Among men, however, it was associated with decreased marital satisfaction and more destructive forms of behavior.[89] The reason for this difference is not clear, but the explanation may lie in the kind of humor women and men generally use. It may be that men are more prone to using sarcastic, belittling, or other negative forms of humor which increase distance from one's spouse, while women use more positive forms of humor that reduce distance and promote intimacy. This gives men an extra incentive for learning to use humor more effectively.

Finally, when negative situations do arise in a marriage, the critical thing is that positive, relationship-enhancing behaviors are the norm, and not negative, disruptive forces that tend to undermine the relationship over time.[90] In fact there is evidence that for a marriage to be successful, you need at least a 5:1 ratio of interactions resulting in positive vs. negative emotions.[91] Boosting your humor skills and building humor into your relationship on a daily basis helps assure that this ratio remains slanted in a positive direction.

It was noted in the Introduction that a 3:1 ratio of positive to negative emotion is the minimal threshold for human flourishing. The need of a more elevated ratio (5:1) for a successful marriage suggests that a flourishing marriage is more difficult to achieve than flourishing as an individual. So adding a daily dose of humor to your marriage may be even more important than building humor into other aspects of your life.

Positive (Adaptive) vs. Negative (Maladaptive) Humor

The above discussion of the link between sense of humor and coping presents a somewhat rosier picture than actually exists in the research findings. I've focused on the studies which document humor's power to help cope with stress. In each of the areas discussed above, however, some research has failed to show any significant impact of humor—or required a more qualified statement of the benefits of humor than I've provided. The discussion to this point does, however, capture the general thrust of the findings.

A major cause of the lack of consistent evidence for humor's coping power (as indicated be sense of humor measures) may be attributed to the fact that virtually all of the studies relating sense of humor to stress and mental health relied upon measures of sense of humor that failed to distinguish between positive and negative forms of humor. We all know from our own experience that some people initiate a great deal of humor—even in stressful situations—but their humor tends to be sarcastic, rude, or simply inappropriate in some way. Such humor certainly was not the basis for the longstanding survival of the familiar phrase, "Laughter is the best medicine."

As you might expect, the tendency to use positive forms of humor and avoid negative ones is associated with such positive personality characteristics as optimism, hope and happiness. In fact these personality characteristics appear to play an important role in accounting for humor's power in coping with stress.[92] (Humor's power to help manage your mood and sustain a more positive frame of mind is emphasized throughout this chapter.)

Both Nicholas Kuiper and Rod Martin have recently developed separate measures which distinguish between positive and negative forms of humor.[93] These new measures reveal that positive and adaptive forms of humor are associated with higher self-esteem, interpersonal competence and overall psychological well-being and lower depression and anxiety. Negative and maladaptive forms of humor are associated with lower interpersonal competence, self-esteem and psychological well-being and higher levels of depression and anxiety—and even more frequent psychiatric symptoms.[94] This makes it clear that *simply having a well-developed sense of humor is not enough to obtain the mental health benefits humor offers, since a well-developed negative sense of humor actually interferes with good psychological health and effectiveness in social interaction.*

Positive forms of humor were also associated with a skilled use of humor. Thus, the positive humor users were good at producing humor that helped them cope, got others to laugh, and strengthened social relationships. Some of their humor tended to be self-enhancing, but not at the expense of others. Their humor helped them deal with difficult situations, while still maintaining a realistic perspective on life. And people using such humor tended to have a humorous outlook on life in general. Other positive forms of humor were more focused on building social relationships, serving to "raise group morale, identity, and cohesiveness by reducing conflicts and increasing others' feelings of well-being. This non-hostile use of humor involves joking and banter to reduce interpersonal tensions and facilitate relationships with others."[95]

Among negative types of humor, rude and aggressive humor included humor that was coarse, vulgar, sarcastic, ridiculing, teasing, or otherwise put others down. Self-defeating humor involved efforts to disparage oneself—often in an effort to gain the approval of others. Continued use of this kind of humor has a high personal cost in terms of one's own self-image. A final negative form of humor was called "belabored" humor. This involved poor skills at either sharing humor or responding to the humor of others. This was described as a "social compensatory style" of humor, because it "represents an inappropriate attempt to fit into social groups, with the individual using laughter and humor as a tool to please others and also mask personal and social anxieties."

Each of these negative forms of humor was found to have a detrimental effect on psychological well-being, while the positive forms were supportive of well-being. This helps make sense out of the failure of measures of sense of humor to consistently predict either physical (as discussed in Chapter 2) or psychological health and well-being (as discussed in this chapter). From this point on, researchers will obviously have to distinguish between these two types of humor if we are to fully understand just how (and how much) humor and laughter contribute to physical and emotional well-being, as well as personal resilience. (It should be noted that all three measures of positive humor in the new sense of humor tests were significantly positively related to the most frequently used measure of using humor to cope with stress, called the Coping Humor Scale.)[96]

It is also worth remembering the commonly accepted wisdom that the ability to laugh at oneself is a good sign of a healthy sense of humor, as well as of good mental health generally. Taken as a whole, the existing research on humor supports this view. But *it is the capacity to laugh at yourself and the occasional use of this capacity that is good for your mental/emotional health. This new evidence suggests that you can go too far with such humor.* Having this as a dominant feature of your sense of humor may actually predispose you to greater risk of depression or anxiety (of course, it could also be a result of such depression or anxiety).

Distinction between Genuine and Non-Genuine Laughter. A similar issue in connection with the health-promoting impact of laughter concerns the distinction between genuine spontaneous laughter and socially driven laughter. Until recently, researchers have not distinguished between these two kinds of laughter. The distinction is made on the basis of specific facial muscles contracting during smiling and laughter (the genuine variety is referred to as "Duchenne" smiling or laughter, named after the person who first made the distinction). However, Willibald Ruch, at the University of Zurich, and others have emphasized that this distinction may be a crucial one for understanding the effects of laughter.[97] Ruch and his colleagues, for example, found that the pain reduction effect we've come to expect from laughter and humor (as discussed in the next chapter) only occurred when the laughter was accompanied by genuine or Duchenne facial expressions. Similarly, only Duchenne laughter was effective in undoing negative emotions and stress.[98] And only genuine, emotionally-driven laughter elicits positive emotion in others.[99] This distinction will clearly be important as researchers in the coming decade try to sort out the relative contributions of humor and the act of laughter to health.

The Chicken/Egg Dilemma: Which Comes First, a Good Sense of Humor or Psychological Well-Being?

There is one basic problem—as we have noted—with all of the sense of humor studies discussed here. It's the old chicken and the egg problem. Do you feel happier (with less negative and more positive emotion) because your sense of humor protects you from negativity and keeps you in a better mood, or does the fact that you're (for other reasons) less anxious, angry or depressed and feeling good cause you to find more to laugh at in everyday life? Does the fact that you use humor to cope with life stress cause the improved psychological well-being, or is it your more positive psychological state that allows you to find humor in life—even in stressful situations?

As we have noted, all of the correlational studies discussed here provide no way to answer this question. Chances are that both directions of cause are operating to some extent. That's where the experimental research comes in. The fact that good experimental research shows that we can generate stress in people and then use humor to reduce it, while boosting positive emotion and reducing negative emotion in the process, makes a convincing argument for the view that the possession of good humor skills does cause the mood improvement and other indices of psychological well-being. Also, the endless examples of people who (successfully) use humor to manage stress and avoid emotional burnout in a wide range of extreme-stress work environments or life circumstances (discussed next) make it difficult to doubt humor's capacity to cause an improved sense of psychological well-being. As noted in the previous section, this is most likely to be true for positive forms of humor and may be the reverse for negative humor.

Using Humor in High-Stress, Real-Life Situations

Newspaper and other mass media reports of unanticipated crisis situations often include comments on spontaneously emerging humor in the midst of the crisis. For example, a couple of years ago, two cable cars which carry thousands of tourists and residents every day between Manhattan and Roosevelt Island in New York City's East River broke down and stranded 69 passengers high above the river—some for up to 11 hours. A baby (and other children) and a dog were among those stranded. Several people in the cars were very afraid of heights. Passengers interviewed after their rescue noted that many people soon fell into joking and singing to ease their anxiety about the car falling.[100]

A private school in Washington was recently faced with an unusual problem. Many of the 12-year-old girls were just beginning to use lipstick and they would put it on in the school bathroom. This was not a problem, but they would then press their lips to the mirror, leaving dozens of lip prints that the night custodian would have to remove every evening. Day after day, he removed the annoying prints.

Finally, the principal developed a plan. She called the suspected girls to the bathroom and met them there with the custodian. She explained that all the lip prints were creating a problem for the custodian, who had to clean the mirrors every night. To demonstrate just how difficult this task was, she asked the custodian to show the girls all the effort he had to go through. He took out a long-handled squeegee, dipped it in the toilet, and cleaned the mirror with it. After that, there were no more incidents of lipstick on the mirrors.

The stress-relieving power of laughter was also evident when a Qantas Airlines jumbo jet carrying 346 passengers experienced an explosive "bang" while cruising at 29,000 feet. The plane suddenly descended rapidly as oxygen masks dropped from the ceiling and debris flew about throughout the cabin from the hole (the size of a small car) that suddenly ripped through the side of the plane allowing a clear view of the ground through the floor in the plane. There was total quiet on the plane (except for a crying baby) until it safely touched down in Manila . . . at which point very loud and relieved laughter erupted throughout the plane. There was clearly no humor here, but the sudden end to the extreme stress (people did not know if they would survive the landing) was reflected in the release provided by laughter.[101]

Coping with Cancer. Later in this chapter, a distinction is made between problem-focused and emotion-focused coping. Problem-focused coping is very effective when the source of stress is under your own control. Emotion-focused coping tends to be more effective when you have no choice but to deal with a situation that seems out of your control. The basic idea here is that you can always take steps—one of which is to find a light side of the situation—to at least control your emotional reaction to the situation, even though you can't fully control the situation itself. (We noted earlier that this is a key component of emotional intelligence.)

Most severe or chronic diseases, such as cancer, Parkinson's, arthritis, etc., are generally placed in this "uncontrollable" category, even though there are often some things you can do (e.g., practice good nutrition, get adequate sleep, and manage everyday stress well) to prevent worsening of the condition. Humor is an effective tool in helping to keep negative emotion from overwhelming you as you receive treatment and otherwise battle the disease.

I have provided many programs on the benefits of humor to cancer patients (usually for National Cancer Survivors Day). After many of these programs, someone comes up to me and says, "You know, what you said is so true. If it hadn't been for my sense of humor, I wouldn't have survived the treatments, let alone the disease!" They say that finding a light side of the situation was essential to keeping going and that their sense of humor helped maintain a sense of hope and determination to fight the disease.

One woman who had had a double mastectomy told me that it wasn't that bad; for a short time after the surgery, it gave her more cleavage than she ever had before (due to the resulting swelling). Bernie Siegel used to frequently talk about one of his patients who went through a mastectomy and a divorce at about the same time. She said she "gave up a tit and an ass." While the remark is crude, it worked well for this patient.

In cancer support groups, patients often talk about how important humor was in getting them through their ordeal. Some even joke about the threat that cancer still poses to their life. I asked members of one support group if they ever told jokes specifically related to their cancer. One man told the following joke to me.

A man was told by his doctor that he had a very advanced cancer. It he was told he only had 24 hours to live. He went home and told the terrible news to

his wife, and they came to grips with it as well as they could. That evening his wife asked him if there was anything special he wanted to do on this, his last night. He said, "I just want to make love to you one last time." So they went upstairs and made passionate love, just the way they did on their Honeymoon.

A couple of hours later, she said, "Honey, you've still got 10 hours left to live. What would you like to do?" Again, he answered, "I just want to make love one more time." So they just took off their clothes and made love again right on the living room floor.

A couple of hours later, she again asked, "Honey, you've still got 8 hours left to live. What would you like to do?" Once again, he said, "Oh I just want to make love to you again before I go." And she said, "Well, that's easy for you to say. You don't have to get up in the morning!"

The entire support group laughed at this joke—except for one man who was new to the group and only had his diagnosis of cancer for a few months. He was not ready for humor along these lines. It elevated his stress, rather than easing it. For anyone who has a diagnosis of a serious illness, it is essential to go through the full gamut of emotions, including the shock, denial, anger . . . and more. Humor only helps you cope when you come out the other side and accept the reality of your disease. "OK, I have cancer. That's the way it is. How can I now go about living my life with as high a quality of life as possible?" Humor is a powerful coping tool once you get to this point of acceptance. If you have any doubts about this, ask any long-term cancer survivor who you know well what they think of the idea.

It is noted in Chapter 2 that laughter increases the activity (and number) of natural killer cells, a part of your immune system whose role is to seek out and destroy tumor (cancer) cells. The fact that Gilda Radner, of *Saturday Night Live* fame, died of cancer shows that while humor may strengthen your immune system, it will probably not be enough to counter the force of the disease itself. But it will help your body mobilize its own healing forces so that your emotions are working for you, and not against you (as is the case when you get swallowed up in chronic negative emotion). And Gilda made it very clear that her sense of humor helped her cope with the disease and *improved the quality of her life while she fought the battle. She knew that even though her body was losing its fight against the disease, she was winning the battle to cope with it.*

In her book, *It's Always Something*, she says, "The important thing is that the days you've had, you will have lived. What I can control is whether I'm going to live a day in fear and depression and panic, or whether I'm going to attack the day and make it as wonderful a day as I can." She knew that humor was her strongest ally in living her days fully. It also can be yours. More recently, comedian Robert Schimmel, Stand-up Comic of the Year in 1999 was diagnosed with stage III non-Hodgkins lymphoma. His 2008 book, *Cancer on $5 a Day*, documents how important humor was for him in battling the disease.

> *"Live each day as if it were the last day of your life; some day you will be right."* (Anonymous)

Michael Landon, starring as Little Joe Cartwright in the long–running TV series *Bonanza*, was a model for us all during his bout with cancer a couple of decades ago. The media marveled at the way he kept up his spirits in the presence of poor odds of survival. His sense of humor played a crucial role in enabling him to do this. It was evident during his last television appearance, on *The Tonight Show*. While discussing his condition, he asked the studio audience if anyone had ever taken a coffee enema. When someone answered "yes," he said, "You must be fun to have breakfast with." At a news conference in which he discussed his health, he said he was especially helped in preparing for his death by a role he had played in *Highway to Heaven*, ". . . since I played a dead guy anyway." In the same interview, he added, "I think you have to have a sense of humor about everything," and that included his illness.

Michael Landon's ability to maintain a positive and fun attitude toward life helped sustain his family, friends, and loved ones throughout his ordeal. There are many Michael Landons across the country today, and *the reason they are able to use humor to maintain a high quality life during their illness is generally that they had developed and used their sense of humor before they ever got a life–threatening illness.* If you're someone who has been pretty serious most of your life, use this insight right now to begin getting back in touch with the playful side of yourself and to exercise your sense of humor at every opportunity. By doing so, you'll build skills that will then be accessible to you on your worst days.

"No matter what your heartache may be, laughing helps you forget it for a few seconds." (Red Skelton, comedian from the 1940's & 1950's)

BUILD YOUR HUMOR SKILLS

[Turn the page for answers. Work on both jokes before checking answers.]

1. A drunk guy staggers out of a bar just as a fire engine races past, with sirens wailing and lights flashing. He immediately starts chasing it, running as fast as he can until he finally collapses, gasping for breath. He looks up as the fire engine and shouts, "Ok if that's the way you want it, keep your _____!"
Clue: He mistakes the fire truck for another kind of truck with something he wants.

2. Psychiatrist to his receptionist: "Just say we're very busy; don't keep saying its _____."
Clue: A familiar phrase, meaning things are very hectic, almost out of control.

Erma Bombeck reported in her book, *I Want to Grow Up, I want to Grow Hair, I Want to Go to Boise,* that when she visited a cancer camp for children and adolescents, she found that they often used humor.

She was amazed at their vitality and ability to retain a playful attitude in life while battling their disease. One girl was waiting to see her doctor and noticed some plants on the window sill that had gone unwatered and were dying. She said, "I certainly hope he's better at taking care of his patients than he is his plants."

A boy who had had a leg amputated developed the habit of draping his artificial leg over his shoulder when in the car, taking great delight in the reactions of people in other cars. A teenager was asked by her friend, "What's your sign?" She answered, "Cancer, of course!" Another teenager noticed two preschoolers staring at her wig (worn because of the chemotherapy–induced hair loss). She suddenly ripped off the wig and said, "See what happens when you don't eat your veggies!" The startled children ran off. While this is not the way anyone wants their teenagers to treat young children, the resulting laughter by the wig-wearer was certainly therapeutic.

Do these remarks mean that these kids are not taking their disease seriously? Absolutely not. It's a sign that they want to keep on living life every day, even though they have cancer. Pediatric cancer patients have the built–in exuberance of childhood and youth, and this enables them to maintain a zest for life during their ordeal. *Joking about cancer is not a form of denial in these kids. It's a reflection of their success in coping with the reality of the disease. They are refusing to lie down and become victims.* The limited research on children with cancer supports the view that humor does help cope with at least some of the ordeals associated with cancer.[102]

My wife used to work in a pediatric oncology unit of a hospital and often found the children using humor to take control of their fears and anxieties. One eight–year–old wrote a letter to her nurse (who had long hair), opening with, "Dear hairy scary nurse, I love spinal taps . . ." In the same letter, she said that if the nurse ever got sick, she (the girl) would help her get better, assuring her that she would "take good care of you and give you lots of shots." Since the girl did not like getting shots herself, this playful remark was a way of coping with that particular source of anxiety.

Many adult cancer patients who successfully fight off the disease later say that getting cancer was the best thing that ever happened to them—that they had been taking life for granted and had never really known how to live. When their survival was in doubt, they learned to live as if they had little time left and to enjoy one day at a time. They came to experience more aliveness in their everyday life and learned to be more present to their experiences. Rediscovering a sense of playfulness and humor will give you this same renewed zest for living and the ability to "be here now." So why wait until you get cancer (or any other life-threatening illness) to learn to live life fully and fill each day with joy and fun?

Recent studies of adult cancer patients have supported the view that humor helps patients manage the distress[103] and depression[104] associated with a diagnosis of cancer. Among women with advanced breast cancer, humor and other active coping strategies (such as use of emotional support from others, religion, positive reframing, or venting) were associated with a higher quality of life, while more avoidant coping strategies (such as using alcohol or drugs) were associated with a lower quality of life.[105] Similarly, among breast cancer patients, women who reported using humor to cope with their ordeal reported less distress than non-humor using patients the day before surgery, three days after surgery and also three months later.[106] Hospital staff can support this coping process by using humor with patients to help them both relax (and manage the understandable anxiety that goes with cancer) and discuss their concerns more openly.[107] Finally, in addition to reducing levels of negative emotion, humor also reduces the degree of neuroendocrine response to stress among breast cancer patients.[108]

ANSWERS TO JOKES

1. lousy ice cream   2. madhouse

An interview-based study of breast cancer survivors provided good insight into the ways in which women think about their use of humor during their daily ordeal with the disease.

"A consensus occurred regarding how the use of **humor is a step to recovery**. Women reported that humor gives hope to survive through the moment. One woman said, 'I just feel anytime you can laugh, it can help, even your spirituality. It is much better than crying or hurting and it keeps you from hurting as much.' . . .

Most of the women felt that their use of humor made them **want to help others**. Many . . . felt it necessary to help their families cope with the diagnosis, which helped the women cope as well. Many joked about their hair loss to put their kids at ease, or they wore different wigs or no wigs at all. . . . One woman said, 'I know they were worried about me dying, but if I could joke with them on things, it would make them think I was more confident . . .'

The use of humor also evolved over time after the diagnosis. Many women did not see any humor at first but later found humor in situations where they would have not seen humor before." [109] (Bold type is original author's.)

Humor, of course, is just one positive coping strategy. The use of religion, emotional support and venting is also associated with a higher quality of life, while avoidant and negative strategies are associated with a lower quality of life among advanced breast cancer patients.[110]

Some cancer patients, of course, are just not comfortable using humor to cope with their cancer. My own conversations with patients following Cancer Survivor Day programs suggest that it is individuals who often used humor *before* their cancer who are able to use it to cope after their diagnosis. The evidence suggests that the percentage of cancer patients who use humor to cope may be anywhere from 21%[111] to 50%.[112]

It is generally even more stressful to have a child come down with a serious disease than for oneself to do so. Can humor help parents as they go through the ordeal of treatments and uncertain outcomes with their children? In the case of mothers whose children were undergoing a bone marrow transplant, those who accepted the reality of their child's disease, and who used humor as a coping strategy, were least likely to become depressed, while those who relied more on alcohol to cope showed more signs of depression.[113]

Consistent with Erma Bombeck's observations of kids with cancer (described above), elementary school cancer patients who scored higher on a measure of using humor to cope showed better psychological adjustment in dealing with their cancer than did children who tended not to use humor as a coping tool.[114] In the case of older kids (9 to 16 years of age) humor was often used in connection with their cancer, but these kids said that they did so only after they had dealt with the realization that they had cancer and had absorbed a lot of information about the disease.[115]

The focus here has been on the use of humor by cancer patients. But there is every reason to assume that the findings discussed also apply to patients with other serious diseases. Just a couple of examples will be provided in support of this notion. Among a group of patients with chronic obstructive pulmonary disease (which places great restrictions on one's quality of life and tends to increase strain in the relationship with one's spouse), those who used humor more often to cope in daily life enjoyed a better quality of life. Just as importantly, their use of humor in connection with their illness served to give their spouse permission to use more humor as well, and this improved the quality of life for the spouse.[116] Even in AIDS-ravaged Africa, the coping power of humor has been noted. One African HIV-infected man said that "Among people who make jokes, you forget. You don't think about death, you enjoy life."[117]

Hospital Staff. Doctors and nurses confront life–threatening tragedy on a regular basis. So if humor does help cope with tragedy, we would it expect to show up in hospitals. And we should find the most humor in those areas of the hospital where the threat and actual occurrence of death is the greatest; namely, in the emergency room, operating room, and critical care units. Surely doctors and nurses in these settings would use humor if it really helps you cope.

"Humor is an important piece of my survival skills. Over time, if I took home the weight of everything that goes on every day here, I wouldn't be able to get out of bed in the morning." [118]

(A hospital physician)

As noted in Chapter 2, this is exactly what happens. While humor is common in all areas of the hospital, it is most common in the emergency room (including psychiatric ERs), operating room, and critical care unit.[119] These also are the areas where humor is the crudest and most macabre. Hospital staff are quite aware that they have this unusual sense of humor. Many are also keenly aware of using humor to manage their own roller coaster emotions. In the keynotes I do for hospitals and healthcare conferences, I always ask those in the audience to describe their own sense of humor in a single word or two. The answer is always the same: "sick," "black," or "macabre." I then ask about the areas of the hospital where this humor is most common. Again, the answer is always the same: "emergency room," "operating room," "intensive care," and "the morgue." It is the emotional turmoil generated by constant exposure to death and serious injury/illness that obliges them to come up with some means of preventing negative emotion from taking over. They learn on the job that humor does this and helps sustain a positive focus in their contact with patients.

Hospital staff are also keenly aware that their gallows humor is to be shared only with other staff—and not with patients. They know they need a dose of humor on a daily basis, but recognize that it will be viewed as inappropriate by anyone who does not share their daily exposure to death and serious illness/injury. Their humor "is used to create camaraderie among the staff in dealing with stressful situations."[120] By finding a way to laugh in the midst of the terrible things that happen to people, they enable themselves to carry on and help the next person in the bed down the hall. As we will see in the next section, police, firemen and other emergency responders who have the same kind of experience with death and dying share a similar sense of humor.

The following jokes would not be unusual in a hospital.

What's the difference between humor and aroma?
Humor is a shift of wit . . .

Did you hear about the nurse who swallowed a razor blade? She performed a tonsillectomy, a hysterectomy, and circumcised an intern.

While the average person can laugh at the first example, the second probably goes beyond your limit. It is crude and grisly and produces imagery most of us prefer not to think about. Of course, hospital staff also laugh at more benign forms of humor, including what patients say. For example, after completing his examination of a young woman, a male gynecologist told her she had acute vaginitis. Her response was, "Why thank you." Another woman was concerned about the dangers of tampons. She asked her doctor if she was at risk for toxic waste (confusing it with "toxic shock") syndrome. The following examples are typical of this more benign form of humor. They relate to the fact that even when a nurse or doctor offers an explanation of a medical condition, patients don't get it quite right. Each of these comments was made by a patient or family member to other family members.

"The doctor said I have sick-as-hell anemia."

"I have micro-orgasms in my blood."

A doctor explained to a woman that her husband had died of a massive myocardial infarction. She was later heard telling family members that he died of a "massive internal fart."

Some staff also frequently share with each other the ambiguous remarks (or mistakes) occasionally written in patients' medical records. Here are a few examples of those.

She has no rigors or shaking chills, but her husband states that she was very hot in bed last night.

Pt. suffers from abdominal cramps, with constipation on the one hand and BM's on the other.

Patient suffers from headaches while menstruating from the top of her head.

Pt. referred by private physician with green stools.

Pt. says he urinates around the clock every two hours.

Vaginal packing out. Dr. Cartwright in.

Rx: Mycostatin vaginal suppositories, #24. Insert daily until exhausted.

In decades past, when tuberculosis was a common health threat, the following jingle was popular in sanitoriums.[121]

T.B. or not T.B. That is congestion. Consumption be done about it? Of corpse! Of corpse!

Staff members who are initially put off by crude hospital humor gradually learn to enjoy it—or find a new career. They realize that this kind of humor helps them live with the emotionally draining things they confront every day by creating a momentary positive focus; it also helps them fight burnout and do their job effectively. Physicians and nurses are routinely in the position of caring for dying patients. Even though it's a daily occurrence, many still find it hard to adjust to. So it is no surprise that they are so often drawn to using humor to cope.[122]

The following letter demonstrates doctors' and nurses' awareness of the importance of humor and laughter in coping with the constant stress of their jobs. It was written by the nurse anesthetist present during the surgery on a man who died during the surgery.

"You saw me laugh after your father died. I was splashing water on my face at a sink midway between the emergency room lobby where you stood and the far green room where his body lay. Someone told a feeble joke and I brayed laughter like a jackass, decorum forgotten until I met your glance . . . your eyes streaming with tears . . .

My laugh was inappropriate, and for that I apologize. But it was, nonetheless, a necessity.

I laughed, nominally, at a corny joke. It's no secret that hospital people seem to enjoy warped humor . . . we're often too morbid: burned patients become crispy critters; Vietnam casualties were Jungle–Burgers. It's not pleasant. Neither is hospital work, at times . . .

While we may appear emotionless behind our various masks, please understand: Much of the stress that health care workers suffer comes about because we <u>do</u> care. We cared about your father . . .

That day you saw me laugh, I knew that another patient was waiting who needed my care and full attention in surgery. As I stood at that sink and washed sweat and vomitus from my face and arms, *my laugh was no less cleansing for me than were your tears for you.*"[123] (Italics are McGhee's.)

If you're the next patient to go under the knife with this team after they've lost a patient, you want them to have a good laugh (at anything; it doesn't matter what) before they begin with you. The laughter relieves the tension and upset that could distract them and prevent them from giving you their best efforts during your surgery.

Doctors and nurses will always need to laugh at things the rest of us would find morbid, cold, and unfeeling (if we knew about it). But *this laughter is essential to fighting burnout on their jobs and keeping them prepared to deal with the next crisis situation——with someone's life on the line.* Consistent with this idea, pediatricians who rated themselves as having a good sense of humor reported lower levels of emotional exhaustion.[124] And nurses who use humor on the job cope better with the high stress that goes with nursing; they're also more satisfied with their jobs.[125]

In some cases, staff direct their humor to patients themselves. (See chapter 2 for additional discussion of this.) Interviews of 22 healthcare providers regarding their experiences in using humor with patients revealed the importance of an occasional lighter style of interaction between hospital staff and patients. Humor was considered to be especially important as a communication option because of the great stress patients are under. "Medical interactions between patients and providers, particularly in the case of severe illness, can be fraught with tension and distress. The threat of serious negative consequences, discomfort, debilitation, and even death frequently shadow such meetings. These tensions can be exacerbated by the awkwardness of nudity and physical examinations and the embarrassment of discussing intimate practices and personal failings. *Patient-provider interactions, therefore, require fairly careful management to avoid generating so much negative emotion that communication becomes impossible.*"[126] (Italics are McGhee's.)

In this study, staff were much more likely to use humor with patients who have long-term or chronic problems. This is probably because staff had a lengthy period of contact with these patients; and a good relationship needs to be established with a patient before using humor as part of one's interaction style. The box on the next page shows the most common reasons given by these staff for their use of humor with patients.

One gynecological oncologist (who supervised the work of residents) in this study described how he deals with the embarrassment built into most gynecological examinations. "The resident does all the [initial procedures], and when I come in the patient is already undressed from at least the waist down and in the stirrups with a speculum sticking out of her vagina. And to have someone just walk in at that point can be really embarrassing. So in introductions I usually crack a joke about how this is a very awkward way to meet someone for the first time, just trying to ease the situation and make it less embarrassing for her."[127]

The sudden outbreak of SARS (Severe Acute Respiratory Syndrome) in 2003 was a major source of stress for hospital staff, since little was known about the disease and the vulnerability of healthcare staff working with SARS patients. Among the many doctors and nurses working with SARS patients in a Singapore hospital in July of 2003, over 20% showed what was referred to as "psychiatric morbidity" after working with these patients. Morbidity refers to gloomy and other negative feelings in connection with the disease—due to a fear of contracting the disease themselves. Those who used humor as an active coping strategy, however, were less likely to experience such feelings.[128]

MOST COMMON REASONS FOR STAFF USE OF HUMOR WITH PATIENTS

1. Build rapport or trust
2. Show a sense of humanity
3. Reduce patient anxiety or stress
4. Reduce embarrassment with awkward procedures

Mental Health Professionals. Like hospital staff, those who work in the mental health field are prone to burnout because of constant immersion in other people's problems. I have done many programs for counselors, therapists, social workers and other mental health professionals, and I am consistently struck by their need to "let go" of the emotional build-up resulting from immersion in others' emotional conflicts and turmoil day after day. They are all at ongoing risk of burnout.

In programs I've done for people working with victims of violent crime (including those who have had family members gruesomely murdered), there is a constant risk of vicarious traumatization because of the extreme suffering by the victims. It is crucial for these professionals to have good skills at protecting themselves against the constant emotional onslaught from others' crises. As one put it in a discussion with me, *"We need an emotional condom, and humor serves that role quite well."*

Those working with child abuse and neglect are especially prone to stress and burnout. And humor has been shown to be a powerful coping tool for them, as well. Paraprofessionals who used humor less often to cope in their work with such victims reported more emotional exhaustion than those who used humor more often. The humor users also reported less job stress than their more serious colleagues, as well as a greater sense of personal accomplishment.[129] In the case of child protection workers, shared humor among co-workers, venting, and support networks (family and co-workers) were all found to be important to their ability to remain effective in their work and cope with the emotional stress of a job that most begin to burn out in after two years.[130]

As noted both here and in Chapter 2, the "sick" sense of humor shared by doctors and nurses is actually very healthy for them; it also helps them provide quality care in the midst of extreme stress. Mental health clinicians who regularly work with others' emotional crises tend to share this sick or gallows humor.[131]

Disasters and Other Emergency Situations. Other jobs also require people to cope with the high stress of exposure to death and serious injury, although on a less frequent basis. But when it does occur, it is typically of an extreme nature. Whenever there is a plane crash, serious auto accident, or natural disaster, emergency response teams come face to face with the human tragedy that results from the disaster. In extreme cases, such as the World Trade Center Towers attack on 9/11/2001 or the massively devastating tsunami that struck from the Indian Ocean in late December, 2004, we were all witness to horror and deaths on an unprecedented scale. For those who have to pull lifeless bodies out of the rubble, the emotional toll can be staggering. Untrained individuals who go through this generally say their life is never the same again. Even those with training often have to go through lengthy periods of "critical incident stress debriefing." Can humor help cope with exposure to such extreme cases of death and injury?

1) Police, Firemen and Other Emergency Responders

Wherever you go in the world, firemen, EMS workers, ambulance drivers, and police officers are generally known for their macabre sense of humor. For example, they may talk about "crispy critters" after fires, or "road pizza" after traffic accidents. Following major disasters, such as plane crashes, hurricanes, tornados, major fires, earthquakes, floods, etc., there is generally a critique among the emergency response team concerning how they handled the situation. There's generally a lot of humor in these discussions, as team members let go of the incredible tension and strain that built up throughout the response to the disaster. It helps them counter the psychological gravity they experience on the job.

Following a recent program I provided at the convention of the National Coordinating Council on Emergency Management, many came up to me afterwards and said that they often look for any excuse to laugh after the emergency is handled, or start laughing for no reason at all. Some have no idea why they laugh so hard for no apparent reason. Others know that belly laughter is very therapeutic for them and will help them work through the emotional residue they carry around following the emergency response.

"Life does not cease to be funny when people die any more than it ceases to be serious when people laugh." (George Bernard Shaw)

Emergency workers are wellprepared to deal with the disaster itself, but they are generally not trained to cope with the emotional trauma they experience after the incident is handled. Critical incident stress debriefing teams are generally available to help them cope with the emotional aftermath of the disaster, but humor and laughter allow them to "let go" of much of the emotional burden even before the CISD team comes in. One fire fighter told me that this laughter provides a much–needed "emotional delousing."

As in hospitals, newcomers to disaster relief teams are often put off by their colleagues' humor, because it seems inconsiderate and inappropriate. But the longer they stay on the job, the more they come to see it as an essential part of staying effective in their work and maintaining their own mental health. They also learn *not* to share this humor with their spouse.

I learned first hand the risk of sharing emergency responders' humor with the uninitiated at a state-level emergency response conference several years ago. I was the keynote speaker, and gave several examples of the humor I knew to be typical of the audience before going on to talk to them about why this "sick" humor was really very healthy for them. No one told me that the governor, his wife, and some other politicians were also in the room. A couple of hours later, I was back in my room preparing for a follow-up workshop. There was a knock on the door. My contact person for the conference had come to tell me that several people were quite offended by the humor, and that there would be no more such examples in the afternoon session.

Doctors, nurses and emergency response teams are the only people I would ever consider presenting such humor to, since I know that they can handle it—because it is typical of their own humor—and it helps clarify the benefits of such humor with a few examples on the table. Since that conference with the governor in the room, I've been very careful to be sure I know who is in the room and to clear the use of sick humor in advance.

A woman (who had never worked "in the field" as a first responder) teaching a class on emergency planning in New Orleans told me about her own initial shock at the "horrible" humor displayed by three Emergency Medical Service workers in her class. She found it totally inappropriate, because "they're supposed to be sympathetic and concerned about these people's well being." She communicated this to them, once she'd taken as much of their humor as she could. At that point, one of the guys who had been joking around all the time got real serious and said,

> "You have to understand, it's our way of coping. It's our way of surviving the job we have. When I first started, the terrible things I saw really bothered me. I tried to act real macho, like it wasn't bothering me, but it really was. I wasn't aware of how much it was eating away at me until I responded to a hit–and–run incident, in which a mother and baby had been hit. The mother was killed outright, but the baby was still alive until just before we got there. I was trying to resuscitate the baby. I just kept going and kept going, trying to get the baby to breathe. My colleague finally put his hand on my shoulder, saying, 'Enough . . . enough.'
>
> From that point on, I always found things to laugh at. Without humor as a means of stress release, I really couldn't handle it. As far as I was concerned, that child was my child. Losing that child made me realize I'd been shoving to the back of my mind all the

upset I had experienced from the things I'd seen. I love my job, and I'd never change it, but I'd never survive it if I didn't find things to laugh at."

Research has documented that this macabre or black humor is a common coping tool among paramedics and emergency medical technicians,[132] police officers[133] and 911 dispatchers. I have not found a study to document this among fire fighters, but every fireman or woman I've ever discussed the subject with has affirmed that such humor is commonly used by them to relieve tension and reduce stress.

The humor initiated by emergency responders—generally spontaneous and related to the situation of the moment—clearly plays a significant role in reducing their stress.[134] Among 79 emergency workers responding to an apartment building explosion, 42% of them said they used humor to cope in such situations. And four out of every five who said they used humor during, or after responding to, emergencies said it did help them cope.[135]

In the case of police officers, they must learn to deal with frequent exposure to sudden death in traffic accidents, suicides, homicides, and the taking of others' lives themselves. In one group of 96 police officers from four states, 97% said they had experienced gallows humor on the job. Interestingly enough, those who used such humor more often did not experience less stress on the job. The humor did, however, produce a stronger group cohesion among officers. This lack of reduced stress among high humor users may be because officers in this particular study who used gallows humor were also more likely to initiate other forms of maladaptive humor (e.g., aggressive and self-depreciating humor).[136]

Since most emergency response teams learn through their own experience that humor is an important coping tool, and since some health care professionals suggested over a decade ago that emergency workers need to develop their sense of humor as an adaptive defense mechanism,[137] it is surprising that no program has been established to enable them to develop these skills. My Humor Skills Training Program, presented in my book, *Humor as Survival Training for a Stressed-Out World*, finally provides such a program.

911 dispatchers are also confronted by emergency situations on a daily basis. They must be able to remain calm regardless of the circumstances of the emergency of the moment. So it is no surprise that they often share humor with colleagues between calls to handle the stress inherent in this work.[138]

One of the funniest jokes/stories I've heard from an emergency responder came from an emergency medical technician. I've learned since that virtually every EMT is familiar with it.

There were these EMT students who were pretty shaky. They were in danger of not passing their training course. But they got through it. After their finals, everyone said, "I don't know how you did it, but you made it." And the two new graduates said, "All right! We did it! We're EMTs! And now we're going to save the world!"

So they go out to a restaurant to celebrate. The guy at the next table suddenly stands up, grabs his throat, and starts turning blue. He's obviously choking. The two guys jump up and say, "Plan B! We're cool, we can handle this."

So the two of them get up take off their pants and start licking each others' butt.

The guy who was choking starts laughing so hard that the lodged food comes flying out, and he's fine. At that point, one of the new EMTs says to the other, "Hey, that Hiney Lick maneuver really works!"

Another wonderful story was shared with me by a British man at a FEMA (Federal Emergency Management Assn.) conference where I was speaking. He assured me this was a true story. During the Margaret Thatcher era, when Britain was dealing with numerous bombings by the Irish Republican Army, a man was working on an electrical problem in a large apartment building very near the place where a major bomb went off, causing widespread damage to numerous buildings. After completing several wiring repairs on different floors, he went down to the basement and flipped the master switch to turn the electricity back on. It was at that same moment that the bomb went off across the street. He heard the explosion and came upstairs and looked out the front door. He was dumbfounded by the damage, and promptly went back downstairs and hid. He did not come out for the next two days. He was convinced that he had caused the explosion and would be sent to jail. He was finally discovered by his panicked wife who feared he was killed in the bomb attack. This is not typical emergency response humor, but how could I leave it out?

BUILD YOUR HUMOR SKILLS

[Turn the page for answers. Work on both jokes before checking answers.]

1. The boss was complaining at a staff meeting that he wasn't getting any respect. The next day, a sign appeared on his office door that read: "I'm the boss!" Later that day, when he got back from lunch, someone had taped a note to the sign that said: "Your wife called. She wants _____."
Clue: He's still not getting any respect. Assume that the staff put the note on the sign.

2. "I was so depressed last night that I called Lifeline. I got their call center in Pakistan. I told them I was suicidal. They got all excited and asked if I could _____."
Clue: This is a bit sick (like the humor of many emergency responders). Think terrorist attack.

Emergency workers' humor generally shows up *after* the emergency has been handled. In some cases, however, it shows up in the middle of efforts to deal with a tragedy. One EMS worker was carrying a dismembered arm, following a suicide committed by jumping in front of a train. He said to his buddy, "Hey, give me a hand, will ya?" An ambulance driver explained to me that a woman he was about to take to the hospital kept saying that she had "brain farts." She repeated it over and over, as if she thought it was important. He restrained his laughter until they were safely in route to the hospital, and he realized that she meant brain "infarcts." (An infarct is an area of dead tissue.)

A colleague of this same ambulance driver described the wonderful laugh he had in thinking back to the reactions of onlookers as he began working on a woman who had been hit by a truck. She had just come from a deli carrying a large sandwich which she was clutching to her chest when she was hit. She was still clutching it when the EMS vehicle arrived. As he pulled away her coat and tugged at the tightly–gripped sandwich, pieces of ham, tomato, cheese, and bread were sent flying in all directions. He could hear the onlookers gasp, thinking that all this stuff was coming from her insides. Again, the belly laugh he had afterwards in describing this relieved the tension of the moment and left him in a better state of preparedness for the next emergency.

While humor is a common coping tool among those who work with death and serious injury as part of their job, it is not restricted to this group. Both experienced and inexperienced people who were asked to work with the bodies of people who had died violently have been found to use humor as a coping strategy.[139]

2) Disaster Victims/Survivors

Dr. Sandy Ritz is a public health specialist who has long helped coordinate relief efforts following major hurricanes, fires and earthquakes. She notes that humor is very common among the survivors of such tragedies,[140] concluding that it helps them cope and gives them hope. It helps strengthen the feeling, "we're all in this together." Ritz argues that the humor shown by survivors reflects the four emotional phases survivors generally go through after experiencing a disaster. During the "Heroic phase" (which lasts about a week), emotions are running strong—especially tension and fear. It is called heroic because of the altruistic efforts that typically show up, with neighbors helping neighbors, etc. If any humor occurs during this period, it is designed to ease this tension and anxiety. If the disaster is one of sudden impact (like a tornado) there is likely to be no humor at all in this brief phase.

The Honeymoon phase follows and typically lasts from the first week to two to four months following the disaster. Humor is most likely to occur in this phase, according to Ritz, and generally reflects feelings of optimism about recovery. Survivor humor in the media also occurs most often during this period.

A Disillusionment phase then follows, typically lasting from two months to between one or two years. Feelings of anger, resentment, disappointment, pessimism, and powerlessness tend to emerge here and are reflected in reduced levels of humor. All this negative emotion is generally the result of dissatisfaction with delays, "red tape," paper work, and government bureaucracy in general. The euphoria of having survived the disaster is long gone, and recovery seems to be delayed by endless things outside of the survivor's control. The humor that does occur takes the bitter form of gallows humor and other forms of humor aimed at putting down disaster workers and the agencies which are blamed for their problems. A "them against us" mentality develops, and the humor tends to be directed at anyone who is not a fellow-survivor.

ANSWERS TO JOKES

1. her sign back   2. drive a truck

Finally, a Reconstruction phase is entered, characterized by acceptance and recovery. This phase can last for several years, and is a time of gradual rebuilding and recovery, both in terms of emotional and physical/financial resources. A greater general receptiveness to humor returns, and it again shifts toward a more positive focus, reflecting a sense of community.

Ritz notes that disaster-survivor humor has its own "you-had-to-be-there" fell to it, and that it is specifically designed to cope and instill hope. As she notes,

"This positive adaptive response to disaster makes fun of the situation, relieves stress, boosts morale, and promotes social bonding. It is a defense mechanism to master anxiety, and serves as a safety valve for *letting out aggression and tension.* As a psychological weapon, it can be used as a means of displaying self-reliance and strength, maintaining dignity, and providing a palatable method of communication and conflict resolution." (p. 172. Italics are McGhee's.)

Ritz has created many cartoons which reflect survivors' concerns and their phase of adjustment to the disaster. These cartoons were published in local newspapers at the time of the disaster, and helped survivors find a light side of their plight. She believes that cartoons and other sources of public humor provide a positive force of healing and empowerment in the communities affected by disasters. Two of her cartoons are included here. The "too tense" cartoon reflects the frustration people felt in the endless delays in getting the promised tents to live in after their home was flattened by Hurricane Iniki. The "hot flash" cartoon was published in the midst of fears about SARS in 2003. The same cartoon could be used to ease tensions related to fear of being quarantined in connection with the swine flu epidemic of 2009 and 2010.

As a reflection of the need for humor, she noted that following hurricane Iniki in Hawaii, many families got together and watched funny videos together. What made this impressive is that the entire island of Kauai was without electricity for over two months. The only way they could do this was by finding someone who had a generator, someone else whose VCR had survived, and yet another family that had salvaged some comedy tapes. They obviously knew they needed a good laugh.

T–shirts reflect another way in which survivors actively use humor to cope. Ritz notes that following Hurricane Iniki, one nurse was seen wearing a T–shirt with the words, "I suffer from PISS: Post–Iniki Stress Syndrome." Many wore T–shirts in Los Angeles following their earthquake in the 1980s saying, "Shift Happens!"

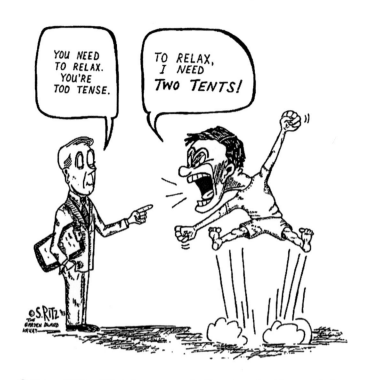

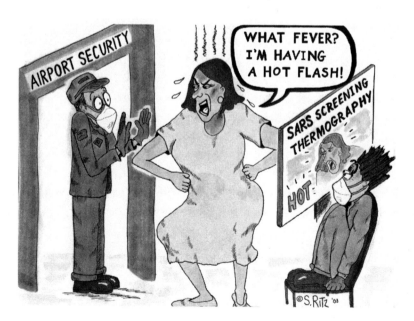

Consistent with Ritz's observations, humor and joking were second only to "talking it out" among the coping strategies adopted by survivors of Hurricane Hugo in the 1980s.[141] My own conversations with disaster relief workers confirm these findings. *The survivors who do best at using humor to cope, however, are those who already had the habit of finding and using humor in their everyday life.* While you will hopefully never have a major disaster to deal with in your own life, improving your sense of humor now will put you in a position to use humor to cope if you do.

House for sale. Half off. (Sign in front of house following California mud slide.)

4 Sale—Skylight included. (In front of house after hurricane.)

House for sale. Some assembly required. (In front of house after hurricane.)

House for sale. Riverfront property. (In front of farm house during major Mississippi river flood.)

New Des Moines (Iowa) zip code: 50H20. (Joke shared among those affected by the same Mississippi river flood.)

One of the best examples I ever saw of this followed a tornado in the Midwest. A man whose house had been destroyed, and whose car was flattened by a fallen tree, put a sign on his car saying, "Compact car!" The sign did nothing to give him back his car or home, but served to say, "This is not going to destroy me; I can deal with this and go on." Another man coped by putting a sign in the place his home used to be saying, "Gone with the wind."

3) General Public

Even the general public finds humor in natural and man–made disasters. It shows up in our laughter at the tasteless jokes that always sweep the country following any national tragedy. Who among us has not at least grinned at jokes like the following, which emerged soon after varying kinds of disasters over the past 25 years?

Did you know that Christa McAulif had "blue" eyes? One "blew" this way and one "blew" that way. (Following the explosion of the Challenger space shuttle in the 1980s; Christa McAulif was the teacher on board.)

Jeffrey Dahmer's mother visits him and has a meal at his apartment. She says, "You know Jeffrey, I really don't care much for your neighbors." Jeffrey says, "OK, then try the veggies." (Dahmer was convicted of cannibalism.)

Following an accident involving Cleveland Indians baseball players Crews and Olin, the autopsy report revealed that the cause of death was "Pier pressure." (The boat in which they were riding ran into a dock.)

How many Branch Davidians can you get in a Volkswagen? Two in the front, two in the back . . . and 181 in the ash tray. (After the fire at the Branch Davidian complex in Waco, Texas.)

What did the devil say when David Koresh arrived in hell? "Well done!" (Koresh was the Branch Davidian leader.)

What did one Florida alligator say to the other alligator? "Hey, those Value Jet meals aren't half bad." (Following the crash of a Value Jet plane into a Florida swamp.)

What's the new area code for Los Angeles? 911. (During a sequence of fires, floods and mud slides in Los Angeles.)

Our urge to joke about disasters does have its limits. Following the 9/11 attacks, there were no jokes related to this event for about a week on late night TV. This tragedy just left the country as a whole too raw emotionally. When the jokes did finally return, they were initially exclusively focused on Osama Bin Laden. This was the only safe target we could allow ourselves to laugh at. After a period of a few weeks, jokes like the second one, below, began to appear.

Why aren't there any tall buildings in Muslim countries?
Because crazy Muslim pilots would try to land on them.

What's the fastest way to the first floor in the World Trade Center? Jump out the window or wait for it to collapse?

Jokes following the great tsunami disaster in the Indian Ocean in late 2004 were much quicker to come around. In spite of the fact that the calamitous loss of lives was many times greater than that of 9/11, it seemed more distant to most people in the USA. We were still horrified at the magnitude of the disaster, but it didn't hit us on a personal, emotional level to the same extent as 9/11. Within a day or two, the following jokes were circulating.

Knock knock. Who's there? Sue. Sue who? Sue NAMI.

What's the least popular detergent in Indonesia? Tide.

I heard the beachfront cities in Thailand had no power. No, no, there's plenty of current running through them.

And, of course, the sick ones always emerge, as well. Here are a couple of examples.

Did you hear that dishwasher manufacturers have stopped sending dishwashers to Asia? A lot of Asians have started washing up on the local beaches.

Why are so many sharks stricken with diarrhea? They've been eating Thai food all week.

Why do we laugh at such jokes? Are we simply cruel and heartless, having no sympathy for the victims of these tragic events? Or does the laughter fill some positive psychological function? Three newspaper reporters have told me that reporters covering such tragedies are responsible for getting many of these jokes going. They often see the tragedy first–hand, or are otherwise closely involved with it. This is very tough on them emotionally, even though they have no personal acquaintance with the victims. The humor helps distance themselves from the situation enough to be able to get their story out without being victimized by their own emotions. It also provides a means of letting go of the feelings that build up as they cover the story.

The rest of us need the same release. *Finding a way to laugh at these tragedies seems to help everyone put them behind them and get on with their lives.* The more intimately involved you are with the tragedy, of course, the more difficult it is to use this source of release. It is healthier to go through the normal grief and anger; it is not healthy or adaptive to force yourself to laugh in the midst of your grief. The time for laughter emerges when you come out the other side and are ready to begin rebuilding some joy into your life. A good laugh (initially at things totally unrelated to the source of your grief) helps you take this first step.

War. Few situations are more stress–inducing than war. It is hard to imagine the spirit of fun and playfulness emerging in the midst of war. And yet jokes and spontaneous humor always seem to proliferate during wartime. The jokes often ridicule the enemy and serve to reduce the terrible tensions, fears, and anger that accompany every war. They provide a momentary rush of positive emotion in the midst of all these negative emotions. They also momentarily reduce the perceived threat posed by the enemy and help generate a sense of control in situations where you're really quite powerless.

As the Iraq war finally draws to a close upon the publication of this book, we can look back on years of comedians' jokes about the war. These jokes typically have some kind of political focus. A few from Jay Leno on *The Tonight Show* are shown below.

"Now there are reports from Baghdad that officials are taking bribes for favors, giving jobs to their relatives, taking money under the table from contractors. You know what this means? The war is less than a week old, and already they have an American-style democracy." Jay Leno

"The war continues in Iraq. They're calling it Operation Iraqi Freedom. They were going to call it Operation Iraqi Liberation until they realized that spells 'Oil.'" Jay Leno

"Saddam Hussein has told his people that U.S. troops will commit suicide when they get to the gates of Baghdad. That's when you know you have a bad army, when your only hope for victory is that the enemy's troops kill themselves." Jay Leno

Just as jokes today commonly poke fun at Barack Obama, many jokes during the height of the Iraq war poked fun at President Bush. The following is typical of the latter. Obviously, this kind of joke is most likely to help you feel less stressed if you are/were against the war to begin with or a democrat. Republicans, similarly, are more likely to feel some stress relief upon hearing jokes ridiculing President Obama. (For example, Q: Why is Barack Obama so thin? A: If he were any heavier, he wouldn't be able to walk on water.)

Donald Rumsfield is briefing George Bush in the Oval Office. "Oh. And finally, sir, three Brazilian soldiers were killed in Iraq today." Bush goes pale, his jaw hanging open in stunned disbelief. He buries his face in his hands muttering, "My God . . . my God." "Mr. President," says Cheney, "We lose soldiers all the time, and it's terrible. But I've never seen you so

upset. What's the matter?" Bush looks up and says, "How many is a Brazilian?"

The following are more representative of jokes that were shared by the general public over the course of the two Iraq wars. These are typical of jokes about the enemy in any war. They ridicule or otherwise poke fun at the enemy.

Q: Did you hear about the Iraqi air force exercise program?
A: Each morning you raise your hands above your head and leave them there.

Q: What do Miss Muffet and Saddam Hussein have in common:
A: They both have Kurds in their whey.

Q: What is the Iraqi air force motto?
A: I came, I saw, Iran.

Q: What is the Iraqi national bird?
A: Duck.

Q: How many Iraqis does it take to screw in a light bulb?
A: None. They can't turn them on anyway.

We know a lot more about the role of joking in wars in the distant past. Citizens joked more than usual in London during the Nazi bombing attacks in WWII, as well as in Czechoslovakia throughout the period of Nazi occupation.[142] Some world leaders even got into the act. When Winston Churchill was told that Mussolini had decided to enter the war in 1939, he announced to the British people, "The Italians have announced that they will fight on the Nazis' side. I think it's only fair. We had to put up with them last time." Humor was also identified as an important coping mechanism among resilient Vietnam combat veterans.[143]

The Jewish people have a greater reputation than any other group for maintaining their sense of humor in the midst of adversity. During the 1991 war with Iraq, Israeli humor immediately began to surface as a means of coping with the threat. The Israelis were in an awkward position in this war, since they were resisting the temptation to be dragged into it—even though they were being attacked. They felt powerless, since their defense was in the hands of the Americans. But this is precisely the kind of situation where humor has real power to help you cope—when you're powerless to act to change your circumstances. They were stuck with a high–stress situation and simply had to deal with it one way or another. As Scud missiles began to fall, people feared for their lives, because they believed that Saddam Hussein would launch a gas attack, as he had against the Kurds in his own country.

The proof of the Israelis' understanding of the coping value of a playful attitude and humor came as the entire world watched the citizens of Jerusalem and Tel Aviv go to their sealed rooms. They sometimes spent hours in these rooms, fearing that a Scud might drop on them at any moment. People were terrified during the early days of the war, still carrying the residues of memories of gas chambers during the Holocaust. What you didn't know was that during the initial attacks, Israeli radio stations sponsored a nation–wide anagrams game to see who could come up with the greatest number of words from the letters composing the name "Saddam Hussein." Government leaders realized that providing the opportunity to have fun in a game would help relieve the tension and anxiety built up while waiting in the closed–off rooms.

"In prehistoric times, mankind often had only two choices in crisis situations; fight or flee. In modern times, humor offers us a third alternative; fight, flee—or laugh." (Robert Orben)

In a study of Israeli humor during the first Gulf War, the researchers pointed out that humor was more prominent in this war than in any other Israeli war, precisely because of the "immense feelings of rage and helplessness and a profound wish to retaliate" that emerged.[144] The Israelis needed to joke more in this war because they weren't in a position to directly retaliate by fighting. Laughing at Saddam helped reduce the feeling of danger.

The following jokes (all reported by the researchers) were typical of those that emerged as the war went on. People sometimes joked directly about the things they were afraid of.

How do you play Israeli roulette?
Give 3 gas masks to 4 people in a sealed room.

Tel Aviv residents are advised to eat plenty of beans during the alert. The reason? To fight gas with gas.

One Tel Aviv resident was said by his neighbors to be immune to chemical missiles; he's such a big fart that he neutralizes them.

Many of the jokes took advantage of the Jewish tradition of playing with language.

What's the new name of Tel Aviv?
Til Aviv. ("Til" is the Hebrew word for missile.)

What's the new name of Israel?
Scudinavia.

What's the reverse of Saddam in English?
Madd ass.

The most common butt of the jokes was Saddam Hussein.

What's the difference between Saddam and the wicked Haman? Haman was hanged, and then we wore the masks. With Saddam, we wear the masks first.

What do Saddam and his father have in common?
Neither one pulled out in time.

Other jokes poked fun at the Iraqis in general.

Every Iraqi tank has five gears, four reverse and one forward. Why does it need the forward gear? In case it's attacked from the rear.

What went wrong with the Iraqi missiles?
They had Soviet bodies, French warheads, and German planning, but local assembly.

The Israeli researcher conducting this study noted that humor was a powerful force in overcoming the anxiety associated with the threat of Scud missiles and also helped rechannel felt anger toward the enemy (as well as some subgroups—especially secular vs. religious Israelis) within Israel. It helped sustain morale through the war, and generally helped the average Israeli cope.

The best known example of this kind of humor, of course, was provided by *M.A.S.H.* This long running television series captured in every episode the way humor helped Hawkeye and the others cope with the traumas of war, especially with the endless strings of wounded and dead sent to their primitive surgical tents.

A nurse who served in the Vietnam war recalled her experiences 24 years later, saying that nurses were exposed to things they had never been exposed to before because helicopters brought in wounded that would have died in the battlefield in the past.[145] Nurses were constantly faced with amputations, mutilations, and terrible wounds throughout the war, "And if you allowed yourself to feel, you could not have continued to do your job."

This nurse noted that it was years before many of her colleagues realized that the war had left them spiritually and emotionally dead. When one nurse returned home after the war, *she discovered that her capacity to enjoy daily life had disappeared. This is one reason why so many who serve in the military during war time intuitively sense that finding something to laugh at is essential to their emotional survival.* The book *Catch 22* shows how many succeed in laughing in the midst of war. It captures the humor of absurd situations that inevitably accompany any military conflict.

I know of only one study that has examined how humor helps cope with the stress of war–like conditions.[146] It focused on 19– and

20–year–old soldiers participating in a training course for combat NCOs in the Israeli Defense Forces. Participants rated each of their fellow members (five people) on how frequently they initiated any kind of humor. Their commanders and peers also rated how well the soldiers coped under stress during the training. Soldiers who joked, told funny stories, or clowned around more were judged by both their peers and commanders to be coping better with the stressful conditions provided in the combat training. As with the Gulf war study described above, the researchers in this study concluded that *joking and funny stories helped the soldiers feel in control.* This sense of being in control helped keep stress levels within reasonable bounds and helped them perform at a higher level.

This is how humor will help in your own life. It will help you take charge of the stress you're under at the moment by keeping your emotional reaction from getting out of hand. This leaves you in a much better position to take action to change the situation.

POW Camps. Bill Cosby once said, "If you can find humor in anything, you can survive it." The ultimate test of this would have been the Nazi concentration camps of World War II. If ever there were a situation incompatible with humor, this was it. And yet the psychiatrist Victor Frankl, a prisoner in the camps himself, noted in his book, *Man's Search for Meaning*, that humor was one of the things that helped people survive in the camps. Finding things to laugh at helped maintain a sense of meaning and purpose in life––even in conditions as extreme as those in the camps.

"I would never have made it if I could not have laughed. Laughing lifted me momentarily . . . out of this horrible situation, just enough to make it livable . . . survivable."   (Victor Frankl)

Many hung on with the thought that they would one day see a loved one again. Others used their imaginations to create humor. Frankl states that he and another prisoner tried to invent a funny story or joke every day. For example, in one joke, a prisoner points toward a Capo (a prisoner who also served as a guard) and said, "Imagine! I knew him when he was only the president of the bank!"

"Humor, more than anything else in the human makeup, affords an aloofness and an ability to rise above any situation, even if only for a few seconds."   (Victor Frankl)

"To become conscious of what is horrifying and to laugh at it is to become master of that which is horrifying." (Eugene Ionesco)

In another frequently told story, a prisoner accidentally bumps into a Nazi guard. The guard turns and shouts, "Schwein!" ("pig" in German). The prisoner bows and says, "Cohen. Pleased to meet you." The joke shows how humor helps reverse who's in control and who is the superior being. Even in the terrible conditions of the camp, the joke provided a means of momentarily overcoming adversity. This same point was made in the 1997 movie, *Life is Beautiful*, in which a Jewish father in a Nazi camp initiated endless humor to protect his son from the tragic reality of the camp.

Captain Gerald Coffee, who spent seven years in a POW camp in Vietnam, said that POWs were kept isolated in an attempt to break their spirit. They kept their spirits up, however, by tapping on the wall of fellow prisoners and telling jokes in Morse code. Again, here is the recognition of the importance of finding some way of generating positive emotion within oneself in the most terrible of conditions. Coffee feels that humor was essential to his survival.

When I interviewed him several years ago, Captain Coffee said that humor was the one thing that was almost constant throughout his stay in the camps, even if it was sometimes a grim humor. For example, the prisoners often were tortured with ropes. When a new POW would appear, they would always explain the daily routines and how they went about communicating with each other. Then they'd say, "It's not so bad once you get to know the ropes." They would look for humor wherever they could find it, including the way they and their captors lived, and even the brutality of the guards.

The POWs often got depressed about their aloneness and feared that they would never get back home. Anything that could break through this depression and anxiety was always welcome. Intuitively, they knew what the research on positive emotion has consistently suggested; they had to be resilient to survive this, and getting a daily dose of positive emotion was a key to their resilience. They recognized that humor did this for them.

In his book, *Beyond Survival*, Coffee describes an old cell that had been converted to a shower. Someone had scratched onto the wall "Smile, you're on Candid Camera." You can imagine the effect discovering this message had on a prisoner standing there with his head bent down, wondering if he'll ever get out alive. In Coffee's case, he said, "I laughed out loud, enjoying not only the pure humor and incongruity of the situation, but also appreciating the beautiful guy who had mustered the moxie to rise above his own dejection and frustration and pain and guilt to inscribe a line of encouragement to those who would come after him . . . he deserved a medal for it."[147]

> "Laughter sets the spirit free to move through even the most tragic circumstances. It helps us shake our heads clear, get our feet back under us and restore our sense of balance and purpose. Humor is integral to our peace of mind and ability to go beyond survival." (Captain Gerald Coffee)

Coffee's stories remind me of an old Shel Silverstein cartoon showing two men being held prisoners in a dungeon. They are clamped to a wall with irons around their wrists and ankles. Below them is a pit containing alligators, and it's 30 feet straight up to the top of the dungeon. So they're against the wall like two insects on a pin. One looks at the other and says, "Now here's my plan."

One of the things that struck me the most in my interview with Coffee was his view that *"having some humor skills before being confronted by the adversity played a very important role"* in being able to use humor in the camps. That's why its important to make the effort now to improve your own humor skills. If you want to have access to your sense of humor under high stress situations, you first need to develop your humor skills in non–stressful situations.

Similar stories were told by hostages held by terrorist groups in the 1980s. Terry Anderson, held captive in Lebanon for 2,454 days, describes in his book, *Den of Lions*, how a sense of humor helped him and his fellow prisoners cope.

"Despite everything, it's amazing sometimes how much laughing we do. Irish hostage Brian Keenan's terrible shaggy–dog stories, John McCarthy's imitations, Tom's [Sutherland] awful puns and drinking songs, Frank's [Reed] tales of Boston. Even the idiotic and frustrating things the guards do set us off in giggles. There's often a bitter touch to it. But not always. Just as often, it's just a relief to be able to laugh at something."[148]

These anecdotal accounts of the importance of humor in coping among POWs have been confirmed in more systematic research. A study of POWs during the Vietnam War was completed on the 25th anniversary of the 1973 release of 566 American POWs. Most of these men experienced extreme levels of torture, starvation and isolation— many for up to seven years. The Navy's own 20-year follow up psychological evaluations of these POWs revealed an incidence of post-traumatic stress disorder (PTSD) that was no higher than that of the general American population.[149]

This was very surprising. What was it that allowed these POWs (mainly highly educated navy pilots) to cope so well? Detailed interviews with 50 of these prisoners showed that *the use of humor played a key role in their resilience in the presence of determined efforts to break their will. Nearly every person interviewed agreed that "humor played a significant role in the survival of the VPOW and in their continued hardiness since the repatriation."* Like Gerald Coffee, those POWs who have written books about their POW experiences have also pointed to the importance of humor in coping.

One of the prisoners interviewed 25 years later recalled an incident which marked a turning point in achieving his own insight about the importance of humor in the camps. Ten months after his capture, he was watching the guards through a hole in the wall. In response to a question by one guard, the other began taking off layers of clothes and a bullet belt in order to reach into an inner pocket. When he pulled out a Baby Ben clock and told the first guard the time, the prisoner began rolling on the floor laughing. The absurdity of having to undress to find out the time led to such strong spontaneous laughter that the prisoner was able from that point on to see the power of laughter in getting him through his ordeal.

> "And I'd been beaten pretty severely every day for most of a month, and I was just absolutely rolling on the floor. When this was all over, I realized, 'I thought I was going to die today; and all I did was have a good laugh.' And so it became apparent to you that humor was going to play a major role."[150]

In most cases, POWs in Vietnam had little opportunity for face-to-face contact with other prisoners; they often spent months, or even years, in isolation. Jokes or funny stories were shared by tapping the walls in Morse code. "Several of the study participants commented that *they considered humor so important that they would literally risk torture to tell a joke through the walls to another prisoner who needed to be cheered up*." (Italics are McGhee's.)

> "Another VPOW, who had been forced to give classified information concerning the maximum airspeed of his airplane, gave an inaccurately low speed that the captors doubted. They pressured him to tell the truth, stating that another prisoner had given a higher airspeed for the same aircraft. Thinking fast, the POW replied, 'Well, that guy is a major. I'm only a lieutenant. They don't let lieutenants fly as fast as they let the majors fly.' The explanation seemed reasonable to the captors; it allowed the lieutenant to avoid further coercion while not giving classified information; and it served as a source of laughter for the POWs for many years."[151]

One Vietnam POW noted in his own book that jokes and poking fun at their captors provided a very effective means of covertly fighting back—of *taking a form of control of your emotions when absolutely everything has been taken away from you.* It was a way of achieving a sense of mastery in powerless circumstances.[152]

This finding for Vietnam POWs in not unique. We have already seen that in World War II, humor helped prisoners in Nazi (and

Japanese) camps survive their ordeal and find purpose in their lives.[153] In the "Pueblo incident" in the 1970s, the crew of the captured ship Pueblo also relied on humor to get through their day. Many of the crew members indicated that it was more helpful than religion.[154]

BUILD YOUR HUMOR SKILLS

[Turn the page for answers. Work on both jokes before checking answers.]

1. The owner of a small deli was being questioned by an IRS agent about his tax return. He had reported a net profit of $80,000 for the year. He complained, "Why don't you people leave me alone? I work like a dog! This place is only closed two days a year and everyone in my family helps out." "It's not your income that bothers us," said the agent. "It's these deductions. You listed six trips to Bermuda for you and your wife." "Oh, that," the owner said, smiling, "Didn't I mention? We _____."
Clue: Sometimes you call out for pizza instead of going to the restaurant.

2. A new hair salon opened up for business right across the street from an old established barber shop. They put up a big sign which read: "WE GIVE $7 HAIRCUTS!" The clever old barber put up his own sign which read: "WE _____."
Clue: What does an auto mechanic do? This clue is a little indirect, but will give you the answer.

Finding humor in the face of death was called "gallows" humor by Freud. His classic example was of a man who was about to be shot by a firing squad and was asked if he wanted a last cigarette. "No thanks," he said, "I'm trying to quit." Again, the joke helped the doomed man turn the tables and take a form of control in the situation. A cartoon I just recently saw showed a man being brought to an electric chair where he was about to be executed. He looked up at his guards and said, "Thanks, I haven't had a chance to sit down all day!"

A sociologist once pointed out that over the centuries, many cultures have used humor as a means of dealing with death.[155] At one time, those doomed to death by fire in India were expected to laugh while climbing up to their own pyre. Parents in ancient Phoenicia often laughed if their children had been committed to death on the pyre. Elderly parents in Sardinia were expected to laugh when being immolated by their own children. All these practices clearly reflect the belief that laughter can help master even the fear of death itself.

You will never face the threat of a pyre or a firing squad in your life, and you will hopefully never wind up in anything comparable to a POW or concentration camp, but you may encounter other kinds of stress that feel just as threatening to you. If humor could help Frankl, Coffee, Anderson, and Sharansky deal with their problems, it can certainly help you deal with yours.

The Importance of Learning to Actively Use Humor

One of the most important questions relating to humor's ability to help you cope with stress is whether you can get any stress–reducing benefits by being a passive enjoyer of humor, or whether you need to be more actively involved in generating humor for it to become an effective coping tool. The evidence presented throughout this chapter suggests that some degree of coping benefit comes from both. Few studies have compared the relative effectiveness of passive exposure to an active use of humor to cope, but the data generally point to the greater importance of actively using humor.

A study completed in Canada did address this issue and found that even if you're someone who finds a lot of humor in everyday life, it doesn't help you cope unless you also make an effort to actively use humor to deal with stress.[156] So you may have a terrific sense of humor when everything is great, but if it abandons you when things go wrong, you'll be just as stressed out as the next person. But we have already seen that other research suggests that even passive exposure to humor offers some help in managing the upset or anxiety of the moment—presumably because of the positive emotion generated by simply seeing a genuinely funny cartoon or funny situation or hearing a joke.

In the 1950s, Eve Arden, star of the popular *Our Miss Brooks* television program, demonstrated this active use of humor when a practical joke was played on her during a stage performance. A fellow actor had arranged to have the phone unexpectedly ring in the middle of a monologue by Eve. She picked up the phone, paused a moment, and handed it to her leading man, saying, "It's for you."

One especially interesting study has good news for everyone (those having either a good or poor sense of humor). Among individuals who were under high stress at the time of the study, those with a poor sense of humor experienced a significantly greater reduction in anxiety after watching a comedy video than after watching a non-humorous video. The comedy video was not, however, more effective than the non-humorous video among the high sense of humor group.[157]

A July 27, 2009 article in the *Washington Post* ("Healing with Humor," by Christian Davenport) noted the many ways in which American soldiers who lost limbs in the Iraq War actively use their sense of humor to cope—as well as make others more comfortable around them. One man is quite aware that people are ill at ease when they see his prosthetic leg. If he sees someone jamming their hand in between closing elevator doors, he says, "Careful, you can lose a limb that way." He finds that this eases their discomfort upon noticing his artificial leg. When children ask about his "robot leg," he tells them that it happened because he didn't eat his veggies.

ANSWERS TO JOKES

1. deliver anywhere   2. fix $7 haircuts

Another soldier who lost both legs in Iraq asks, "What's an amputee's favorite restaurant? IHOP." Davenport notes that "Although doctors [at Walter Reed Medical Center] and therapists can patch up the physical wounds of war, it is often the humor—soldier to soldier, Marine to Marine, patient to patient—that in the space of a punch line can heal as well as the best medicine." While many amputee veterans can't manage this kind of humor, for those that do, "it's the ultimate palliative as they move from denial to anger to acceptance."

Yet another soldier stabbed his prosthetic foot with a steak knife and pretended to howl in pain. Another removed his prosthetic leg before getting on a roller coaster ride, and as the coaster came to a stop, he yelled to the next group, "Don't get on that ride! It'll rip your legs off!" Another was pushing himself up a steep hill when someone asked if he needed a hand. He answered, "No, man, my hands are good. Can you give me a couple of feet?" For some, the article notes, the jokes are a "way of saying he has accepted the way he is, has moved on and wishes others would too." "That's how I make it though the day, especially here at Walter Reed," said one. "To be in this place, you have to have a sense of humor or you'll lose your mind." (This is very similar to McMurphy's comment noted at the beginning of this chapter.)

Luckily, most of us do not have to find ways of dealing with this level of stress. But we still must find ways of coping with our own daily stressors and hassles. In spite of their milder nature, many of us find that we simply cannot find a way of lightening up in the midst of normal daily challenges.

The good news for the humor-impaired is that watching your favorite sit com may be a good way to ease anxiety under stress. But if you have a great sense of humor, you don't need to rely on sit coms or other outside sources of humor. Your own sense of humor gives you all the anxiety-reducing and positive emotion-inducing power you need to manage stress. For individuals with a poorly developed sense of humor, then, the best advice may turn out to be to regularly expose yourself to humor at home, on the way to work, in the office, etc.—wherever you can find it. *Think of humor as a stress deodorant.* If you have a good sense of humor, you have built-in protection all day long. If you have a poor sense of humor, you'll need repeated (external) applications throughout the day (at least on high stress days).

Other studies also suggest that while exposure to humor from any outside source (a comedy DVD, print cartoon, a funny friend, etc.) can help manage stress, it is under conditions of high stress that having a good sense of humor becomes a powerful ally in getting through your day.[158] The ideal stress management strategy in terms of humor, then, is to build your humor skills when things are going well so that you'll have access to your sense of humor when you need it the most. If you consider yourself to have a poorly developed (or even average) sense of humor which abandons you under stress, you might start by building a "mirth aid kit" and keep it handy in your car, your office, and at home so that you have access to it on high stress days. This kit could include print cartoons (*The Far Side* and *Dilbert* work well for me), audio clips of your favorite comedians, comedy DVDs, etc. Of course, you'll also need to put up a reminder in a visible place to actually use it, since you won't be in a mood for humor at that point.

Research on Positive Emotion in General

Humor, of course, is just one source of positive emotion. As noted in the Introduction, there has been an explosive increase in research on positive emotion in general since the turn of the new century. Throughout the 20th century, psychologists paid very little attention to positive emotion. (The resurgence of research on humor, beginning in the 1970s, was the exception to this general trend.) This has all changed, however, as evidence has demonstrated that positive emotion replenishes depleted emotional resources[159] and makes a significant contribution to both our physical and psychological health and well-being.[160]

Among a group of elderly patients with cardiovascular disease, for example, those who reported greater happiness over the 90-day period following their release had lower readmission rates to the hospital—even when health status at initial release and length of initial hospital stay were controlled for.[161] In a well-known study generally referred to as the "nun study," positive emotional content in the autobiographies of nuns written during their early adult years predicted who was still alive six decades later.[162] Positive emotion even appears to protect elderly adults against physical disability (e.g., due to strokes).[163]

"Sometimes a laugh is the only weapon we have." (Roger Rabbit)

There is also a great deal of evidence that positive emotion facilitates effective coping with both acute and chronic stress and is associated with psychological health.[164] Common examples of coping strategies associated with maintaining positive emotions include positive reappraisals of the situation, problem-focused coping, and infusing ordinary events with meaning.[165] Humor, of course, is another.

There are many ways to achieve a daily diet of positive emotion (e.g., music, a good love relationship, playing with children, engaging in any activity you enjoy, satisfying work, prayer or meditation—and, of course, a good laugh[166]). The emotional state generally considered to result from humor and laughter is joy, although the most prolific current humor researcher, Willibald Ruch, has long argued that "exhilaration" is the term that best fits this emotional experience.[167]

In the next section, I offer several possible mechanisms through which humor helps cope and contributes to emotional well-being. As noted in the Introduction, Barbara Fredrickson, a prominent researcher in the area of positive emotions, has offered a very promising explanation of how positive emotions contribute to beneficial health outcomes. She calls her explanation the "broaden-and-build" theory.[168] Negative emotions, she argues, arouse the autonomic nervous system and narrow our attention, directing us to act in very focused or specific ways (e.g., ways to escape, attack, defend, etc.). Positive emotions, on the other hand, counter the arousal generated by the autonomic nervous system and broaden the range of behaviors and thoughts we exhibit. Thus, positive emotions produce more flexible, creative, and integrative thoughts and actions[169] and allow a more flexible range of attention to our thoughts and to the world generally. These benefits are all crucial to effective coping. Again, this is consistent with findings for humor. Exposure to humor, for example has been shown to increase creativity.[170]

Fredrickson argues that *positive emotions undo the lingering physiological reactivity that goes along with negative emotion.* She has completed a series of three experiments which support this view. In each case, a high–arousal negative emotion was first produced (activating the sympathetic nervous system). Subjects then watched a film that induced joy (high–activation positive emotion), contentment (low–activation positive emotion), neutrality, or sadness. In three different samples, subjects in both the high– and low–activation positive emotion conditions showed more rapid cardiovascular recovery from negative emotional arousal than subjects in the other two groups.[171]

In one of these studies, a humor video was used as the high–activation source of positive emotion.[172] Subjects who watched the humor video showed faster cardiovascular recovery than those who watched either a neutral or sadness-inducing video. So the positive emotion associated with humor does have "the ability to regulate lingering negative emotional arousal." In everyday language, this means that *humor does have the power to de-stress you, just as meditation and other kinds of relaxation procedures do.*

Fredrickson and her colleagues extended this finding that experimentally-induced positive emotion facilitates cardiovascular recovery to the notion that *the tendency of positive emotion to speed up recovery (from stress) at the physiological level may be the key factor that provides resilient individuals with their resilience.* They used a measure of trait resilience (a trait is an enduring quality of one's personality) to obtain high- and low-resilience groups of individuals. They first established a base line for six different measures of cardiovascular activity and blood pressure and then induced anxiety by telling each person they would have 60 seconds to prepare a speech. Heart rate and blood pressure both increased during this task. (Other cardiovascular measures also changed significantly.) Self-reports of their subjective emotional experience (using a mood scale) three minutes later indicated that they did, in fact, feel more anxious as a result of this request.[173]

Three findings of central importance for humor were obtained in this study. First, the high-resilience subjects showed a significantly higher positive mood during the anxiety-arousing task than low-resilience subjects. They also appraised the task as less threatening. This is consistent with findings discussed earlier showing that individuals with a good sense of humor are better able to sustain positive emotion in the midst of stress, and supports the notion that having a good sense of humor makes an important contribution to one's emotional resilience.

The second important finding was that high-resilience individuals took less time than low-resilience subjects to return to their baseline on the cardiovascular measures. They overcame the negative emotional arousal more quickly. This left one question. Was it the level of positive emotion sustained during the anxiety-arousing task that was responsible for this faster return to the original cardiovascular state? When the researchers statistically controlled for the level of positive emotion experienced during the task, the relationship between resilience and length of time required to return to the cardiovascular baseline disappeared. This suggests that *the positive emotion experienced was responsible for a quicker return to cardiovascular baseline.*

The physical health implications of this finding are clear. Whether it is through humor or any other means you use to sustain a positive mood in tough times, *a faster return to the physiological state you had prior to the stressful event should reduce the health-damaging effects of stress.* As noted in Chapter 2, there is ample evidence that the kind of cardiovascular reactivity measured in this study—and that commonly occurs in connection with anger and anxiety—plays an important role in such cardiovascular diseases as coronary heart disease and hypertension.[174] In cases (which are becoming more and more common on the job and elsewhere in our lives) where we encounter repeated stressors throughout a typical day, a quicker return to a state of relative physiological equilibrium should allow the body to restore itself in preparation to respond to the next emotionally-arousing event.[175]

How Does Humor Help You Cope?

We all know people who suffer more than their share of traumas, but who manage to draw from some inner strength that enables them to not only go on, but to do so with an upbeat, positive attitude. A strong religious faith can provide this; and, as we have seen, your sense of humor can do so as well. But what is it about humor and laughter that enables a person to get through either a single extremely stressful event or chronic stress day after day and remain in good mental health? How does a good sense of humor help you to bend without breaking? To hang on? Or as McMurphy put it at the beginning of this chapter, how does your sense of humor help you keep from losing your footing? Psychologists, psychiatrists and researchers dealing with this question have not been able to agree on the answer, although—as we have seen—humor's capacity to generate positive emotion in the most difficult of circumstances now appears to be the strongest candidate for its resilience-promoting and coping power.

"The world breaks all of us, but some of us become stronger in the broken places." (Ernest Hemingway)

Other qualities of humor and laughter (discussed next), however, combine with the positive emotion generated to help you cope. It may be any combination of these qualities that are most important in helping a given individual get through a stressful time.

Emotion-Focused vs. Problem-Focused Coping

Researchers drew a fundamental distinction between problem-focused and emotion-focused coping a quarter century ago.[176] Problem-focused coping is very effective when the problem causing you stress is under your control. If your health is being threatened by high cholesterol, effective steps would be to sharply reduce your eating of high cholesterol foods, exercise more and see your doctor. But we all sometimes find ourselves in situations we are stuck with; we have no choice to learn to live with them. Many kinds of job stress fall into this category. We simply have to get our jobs done even though our work load is doubled or we have some impossible deadline to meet. Or we are diagnosed with cancer. In emotion-focused coping, the emphasis is on doing something to change our mood or frame of mind; the goal is to pull ourselves out of our anger, anxiety or depression and substitute a more positive frame of mind conducive to getting done what must be done—to getting through it. Humor is an effective tool in achieving this positive transformation.

As we have seen, disaster survivors often joke in the midst of heavy losses in the aftermath of hurricanes, tornados, etc. People who keep their sense of humor during such ordeals realize that this doesn't change the reality of the fact that they've lost their home and most of their possessions. But they are glad to be alive and use their sense of humor to keep an upbeat, positive attitude that enables them to get on with reconstructing their lives. They intuitively know that finding a light side somehow helps them do this.

In the aftermath of the great tsunami that struck a dozen countries surrounding the Indian Ocean on December 26, 2004, there was no levity to be found in the affected countries (although, as noted earlier, jokes about the disaster were quickly circulating in the United States). The loss of tens of thousands of lives and unparalleled destruction resulting from the giant wave made it impossible for those directly affected to use humor to cope. This was entirely understandable. In fact, it was healthy and appropriate since it is essential to express the grief, sadness and despair experienced in this circumstance. The use of humor to cope here only becomes appropriate months down the road as people try to create a more positive focus that helps them reconstruct their lives and learn to live with the tragedy.

One group of investigators asked individuals to engage in a task which obliged them to focus on their own mortality. While most people felt more depressed (or some other form of negative emotion) following the task, those scoring higher on a measure of sense of humor showed no change in emotional state.[177] The researchers concluded that *it is precisely this protection against the onset of negative emotion that is responsible for humor's power to help you cope.* Humor here was considered by the researchers to be a form of emotion-focused coping.

Substitution of a Positive Emotion
that is Incompatible with Stress

Humor has often been described as providing a "cognitive-affective shift." That is, we restructure the way we think about a situation, and there is an accompanying emotional shift in a more positive direction. Knowing that this shift occurs as a result of humor is crucial if you want to consciously use it to manage your own emotional state.[178]

The most important dimension of humor's coping power, in my view, is its capacity to generate a positive emotional state that is simply incompatible with the negative emotions experienced under stress. It is almost impossible to feel genuinely happy and sad, angry, or anxious at the same time. Even if your intellect tells you there is a positive and negative side of the situation, one of these feelings will dominate. But humor has the power to pull you out of your anger, anxiety or depression and insert a more positive emotion in its place.

The extent to which humor can do this is best viewed as being on a continuum. In the case of extreme stress (as in the 9/11 tragedy), the negative emotion is much too strong for humor to overcome it. In most such cases, it not adaptive to even try to do so. For example, I know of one woman who received a serious cancer diagnosis. The next day, she told her co-workers, "The bad news is I have cancer; the good news is I'm bio-degradable." This was an effort to joke about her situation. But the problem with joking so soon after the diagnosis is that it is often a form of denial—a way to emotionally close yourself off from the shock of what you've just heard. In subsequent days and weeks, she did experience the expected gamut of negative emotions that goes with a cancer diagnosis and joked less about it. Months later, she was again able to use humor in a more adaptive way to sustain a positive daily frame of mind.

The next four sections consider different means by which humor substitutes a positive emotion that is incompatible with stress.

Reduced Feelings of Anger, Anxiety and Depression. There is plenty of evidence, as we have seen, that humor reduces the feelings of anger, anxiety, and depression that generally accompany

96

stress. This has been shown in experimental studies, as well as in studies of people who show a good sense of humor (as measured by paper-and-pencil sense of humor tests). As these feelings are eased, people feel less stressed. The positive feelings generated by laughter and the experience of humor are simply incompatible with feeling angry or anxious.

Have you ever noticed how your own emotions gradually escalate during a typical high stress day? You can feel the tension, anxiety, anger, or general upset build as the day goes on. The growing upset may reflect a few key events or an accumulated effect of simply having too many things to do, with too little time to do them. The longer this goes on, the greater the build-up of emotional tension. If you have no way to release this tension, you soon feel like you're going to explode. Maybe you do explode. You kick the dog, slam your fist against the wall, shout insults at colleagues, or just scream! These reactions generally aren't very adaptive, even if you feel better.

> *"Humor is the great thing, the saving thing after all. The minute it crops up, all our hardnesses yield, all our irritations and resentments slip away, and a sunny spirit takes their place."*
>
> (Mark Twain)

Therapists offer one source of release by providing an environment in which you can talk about the causes of your stress and develop better ways of dealing with it. Humor is certainly no substitute for therapy, but you don't always have access to a therapist, and you may not have anyone else available with whom you can talk it out. *Laughter provides an immediate release of tension. It helps you laugh yourself loose.* You feel a tremendous weight being removed from your shoulders when you have a good belly laugh. It's simply hard to hang on to your anger and anxiety when you're laughing. That's one reason most people say they just feel better after a good laugh.

You can obtain this cathartic release of anger and tension to some extent by forcing yourself to have a good laugh. That's one reason that "laughter clubs," in which groups of people get together and laugh "for no reason," have become so popular around the world. The greatest release occurs, however, when you find or create something to laugh at that you find genuinely funny.

THE IMPORTANCE OF "LETTING GO"

Try this at home. Take a can of soup, a hammer, or any other object that weighs a pound of two. Hold you arm straight out in front of you while holding it. You'll see that this is not hard to do at first. But as the minutes pass, you'll notice some strain on your arm. Continuing to hold it becomes physically stressful, and the object seems to get heavier and heavier the longer you hold it. Eventually, you may even experience pain from the simple act of holding something that was very easy to hold initially. You simply have to put it down for a while to let your body recover.

This same phenomenon occurs with everyday stress. Regardless of whether the stress is related to your job, a personal relationship, your health or a financial crisis, the emotional weight (anger, anxiety or depression) which was initially easy to carry gradually gets heavier and heavier. This was referred to earlier as the Law of Psychological Gravity. You have no choice but to find a way to put the emotional weight down for a bit while your body and mind recover. Your sense of humor gives you a good (and fun!) tool for letting go of these negative emotions for at least a while. You lighten up emotionally as the positive emotion that goes with humor and laughter fills your body/mind and lifts your spirits. This process plays a key role in boosting your emotional resilience. Once in this more positive frame of mind, you are better equipped emotionally to take active steps to deal with the situation causing you stress.

John Glenn was the first American astronaut in space, and there was a great deal of nervousness before the flight. When he was later asked what he was thinking about before the launch, he said: "I looked around me and suddenly realized that everything had been built by the lowest bidder." This joke to himself eased his pre-launch nervousness.

As noted earlier in this chapter, hospital nurses work in a very high stress environment. Most nurses quickly learn that they need a good laugh several times a day, just to release the emotional build-up that goes along with confronting one life-threatening situation after another all day long. They often tell each other jokes like the following just to keep stress levels manageable.

> **Three people died and went to hell. When they got there, the devil gave them a choice of the room in which they would spend eternity. All the rooms were bad, but one was less bad than the others. It was a room in which people were standing in sewage up to their knees. So they all three chose this room. As they were walking away, the devil said, "OK, coffee break's over, back on your heads."**

The reason nurses love this joke is that it pretty much sums up their job. Laughing at such jokes, or at other unplanned funny events, provides a release for their frustrations and allows them to stay positive and focused on doing their usual good job.

This cathartic release of negative emotions provides a kind of emotional cleansing, allowing you to leave the past in the past—instead of carrying it up front in the present. Hospitals often give patients a cathartic to induce a bowel movement. It purges the system, removing poisons from the body. Laughter does the same thing—emotionally. Unexpressed negative emotions become poisons if you let them build up. They sour your attitude toward life and your job and kill your ability to experience joy, spontaneity, aliveness and fun. So think of laughter as an "emotional movement." And just as you need a good BM every day to stay healthy, you also need a good EM.

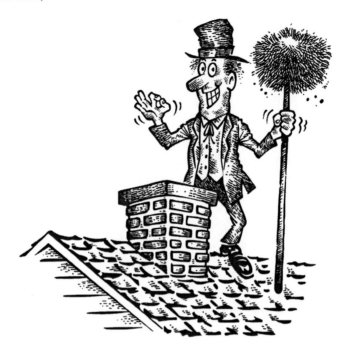

LET ME HELP YOU SWEEP OUT THAT NASTY BUILD-UP OF UNWANTED NEGATIVE EMOTIONS.

In the case of anger and aggressive behavior, we know that humor is not alone in its power to reduce angry feelings. Doing something to arouse sexual feelings or empathy can also make us feel less angry by substituting an incompatible (positive) feeling. In a classic study demonstrating this, Robert Baron used a naturalistic setting to study how male motorists responded to a situation where they were prevented from proceeding for a full 15 seconds after a traffic light (at which they were stopped) changed from red to green.[179] In the empathy condition, a woman (working with the researcher) who was normally dressed walked in front of the stopped car with a bandaged leg and on crutches. In the sexual arousal condition, the same woman walked in front of the car while skimpily dressed in a revealing outfit. Finally, in the humor condition, she walked in front of the car dressed normally, but wearing an outlandish clown mask. Aggressive behavior was defined as horn honking by the blocked motorist. In each case, waiting motorists waited longer before honking than they did when the woman walked in front of the car in normal attire. While the emotions aroused in the three conditions were quite different, they all served to reduce the level of anger experienced by the waiting motorist, presumably substituting a more positive emotion in its place.

In the case of clinical depression, the reappearance of laughter (strikingly absent in heavily depressed individuals) in social contexts is commonly viewed as evidence that recovery is progressing.[180]

Many people are aware of humor's power to manage their mood and consciously seek it out to give themselves a positive boost. In one study, 34% of people surveyed said that they sometimes purposefully use humor or laughter to pull themselves out of a bad mood or reduce feelings of nervousness, anxiety or tension.[181]

Distraction. Distraction is one mechanism by which humor pulls you out of a negative mood and puts a positive one in its place. Humor and other playful activities draw you in and literally cause you to forget your troubles for a while. They keep you from ruminating about your situation. Ruminating keeps you immersed in the details of the stressor and sets you up to wallow in negativity as long as the problem is on the front burner of your mind. *Finding something to laugh at breaks through the cycle of negative thoughts that lead to negative emotions, which trigger even more negative thoughts, and so forth.* This, in turn, enables you to focus your attention in a more positive direction and leaves you in a better state of mind to take action. Instead of thinking, "Ok, this is it; I'm in big trouble now," "I'll never have enough money," "I always have bad luck," or "No one likes me," you are more likely to think, "Ok, that's the way it is; now what? How do I deal with this?"

Humor, in my view, is—at its core—a form of intellectual play or play with ideas. And one of the most fundamental characteristics of play is its tendency to fully engage you in the activity itself. In play, you become fully immersed in things that are intrinsically enjoyable or fun—and which, of course, generate positive emotion. So it's not surprising that humor helps you (at least momentarily) forget your worries and concerns.

The power of humor to distract can also help in connection with threats to physical health. Norman Cousins used to tell the story of a man who suddenly developed a wildly beating heart (paroxysmal tachycardia), a condition that sometimes requires immediate medical attention.[182] His wife phoned the family doctor, who instructed her to do anything she could to keep him from panicking, because that could make the problem worse and cause complications. She immediately played an old *Candid Camera* videotape, in which Buster Keaton is seated at a lunchroom counter and having a difficult time keeping his glasses and toupee from repeatedly falling into his soup. Her husband laughed and laughed, and when the doctor arrived, his pulse was back to normal. The doctor said that the wife's quick thinking averted a potentially serious situation.

Production/Maintenance of a Positive Mood. It has been repeatedly noted that humor is capable of sustaining a positive mood and of increasing the level of positive emotion when you're already in a negative emotional state. This power to substitute a positive for a negative emotion may be the most important source of humor's ability to help you cope. Anything which helps you maintain a more positive, upbeat, optimistic outlook in life puts you in a better position to cope with life's trials. But extended periods of stress can cause anyone to fall into a persistent negative mood. This adds to your stress by making you less efficient in dealing with it. If you can find a light side of the situation, it helps prevent this mood disturbance from occurring.[183]

Negative moods (especially depression) also weaken your motivation to take action. You feel there's no point, since you'll fail anyway. You're more likely to feel powerless and decide that things are hopeless. The more positive mood generated by humor stimulates hope and motivates you to take action. Even if you're not very good at actively using your sense of humor to cope, but really enjoy humor and often find humor in everyday situations when you're not under stress, then these two aspects of your sense of humor may be enough to help keep you in a more upbeat, positive mood.[184]

For many people, a bad mood from stress shows up as depression. The power of humor to counter depression was evident in a patient in a hospital who was given limited chances of survival. One day a clown visited the hospital, gave her several good laughs, and raised her spirits. She decided then and there that "They're going to take me out of here in a wheel chair, not in a box." Ten years later, she continued to avoid the box and loved life.

> *"[Humor] does put you in a good mood . . . Usually when people are sick, or have something wrong, they get depressed. They can't do this, they can't do that . . . But if you start to laugh, it'll change your mood. It's a feeling of 'I can, I can,' instead of 'I can't.' Because depression is 'I can't,' and laughing is 'I can.'"*[185]

(Sid Caesar)

As we have seen, humor is an effective means of staving off, and bringing you out of, mild (non-clinical) levels of depression.[186] And finding humor in a situation when you're under high stress helps keep you from getting depressed.[187] So this again demonstrates the importance of developing your humor skills.

In one innovative study, young women in different phases of their menstrual cycle were asked to select from among comedy, drama, and game show programs for an evening of television viewing. Premenstrual and menstrual women preferred comedy over the other choices to a greater extent than did women mid-way through their menstrual cycle.[188] The researchers conducting the study concluded that this choice was due to "a desire to overcome the hormonally-mediated noxious mood states that are characteristically associated with the premenstrual and menstrual phases of the cycle."

Finally, among a group of 35 patients in a rehabilitation hospital, 91% said that laughter puts them in a good mood.[189] If laughter can improve the mood of patients with brain or spinal cord injuries, severe arthritis, neurological disorders, and amputations, it can improve your mood in the midst of common everyday stressors. At the neurological level, you will see in Chapter 3 that humor and laughter stimulate known dopamine-based pleasure centers in the brain. This may well be central to humor's ability to generate and sustain a positive mood.

BUILD YOUR HUMOR SKILLS

[Turn the page for answers. Work on both jokes before checking answers.]

1. A woman went with her husband to the doctor's office. After his checkup, the doctor called her into his office alone. He said, "Your husband is suffering from a severe stress disorder. Unless you do the following, he will surely die. Each morning, fix him a healthy breakfast and be pleasant at all times. Make him a nutritious lunch and dinner, and be especially nice to him in the evening. Don't burden him with chores. Don't discuss your problems with him, since this only makes the stress worse. No nagging. And most importantly, make love to him several times a week. If you can do this for 9 or 10 months, I think your husband will regain his health

On the way home, the husband asked what the doctor said. She answered, "He said _____."

Clue: Would you be able to do all the things the doctor suggested?

2. Tom and Mary were patients in a mental hospital. One day, as they walked past the hospital swimming pool, Tom suddenly jumped into the deep end and just sank to the bottom. Mary quickly jumped in, swam to the bottom and pulled Tom out.

When the hospital director learned about Mary's heroic act, she immediately ordered that Mary be discharged from the hospital. This act clearly pointed to Mary's mental stability. When she went to see Mary, she said, "Mary, the good news is that you're being discharged, since you were able to rationally respond to a crisis by jumping in the pool and saving the life of another patient. This tells me that you are now very sound minded. The bad news is that Tom, the patient you saved, hung himself in the bathroom with his bathrobe right after you saved him. I'm so sorry, but he's dead."

Mary promptly answered, "Oh, he didn't hang himself, I _____. How soon can I go home?"

Clue: She's not as sound-minded as the director thought.

Hope and Optimism. Among patients coping with serious diseases, hope is one form of positive mood that is of special interest. Bernie Siegel, a surgeon specializing in cancer, noted more than two decades ago that hope, optimism and determination to beat the disease were much more common among his "exceptional cancer patients" (patients who beat strong odds against their survival), than among those who succumbed to the disease when having the same odds. I have had many cancer patients tell me that keeping the ability to laugh in the midst of their cancer helps sustain a sense of hope that they can beat the disease. In a national survey of 649 oncologists conducted in the 1980s regarding the importance of different psychosocial factors in battling cancer, "more than 90% of the physicians surveyed said they attached the highest value to the attitudes of hope and optimism."[190]

Little research has been conducted on humor and hope, but the evidence is growing to support the view that they are closely connected.[191] For example, high-hope people have been found to use humor more often than low-hope people to cope with everyday problems.[192] Among breast cancer patients, the use of humor by patients was positively related to optimism both prior to surgery and at 3, 6 and 12 months after surgery.[193] In one group of older adults, 94% of "high-hope" seniors said that "lightheartedness" is a necessary component in dealing with the stresses of life.[194]

"Most folks are about as happy as they make up their minds to be."
(Abraham Lincoln)

These studies suggest that high-hope individuals are more likely to use humor to cope. But can the use of humor actually increase one's current feelings of hope in connection with a difficult life circumstance? Since genuine humor and laughter are accompanied by strong feelings of exhilaration and joy, can these feelings elevate hope? If so, can a single experience of humor strengthen feelings of hope, or is a regular diet of humor over an extended period of time required? At this point, we don't know. Watching a comedy videotape has been shown to increases feelings of hopefulness,[195] but asking people to sort *Far Side* cartoons into "funny" and "unfunny" had no impact on feelings of hope.[196] This could be due to the specific form of humor used, or it may be that the sorting task interfered with the simple enjoyment that usually accompanies humor. Or perhaps static cartoons simply do not generate a strong enough humor experience to generate feelings of hope. In any case, the effectiveness of a comedy video in boosting hopefulness has been replicated in another study.[197]

Finally, only weak positive relationships have been found between sense of humor and optimism,[198] probably because the measures used failed to distinguish between positive and negative forms of humor (see discussion earlier in this chapter). There is every reason to think that only positive, adaptive forms of humor would be associated with optimism, while hostile, sarcastic, self-put-down, and other forms of negative humor would be associated with a more pessimistic outlook on life. In any humor test that fails to make this distinction, these opposing influences would cancel each other out, leaving the low positive relationship that was found.

ANSWERS TO JOKES

1. you're going to die (other similar answers will work)

2. put him there to dry

One promising finding concerning humor and optimism is that completion of the Humor Skills Training Program I've developed as a means of learning to use humor to cope with stress has been shown to boost levels of optimism among adults. This research is discussed toward the end of this chapter.

Physiological Undoing

The reduced negative emotion and increased positive emotion resulting from humor is, in part, a reflection of humor's ability to put your mind at ease. It also puts your body at ease. Three lines of recent evidence support this view. We have known for years that when you're angry, fearful or anxious, your autonomic nervous system is activated. Blood pressure and heart rate increase, and stress hormones are released in the body. The damaging effects of these changes when they are chronically present are well known. However, research discussed above (and in Chapter 2) has shown that humor is an effective means of counteracting or "undoing" the lingering cardiovascular effects of these negative emotions.[199] Humor, then, helps restore physiological equilibrium and puts one in a better position to meet the challenges posed by the next stressor.

Reduction of Stress Hormones. It was noted earlier in this chapter that circulating levels of cortisol are reduced following exposure to humor. The presence of cortisol and other stress-related hormones contribute to the elevated negative emotion we feel when under stress, so the experience of stress should be reduced as a result of this drop in level of stress hormones.

The Relaxation Response (tension release). Stress causes you to get upset or anxious; you become more physiologically aroused in general. This arousal and these feelings, in turn, increase muscle tension. This increased muscle tension can, in turn, help sustain—or even increase—your anger or anxiety. A vicious cycle is created in which your upset feeds on itself. Relaxing the body reduces arousal and produces calmer thoughts and emotions (while reducing levels of circulating stress hormones at the same time).

"Humor is an affirmation of dignity, a declaration of man's superiority to all that befalls him." (Romain Gary)

As noted in Chapter 2, laughter produces muscle relaxation automatically and naturally. You don't have to learn to produce this relaxation effect. Nature has built it into your body. As you learn to laugh more heartily and more often, you become more relaxed—whether you're trying to or not. This makes laughter an effective stress-reducing tool when you really need it. Of course, there are some risks in being a good belly laugher. Muscles may relax that you don't want to relax. If you've ever fallen into hysterical laughter after two or three beers at a party, you know what I mean.

Some researchers have argued that simply substituting an emotion that is incompatible with anger or anxiety is not enough to assure reduced feelings of distress.[200] They note that it is also important that feelings of arousal or tension are reduced. Those who work in the field of stress management universally recognize this, as can be seen in the fact that the number one goal of all stress management techniques (including biofeedback training, deep breathing, meditation, massage, and more) is muscle relaxation and increased feelings of being relaxed. When muscle tension is reduced, a drop in psychological tension generally follows. People feel less stressed and in a better frame of mind to deal with their problem when they are in this more relaxed state.

More Accurate and Positive Appraisal of Stressful Situations

While some explanations of humor's coping power focus on the impact of humor and laughter on our emotional state (we are less stressed because we experience positive emotions that are generally incompatible with stress), humor may also help us cope by causing us to view the potentially stress-inducing situation as being less threatening. For example, among female executives, those scoring higher on a sense of humor test were more capable than their low sense of humor peers of restructuring and reappraising stressful situations in a more positive way.[201] They also were more likely to perceive the stressful event as a challenge to their personal growth, expecting some form of gain in the long run.

Of course, these two explanations are not independent, since it could be the lowered negative affect and heightened positive affect associated with humor that leads us to view the situation as less threatening. But the basic idea here is that it is our interpretation or appraisal of a situation that makes it stressful, and not the situation itself. Seeing a light side of a stressful situation helps us reframe it and view it in a less threatening manner. We have already discussed evidence above that a sense of humor helps individuals appraise a situation as more of a challenge, rather than a threat.

One pair of researchers, who have conducted a great deal of research on humor and stress concluded that "the stress–moderating effects of sense of humor appear to operate, at least in part, through more positive appraisals and more realistic cognitive processing of environmental information." By pulling us out of the negative emotion of the moment, humor helps us see a positive side of things and substitutes a frame of mind in which we can more accurately assess the situation.[202] Consistent with this view, college students ". . . with a good sense of humor [were found to] more accurately and realistically appraise the stress in their lives than those with a poor sense of humor."[203]

One of the effects of high stress (especially the chronic sort) is that judgments and behavior tend to be determined mainly by the emotion of the moment, not by a well thought-out appraisal of the situation. Normally, we go through our lives with a balanced interplay between our emotional brain and cognitive (thinking) brain. We have our emotional ups and downs, but our rational side continues to exert the more dominant influence on our behavior. But we've all had the experience at some time of doing or saying something in a fit of anger, jealousy or anxiety that we would normally never do/say. We hear phrases like, "I don't know what came over me; that's not like me," "I lost control," or "I just lost my head." Our cerebral cortex, which is responsible for rational behavior somehow gets put on the back burner, and the older emotional brain takes over.

People who have panic attacks can have this experience for an extended period of time. The extreme panic makes it impossible for them to think clearly or behave in a typical fashion. Some researchers have recently referred to this phenomenon as "neural hijacking" or "emotional hijacking."[204] Neural hijacking involves an explosive emotional reaction that originates in the amygdala—an old brain center known to be very important for emotion. These reactions occur in an instant, triggering an emotional verbal outburst or other behavior before our thinking brain is activated and can regulate the behavior.

Such neural hijacking typically involves negative emotion, but it may be that strong belly laughter is also be a form of neural hijacking.[205]

It simply takes a positive rather than a negative form. When we find something hysterically funny, we cannot contain ourselves. We have to have the emotional release that laughter provides. The subjective experience is one of joy and exhilaration. In extreme levels of this state, we may engage in unusual or inappropriate behaviors, just as we do in negative forms of neural hijacking. In most cases, however, the resulting behavior is simply silly and exaggerated, which generally does not pose a major problem—unless it is clearly totally inappropriate to the situation (weddings, funerals, etc.).

It may be this positive neural hijacking that is the key to humor's power to pull us out of a negative emotional state (such as anger, anxiety or depression) and catapult us into a more positive mood and frame of mind. This is consistent with the suggestion that humor triggers a "cognitive-affective shift," or a restructuring of the situation in a way that makes it less threatening.[206]

Maintenance of Perspective on Problems

Roseanne Roseanna Danna (Gilda Radner), of original *Saturday Night Live* fame, used to say, "It's always something; if it's not one thing, it's another!" If this sums up your life, you may be getting too caught up in minor hassles, while losing sight of the big picture. Your battery is dead! The photocopy machine at work is jammed! You're out of coffee! Your I Pod or computer is not working! Someone cut in front of you in line. Your suit/dress isn't ready when it's supposed to be. You got in the shortest line, and the long line is moving faster.

As you learn to lighten up in life, you realize that these problems are just not worth the toll taken by getting all bent out of shape by them. Humor enables you to take an emotional step back from them; and from this more distant vantage point, they lose their emotional control over you, leaving you in a better position to take effective action to deal with them.

Do you catastrophize your problems, acting as if each one is the end of the world? During my years as a university teacher, I once had a student who was in the last semester of her senior year, and she had to pass my course to graduate. The problem was that she had an "F" going into the final exam. She came into my office, burst into tears, and blurted out: "If I don't pass your test, I won't graduate! And if I don't graduate, I won't get a job! And if I don't get a job, I'll become a bag lady and live in the streets and be miserable for the rest of my life!" It was all I could do to resist laughing at this spectacle, but she failed to see the humor of it. She had completely lost perspective, and was pinning her entire life on the outcome of that course.

"Humor is the healthy way of feeling a 'distance' between one's self and the problem, a way of standing off and looking at one's problem with perspective." (Rollo May)

Dr. Robert Elliott, former Director of the National Center of Preventive and Stress Medicine, said in 1983 that we all need to develop some means of maintaining a broader perspective on our problems. Your sense of humor is one of the best tools you'll find for doing this. As you learn to lighten up, you automatically become more adept at keeping your focus on the big picture as you see your daily hassles for what they are—problems to be dealt with in the most effective way possible.

We've all heard the phrase, "Don't sweat the small stuff." It was noted earlier that many cancer patients who have defeated their cancer are very good at doing this. Their cancer has given them a different perspective on the daily hassles that used to cause them stress. They don't deny these hassles. They just accept them for what they are and get on to dealing with them. They've learned that life is too important to be in a stew all the time about minor matters. Why wait until you get cancer to learn this lesson? Developing your sense of humor helps you become someone who no longer sweats the small stuff.

The letter reproduced below (written before the onset of instant e-mail) clearly demonstrates the importance of perspective.

Dear Mom and Dad,

I'm sorry for not writing, but hope you will understand. Please sit down before you read further.

I'm doing much better now after recovering from the concussion I received jumping from my dorm window when it caught fire last month. I can almost see normally now, thanks to the loving care of Norman, the janitor who pulled me from the flames. He more than saved me; he's become my entire life. I've been living with him since the fire. We're planning to get married. We haven't set a date yet, but plan to have one soon, before my pregnancy shows.

Yes, I'm pregnant. I knew how excited you'd be for me, given how much you wanted to be grandparents. We'd be married by now, if it weren't for Norman's infection that prevented him from passing the blood test. I caught it from him, but the doctors are sure it won't affect the child.

Although he's not well educated, I know your own tolerance will make it easy for you to accept Norm.

Your Loving Daughter,

Mary

P.S. There was no fire. I had no concussion. I'm not pregnant. And there is no Norman. But I'm getting an "F" in biology, and I wanted you to see that grade in its proper perspective.

The notion of keeping daily problems in perspective is closely related to the just-discussed idea that humor supports the ability to appraise a potentially stressful situation in a more accurate and less threatening way. Part of humor's ability to do this is a result of its tendency to emotionally distance you from the source of stress.[207] It achieves this, in part, by substituting a more positive for a negative frame of mind. Also, by taking either oneself or the situation less seriously, the situation becomes less threatening; and this, in turn, helps keep negative emotional reactions in check and sustains a more effective frame of mind for dealing with the source of stress.

Increased Sense of Control

A perceived lack of control, or a sense of helplessness, may well be most important single cause of stress. An unwanted event occurs, but you feel powerless to change it—possibly because several problems emerge at the same time. Finding something to laugh at in the midst of the problem helps you feel more in control, because you really are taking a form of control—control over your emotional reaction to the situation. Rather than allowing the circumstances to generate feelings of frustration/anger, tension/anxiety, or depression, you create a positive mood which supports dealing with them.

A recovering alcoholic put it this way:

"I take control by looking in the mirror and having a good laugh before I walk out the door in the morning. I leave with the intent of passing on a smile to whoever I meet. It changes everything . . . A good laugh helps me take charge of the things that used to upset me. I can get into the nuttiest traffic situation now, and it doesn't bother me. I just let them be who they are, and I go on my way. Before, every little thing that happened on the road upset me. But if I can manage to find a bit of humor in things, it keeps me in a good mood. By the time I get home, I may be tired, but I'm not beaten or depressed or angry. And it's all under my control."

Are you a thermostat or a thermometer? A thermometer just reflects temperature as a function of what's happening around it. Something happens that you don't like, and your temperature goes up. You get angry. A thermostat can be set in advance to operate at a given temperature. Learning to lighten up in difficult situations gives you skill that enables you stay cool, while the thermometers around you are heating up.

Carol Burnett grew up in an alcoholic family, and her parents argued all the time. One day she began giving points during the arguments, depending on how well each was doing (similar to the way judges give points to skaters in the Olympics). By making a game of it, she managed to take a measure of control over a very stressful situation. She stopped being a passive victim of the violent emotions around her and took charge of at least her own emotional reactions.

At a national level, when an Israeli radio station set up an anagrams game for listeners to play (make up as many words as possible from the letters composing the name "Saddam Husein) while they waited in their sealed rooms for the gas-carrying Scud missiles that might land nearby, it provided listeners a means of taking some measure of control over their fear in that moment.

A very old theory of humor argues that we laugh at situations, events, and jokes which make us feel superior. The enjoyment of put-down jokes can, in part, be explained in this way. We feel superior to the person or group put down in the joke. But the same idea applies to stressful situations. When you find something to laugh at in the midst of difficult circumstances, you will notice a change in yourself. You'll feel like you've beaten it, like you've risen above it.

In support of this view, researchers conducting a study (described earlier) of Israeli soldiers concluded that humor increased the soldiers' feeling that they were in control of whatever situations came up, and that this enabled them to perform at a higher level.[208] It will work the same way for you on your job. Consistent with this idea, a humor training workshop has been shown to strengthen the general belief that important events in our lives are under our own control, rather than a result of outside forces or luck.[209]

There is also evidence that people with a good sense of humor are more likely to make effective attempts to solve the stress-causing problem. In a study of college students, *"Both men and women with a stronger sense of humor were significantly more likely to use positive coping strategies such as deliberate efforts at resolving the problem causing stress . . ."*[210] (Italics are McGhee's.)

Finally, feeling a sense of control also contributes to the activation of your healing systems when you are physically sick. Along with humor, this feeling can also come from love, faith (in your doctor, a medicine, or God), meditation, exercise, good nutrition, or other coping skills.[211] If you believe you can have impact on a stress-inducing situation, this enhances the operation of the body's self-healing mechanisms.

Increased Energy/Decreased Burnout

Anger and anxiety are energy-sapping emotions. If your job causes you stress day after day, week after week, the anger, anxiety, or depression—and general tension—you live with drains the energy you need to be perform effectively. It also lowers your morale and job satisfaction and sets you up for burnout.

As you learn to lighten up on the job, in your relationships, on the way to work, etc., you'll have more energy and experience less burnout. Laughter recharges your batteries. It fights burnout by giving you back the energy you're supposed to have, and by making work more enjoyable. It restores energy by cutting through energy-sapping emotions and replacing them with energizing ones. In short, it revitalizes you. People who are able to incorporate humor and a sense of fun into their job look forward to going to work and are more effective when they get there. This alone reduces job stress.

"I've developed a new philosophy . . . I only dread one day at a time." (Charlie Brown)

I noted earlier in this book that in my keynote addresses there is one point at which I always go through a funny routine in which the entire audience and I break laughter down into five basic steps and relearn how to do real belly laughter (for those who are too busy, too stressed out—or have just forgotten how—to laugh during the day). I get several people up front to model this, but the entire group does it together. It winds up with the entire room doing 30 seconds or more of real belly laughter. Afterwards, I ask people to shout out any differences they notice in how they feel (or physical changes in their body), relative to how they felt before the laughter. Most of the time, someone says that they feel more alert or energized.

I have asked entire audiences to vote on this issue several hundred times. I give them three choices: they should categorize themselves as feeling 1) more tired and having less energy, 2) no significant change in energy level or 3) more energized. With rare exceptions, about 75% of the audience say they have more energy. Roughly 15–20% say they notice no significant change in energy and about

5% report less energy. I have never found as many as 20% reporting less energy, and never less than 60% reporting more energy. (Well, there was one exception when I did an early Saturday morning presentation in a hotel; I found out later that most of those present had been out late the previous night partying.)

This increased energy is surprising, because belly laughter is a real physical workout. Your heart rate goes up, you start sweating, and you may even get sore muscles. This should leave you tired and less energetic; but most people report the opposite. My guess is that this energizing effect would be most noticeable when you actively find humor in a situation yourself, but there is no research on this. In fact only one study has given any attention at all to this topic. Consistent with my own observations with audiences over the past 15 years, watching a video of a Bill Cosby comedy routine sharply increased viewers' feelings of energy.[212]

Stronger Social Support Network

Another way in which humor may facilitate coping is by proving a stronger social network.[213] A good sense of humor is generally seen as a desirable quality in the people we develop friendships with, work with, and marry. People who love humor and who are able to make others laugh are more likely, in return, to be liked and sought out as friends. In short, those who have good humor skills tend to be better at initiating and maintaining positive social interactions, and these interactions gradually build up a strong social support network that one can draw on in times of stress. The role of such a support network in helping cope with life stress is well established.

Consistent with this view, individuals with a more developed sense of humor have been found to show less social isolation and greater interpersonal intimacy than their low sense of humor peers.[214] Of course, having an outgoing personality makes it easier to make social connections with others, so it comes as no surprise that more extraverted individuals tend to score higher on sense of humor measures.[215] This may well be one of the main underlying reasons why people with a stronger sense of humor develop stronger social networks. Similarly, the finding that those scoring higher on humor tests tend to have a more cheerful general demeanor[216] would lead them to be sought out more often as friends .

"A smile confuses an approaching frown." (Anonymous)

People who score low on several different measures of sense of humor show greater avoidance of social situations, and more distress when in a social situation, than high sense of humor individuals.[217] Having a better sense of humor, then, also goes along with having less social anxiety. This same study showed that high sense of humor individuals also viewed themselves as being very sociable. A higher level of self-esteem (discussed earlier) would similarly boost high sense of humor individuals' comfort level in social situations.

Which is More Important, Humor or Laughter?

The main focus of this chapter has been the mental/emotional experience of humor, not the act of laughter that usually (but not necessarily) accompanies it. It's difficult to isolate the separate influence on stress reduction of these two aspects experiencing humor, since they occur together. It seems likely, however, that they work together in helping us cope, having a combined effect that is more powerful effect than either would have alone.

At this point, the research that has been done does not allow a conclusion about the relative benefits of humor vs. laughter. I have emphasized the ways in which the experience of humor a) reduces or prevents negative emotion and b) produces or sustains positive emotion, provides a sense of control and helps maintain perspective on daily problems. But the act of laughter surely plays just as important a role in producing muscle relaxation (the main goal of all stress management techniques) and may also be crucial in reducing negative emotion and increasing positive emotion.

There is already some support this view. For example, in a study in which exposure to humor generated a more positive mood, greater increases in positive mood were associated with greater amounts of laughter.[218] (Of course, greater perceived funniness of the materials presented may well have been responsible for both the more elevated mood and elevated laughter.) The strongest case for the resilience-boosting power of laughter comes from the finding that even forced, non-humorous laughter in a laboratory setting leads to higher levels of positive mood.[219]

Again, Emotional Resilience is the Key to Good Mental Health

The central idea presented in this chapter is that your sense of humor is a powerful ally in providing the emotional resilience you need to cope well and maintain good mental health in today's high-stress world. So I'll elaborate a bit more here on the general notion of resilience.

Resilience is generally viewed as the ability to cope well in the midst of some personal adversity, hardship or loss.[220] Researchers in the Positive Psychology have argued that "emotional flexibility" is important in boosting emotional resilience. An emotionally flexible person is able to manage their mood or emotional state to more effectively meet the demands of the current difficult situation,[221] and humor—as we have seen—is a potent mood management tool.

The presence of emotional flexibility has been demonstrated at the neurological level in people independently identified as having high "trait resilience." The amygdala is an area of the brain long known to play a key role in emotion. It is activated in response to threat[222] and shows sustained activation in depression.[223] Both high and low resilience individuals show increased activation of key areas of the amygdala (as indicated in an fMRI study) when a threat is present. Among low resilience individuals, however, this increased activation persists even when the threat is gone. Among high resilience people, activation of the amygdala stops when the threat is not present.[224] So *part of what provides increased resilience is this ability to manage your emotional state to fit the situation of the moment.* This finding is directly related to the importance of having skills that keep you from "stewing in your emotional juices" after the stressful event has ended.

One of these skills, of course, is your sense of humor. As noted in the Introduction, people with high levels of trait resilience often use humor as a coping strategy.[225] Even children with high trait resilience initiate more humor when under stress than children with low trait resilience.[226] Increased use or appreciation of humor is also associated with greater resilience among cancer patients,[227] surgical patients[228] and even combat veterans.[229]

According to Fredrickson's "broaden-and-build" theory of positive emotions (discussed above), negative emotions typically narrow the range of thoughts and actions that are considered in dealing with any stressful (or non-stressful) situation, while positive emotions generate a broader range of thoughts and actions related to how to respond to the situation. This is precisely what enables positive emotions to serve us so well when we have to adapt to difficult situations. The broadened repertoire of thoughts/actions associated with positive emotion is central to developing a greater variety of intellectual, physical, emotional and social resources.[230] Most importantly, the coping resources acquired during states of positive emotion tend to last long beyond the transient positive emotion of the moment during their acquisition.[231]

There is evidence of a reciprocal spiraling effect when it comes to positive emotion and coping. That is, increased levels of positive emotion support improved coping; and this better coping, in turn, contributes to still more positive emotion.[232] This process is crucial to sustaining long-term emotional resilience.

The key question here is, how much positive emotion is required to sustain this resilience-inducing spiraling effect? According to Fredrickson, "What matters most is the ratio of your positive emotions to your negative emotions. This is what I've called your positivity ratio. Just as ice melts into water when it passes a certain temperature, people who are languishing in life can move to flourishing in life if their positivity ratio is 3:1. We need three positive emotions to lift us up for every negative emotion that drags us down. The sad part is that my research shows that most people clock in at ratios of 2:1, and many people are worse off still."[233]

She advises people to use a daily log to track positivity ratios. "Discover what makes you come alive and give those activities a higher priority." For most people, shared humor and laugher makes you feel more alive and energized. She notes that although a lot of things that increase aliveness are viewed as frivolous (humor certainly qualifies here), it is crucial to invest in your own well being by building these into your daily life.

Fredrickson has also suggested that positive emotion has contributed to our resilience and survival as a species.

"Whereas the narrowed mindsets sparked by negative emotions were adaptive in instances that threatened survival in some way, the broadened mindsets sparked by positive emotions were adaptive in different ways and over longer time frames: Broadened mindsets were adaptive because over time such expansive awareness served to build our human ancestor's resources, spurring on their development, and equipping them to better handle subsequent threats to survival.

. . . positive emotions were adaptive to our human ancestors because, over time, positive states and their associated broadened mindsets could accumulate and compound in ways that transformed individuals for the better, leaving them with more social, psychological, intellectual, and physical resources than they would have otherwise had. When these ancestors later faced inevitable threats to life and limb, their greater resources would have translated into better odds of survival, and of living long enough to reproduce."[234]

Are You Born with/without a Sense of Humor? Can it be Developed as an Adult?

I often hear people say, "You're either born with a good sense of humor or you're not; and I wasn't, so there's not much I can do about it." This is clearly not the case. Most people come to this conclusion after watching the amazing skills some people have of coming up with witty remarks on the spot, with no apparent effort at all. It's so easy for them that it is assumed to have always been there and have a genetic basis. In fact, these skilled humorists have been practicing humor for many years; they've had humor on the front burner for so long that funny remarks just pop into their mind with no effort at all. The thing to remember is that if you were to spend 10, 20 or 30 years cultivating your sense of humor you'd be really good at it too! Luckily, it doesn't take 10 years—or even one year.

In two of my earlier books on the development of children's humor, I argued that we all have the same basic foundation for the development of our sense of humor when we are born.[235] This includes a general predisposition to play, which is extended to both physical and intellectual skills as we develop during childhood. In fact, developmental changes in children's humor are the same around the world, since they reflect basic underlying changes in children's intellectual development. (For a discussion of the development of children's humor, see my book, *Understanding and Promoting the Development of Children's Humor.*) As new mental abilities emerge over the preschool and elementary school years, kids play with those skills. As children become capable of thinking at more complex and abstract levels, these features enter into their humor.

In certain ways, then, all children show the same kind of humor at a given developmental level. There are many other ways, though, in which every child's sense of humor is unique. Any parent who has had more than one child can tell you this. As we get older, our environment starts to have a growing impact on our sense of humor. Some parents strongly support their children's sense of humor, while others just find their kids' silly antics tiresome and annoying. I've also had many adults tell me that they were physically punished for their efforts at humor when they were kids—even when their humor wasn't harmful to others. All of these experiences during childhood and adolescence serve to form the unique sense of humor we have by the time we become adults.

In spite of the strong drive to play and enjoy humor that we all had as kids, some of us became adults who are *terminally serious* and *humor impaired.* We all know someone like this; you've known them for years, and you've never once seen them laugh or come up with any kind of funny comment. There is no research on whether such humor-impaired people can learn to improve their sense of humor as an adult, and perhaps even use it to cope with the stress in their lives. There is evidence (discussed following the next section), however, that you can take an average group of adults and boost their humor skills.

The Role of Temperament

Infants differ in temperament from birth. For example, some are irritable, unresponsive, prone to crying, or physically inactive while others have a generally good disposition, are more extroverted and responsive, and very active. Research on adults has determined that certain temperaments (as defined in adulthood) predispose some individuals to have a better sense of humor than others; this should make it easier for them to learn to use humor to cope with life stress.

Willibald Ruch, now at the University of Zurich in Switzerland, has determined that there are three basic personality traits (enduring behaviors, dispositions, or emotional tendencies) that amount to a temperamental basis for humor. He calls them cheerfulness, seriousness, and bad mood.[236] We all have times when we're in a state of being cheerful, serious or in a bad mood as a result of things that are happening at the moment. People with any of these qualities as a temperament have them as a habitual starting point into which daily experience feeds. While a cheerful temperament provides a general disposition that is very favorable to enjoying and initiating humor, a bad mood and serious temperament produce a frame of mind that is much less conducive to enjoying or producing humor—in fact, as we have seen, it is typically a major obstacle to humor.

Most pertinent to our concerns in this chapter is Ruch's suggestion that "trait cheerfulness might account for the phenomenon of *keeping* or *losing* humor when facing adversity." This is due to the fact that it is more difficult for people who have cheerfulness as an enduring feature of their personality to be pulled out of a cheerful state because they're having a bad day. Even if humor skills can be effectively trained among adults, people who have seriousness or a bad mood as an personality trait would pose the most difficult training challenge.

Humor Intervention for the Humor Impaired

Leaders in the field of Positive Psychology have emphasized the importance of developing positive emotion interventions that are effective and last over time.[237]   Very few such interventions have been developed at this point, although counting one's blessings and expressing gratitude have been shown to be effective strategies.[238] Practicing already-established character strengths is another.[239]

In this latter case, the idea is to strengthen a resource that already exists. One area of emphasis within applied Positive Psychology has been to support the use of one's own "signature strengths." This is an important endeavor, but as an intervention, it might be viewed as "stacking the cards in your favor," since you are adding to an already-established strength. A much tougher test would be an intervention program that builds a character strength which has not already been determined to be a personal strength. *Can a character strength that does not already exist as a signature strength be effectively cultivated and used to promote happiness and well-being?*

As already discussed, a 3:1 ratio of positive to negative emotion is needed to support personal flourishing, and most people fall below this optimal ratio.[240] As this chapter has shown, humor provides one effective means of generating a quick boost in positive emotion. In the 1990's, I developed a hands-on Humor Skills Training Program for individuals who do not have a well-developed sense of humor. The program is designed to build the basic foundation skills of humor that might then be used to cope with any form of life stress. The latest version of this program is presented in my book *Humor as Survival Training for a Stressed-Out World* (also published by Author House in 2010). The research documenting the programs effectiveness in both boosting humor skills and increasing positive emotion is also discussed in detail in that book.

Each step of the program focuses on a separate skill and is accompanied by a set of skill-developing activities to practice for one or (preferably) two weeks. This "homeplay" is provided for each step, showing things you need to do in order to build skills associated with the step. The lengthy period of practice is considered to be crucial in generating a lasting boost in skills. (Similarly, positive psychologists studying happiness have emphasized the importance of habitually practicing the happiness-inducing technique in order to avoid the "hedonic adaptation effect" that commonly occurs with positive emotion.[241]) Using humor to cope is not practiced until the end. The key idea is to first build up humor habits on the good days, when all is going well, and then extend those habits to the stressful situations you encounter. The box on the next page lists the steps in the program.

The first thing this program does is help you better understand both the nature of your own sense of humor and early influences that may have caused your sense of humor to move in this direction. As part of the process, you are encouraged to immerse yourself in many different kinds of humor for a couple of weeks. The next step is to practice getting back in touch with the playful side of yourself in a general sense. Don't worry about humor per se yet; just get more comfortable with being playful and having fun. The reason for this is that most people's own natural sense of humor (which may have been lost for years due to stress and other factors) surprisingly re-emerges once the spirit of play is recaptured.

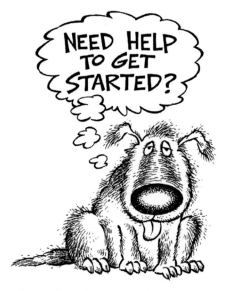

The next two steps begin building humor skills by focusing on verbal humor—first jokes and then spontaneous verbal humor that you create yourself. (For those who are not comfortable with hearty laughter, guidelines are also offered for how to become a good belly laugher.) You are then shown how to find more humor in your own everyday life, followed by learning to poke fun at yourself. Only then does the focus shift to using humor to cope with stress. Finally, a week or two is used to practice putting all these habits together, strengthening the whole package of your new sense of humor.

Several studies have now tested the effectiveness of this program in Europe, the United States and Australia. They confirm the notion that *it's never too late to improve your sense of humor.* The first test of the program was completed in the USA using seniors living in several retirement communities. While some seniors went through the

8-Step Program (spending a week on each step) and actively worked on improving their sense of humor, others got together weekly and just watched their favorite old comedy programs together (passive exposure to humor, with no focus on building humor skills).

PAUL MCGHEE'S HUMOR SKILLS TRAINING PROGRAM

1. A. Surround yourself with humor you enjoy.
   B. Determine the nature of your sense of humor.

2. Cultivate a playful attitude: Overcome terminal seriousness.

3. A. Laugh more often and more heartily.
   B. Begin telling jokes and funny stories.

4. Play with language: Puns and other verbal humor.

5. Find humor in everyday life.

6. Take yourself lightly: Laugh at yourself.

7. Find humor in the midst of stress

8. Put it all together: Use humor to cope.

While the two groups showed similar coping abilities at the beginning of the study, the groups making an active effort to boost their humor skills scored significantly higher than the passive humor group on two different measures of coping at the end of the eight weeks. The humor training group also scored higher than the passive group on the "Humor under stress" subscale of the Sense of Humor Scale associated with the 8-Step Program. There were no group differences in this subscale at the beginning of the study.[242]

So going through the skills training program not only helped these seniors cope better with the stress in their lives; they also got better at learning to use humor to cope during their own high stress days. This suggests that *you're never too old to learn to lighten up.*

Separate studies of Austrian, Swiss and Australian adults have demonstrated this programs effectiveness in improving one's humor skills, with sense of humor improvement continuing to be shown as long as three months after completion of the program—including the use of humor to cope with stress.[243] One of these studies also showed a significant increase in life satisfaction as a result of the humor training program.[244] The program also produced increases (which remained present three months later) in positive emotion, optimism and the ability to control one's own internal states (recall that the ability to manage one's emotional state is a key part of emotional intelligence) and decreases in stress, depression and negative emotion generally.[245] Additional discussion of research related to assessments of this Humor Skills Training Program is provided in *Humor as Survival Training for a Stressed-Out World.*[246] Other approaches to improving one's sense of humor have met with mixed success.[247]

Use of Humor by Therapists

Given the tremendous amount of evidence supporting humor's contribution to psychological well-being, along with its effectiveness as a coping tool, it should also be a helpful ally in therapy. And this is, indeed, the case. Over the past quarter century, there has been a slow, but steady, movement among therapists around the world to use humor as a therapeutic technique. I will not describe here the many approaches therapists have developed for using humor in therapy. Other books do that quite effectively.[248] The goal here is to simply discuss some of the evidence documenting that humor does help people deal with the kinds of stress that caused them to seek therapy in the first place. As you would expect, *humor has been shown to be an effective tool for helping patients let go of pent-up emotions in a therapeutic context.*[249]

"You don't stop laughing because you grow old; you grow old because you stop laughing."   Michael Pritchard

We've all heard the phrase, "Some day, we'll look back at this and laugh." We're aware that there is an absurd or comical side of a stressful event, but our emotional upheaval at that moment denies us any real experience of humor in connection with it. With time, the difficult emotions subside, and we can appreciate the light side that was there all along. Some therapists purposefully use this notion to help patients focus their attention on some incongruous or bizarre incident connected with their trauma. A therapist told me more than a decade ago the following (true) story about a way in which humor provided a turning point in a patient's therapy.

A woman whose husband had died spent a couple of years in therapy, with no real progress. She felt guilty about her husband's death, and could not get past this. She had insisted that her husband do some outside yard work when he preferred to putter around inside. He died of a heart attack while working in the yard. She constantly said to herself, "If I hadn't insisted he work outside, he'd be alive today." She went from therapist to therapist, but no one seemed to be able to help her.

Finally, one therapist who had had several sessions with her said to her one day, "You know, I've been thinking about it, and I've decided you're right. You killed him. I think you should march right down to the police station and turn yourself in."

The shocked patient suddenly sat up straight and stared at him. After a brief puzzled look, a smile came across her face, and then a short laugh. That laugh was the turning point in her therapy. From that point on, she continued to improve.

This is a wonderful example of how a therapist can use exaggeration to help a patient achieve a fundamental insight—in this case that she was not responsible for the conditions within his body that actually triggered the heart attack. If it were not this specific work that her husband was doing, some other minor physical activity could just as well have triggered the attack.

A man goes to a doctor and says he's very depressed. He is saddened by the terrorist threats, global financial crisis, people losing their jobs, inability to afford healthcare, and general madness he sees in the world. He is afraid we're in a permanent recession and things just aren't going to get any better. The therapist says the treatment is simple. The great clown Rinaldi is in town. He is fantastic. Just go and see him; that will boost anybody's spirits.

The man bursts into tears and says, "But doctor, I am Rinaldi"

There are many kinds of therapy, but therapists generally focus on changing their clients' thoughts, behaviors, or emotions (and underlying physiological changes that go along with these)—or all three. In the example just cited regarding the woman who felt guilty about her husband's death, emotions and thoughts were clearly the target. The intellectual insight regarding the absurdity of turning herself in for murder generated the positive emotion of joy and exhilaration via the laughter, which in turn helped her begin to unload the heavy burden of guilt she had been carrying. Therapists often use humor to help clients achieve a sense of perspective regarding their thoughts and behaviors. This new perspective helps the individual see just how distorted their thinking pattern has been.

Several years ago, while preparing for a presentation to an Alcoholics Anonymous group, I came across a man who shared a story about the lengths he would go to in order to get some alcohol. He lived in a near-suburb of a city and there was a liquor store just a few hundred yards from his apartment. The only problem was that it was on the other side of a major freeway, and there was no road crossing the freeway near where he lived. So he regularly walked across the freeway—sometimes during rush hour—when he ran out of beer. It wasn't until months later in his AA meetings that he finally saw the absurdity of his behavior. Once he had a good laugh at the ways in which he put his life at risk for alcohol, he made a giant leap forward in battling his addiction.

BUILD YOUR HUMOR SKILLS

[Turn the page for answers. Work on both jokes before checking answers.]

1. A little girl was talking to her teacher about Jonah being swallowed by a whale. The teacher said it was physically impossible for a whale to swallow a human, because even though a whale is very large its throat is very small. When the girls persisted in saying that Johan was swallowed by a whale, the teacher became irritated and repeated that a whale could not possibly swallow a person. Finally, the girl said, "When I get to Heaven, I'll ask Jonah." At that point, the teacher asked, "What if Jonah went to Hell?" The girl answered, "Then _____."
Clue: Given what she's seen of this teacher, she doesn't expect him to go to Heaven.

2. The hypochondriac was a regular in the emergency room—so much so that when he didn't show up for a week, the staff took notice of his absence. When he finally did show up again, one doctor said, "Long time no see. Where have you been?" "Sorry, I couldn't make it in," the hypochondriac said. "I was _____."
Clue: What is the one thing that normally *would* lead you to seek medical attention?

I heard a similar story recently as I interviewed two clinical staff (in connection with an upcoming presentation) involved in smoking prevention/cessation programs in a hospital. A tobacco-addicted patient was in the hospital following surgery. He was seen (by a nurse and the doctor who performed his surgery) running out of the (Florida) hospital and crossing a busy intersection to get a pack of cigarettes in a restaurant where the doctor and nurse were eating. The funny part of this was that he was still in his hospital gown! In nothing but the gown, with a $10 bill in his hand, he dodged traffic in order to get into the restaurant as quickly as possible—with the single-tie (in the back) gown flapping in the breeze. The doctor ran over and shouted, "What are you doing!" To the patient, whose nicotine addiction colored his good judgment, this seemed like a perfectly reasonable thing to do, since he really needed a smoke.

A common goal of therapists' use of humor is to help patients manage their emotions. (Remember, this is a skill that is central to emotional intelligence.)

"Since humor directly changes one's emotional state, it can be used as a treatment modality to relieve distressing emotions. Clients can be taught to use humor to relieve anxiety, depression, and anger. Through the purposeful use of humor, clients can learn that they can both *relieve their emotional distress* and also be empowered to *manage their emotional reactions*. For example, a client who was 'dedicated' to maintaining her depression insisted that she wanted to feel less depressed. As part of her treatment, her therapist integrated humorous interventions. After each of the first few humorous interventions (presented over several sessions), she responded to her therapist, 'I hate when you do that (say something humorous).' She became increasingly annoyed with her therapist's use of humor until finally the therapist inquired, 'What is it about my use of humor that bothers you?' Instantly she emphatically replied, 'When you make me laugh, I don't feel depressed!'. . .

A depressed client who experiences and is receptive to humor in therapy can learn *experientially* that, for at least that moment in time, the intensity of the depression fades. Clients can be taught to consciously seek out humorous experiences outside of therapy sessions as ways of managing their emotional distress. A cognitive psychotherapist can use humor to explore and/or test a client's faulty assumptions by exaggerating the client's perception leading to a ludicrous conclusion. For example, if a therapist knows a client experiences test anxiety, the therapist can exaggerate the client's 'failure' on a test to resulting in the client having to drop out of school, then being unemployed, and then being destitute. The absurdity of this illogical progress of events—starting with "failure" on a test and leading to being destitute—can result in a reframing for the client. When clients realize that they have illogically distorted their situation, they are better able to regain a healthier, more realistic perspective."[250]

Although my Humor Skills Training Program (discussed in the previous section) was not designed for individuals diagnosed with clinical depression or anxiety, evidence has been obtained showing that this program is very effective in reducing both depression and anxiety levels of individuals known to be clinically depressed or anxious.[251] This finding confirms the conclusions of the clinical psychologist providing the lengthy quote in the previous paragraph. When the length of the Training Program was reduced from eight to four weeks with a group of patients diagnosed with clinical depression, however, it had no significant impact on symptoms of depression (although it did improve responsiveness among these patients to a procedure specifically designed to induce a positive mood).[252] It is clearly too early to draw any conclusions about the program's effectiveness with any clinical population, although there is every reason to think that for the program to be effective with such a group, a longer—not shorter—period of training is in order.

ANSWERS TO JOKES

1. you ask him   2. sick

Throughout this chapter, frequent reference has been made to people who (as indicated by a sense of humor test) often use humor to cope. These individuals have learned how effective humor is in managing their emotions and are able to use their sense of humor when it matters most. Most people in therapy have not learned this . . . at least not in the area of their problems. So certain therapists help them develop such skills so that they can use humor on their own in the same way that a therapist uses it in a therapy session. The finding that even highly depressed or anxious individuals can benefit from a Humor Skills Program is an especially promising finding, suggesting that some individuals may be able to avoid going to a therapist to find ways of keeping their depression or anxiety within manageable limits. This should be expected, however, for individuals with high levels of clinical depression or anxiety.

To provide one example of how a therapist uses humor, Steve Sultanoff, former President of the Association for Applied and Therapeutic Humor (www.aath.org) often asks a client to share an event that was so funny that s/he wet her/his pants. Patients dealing with anxiety issues are asked to rate their own anxiety level before and after this visualization. Even when the humor is not directly related to the source of anxiety, patients generally report that they feel less anxious afterwards. This realization that humor can be used to reduce anxiety is crucial to many who are plagued by anxiety or panic attacks, since it gives them a sense of control over the emotions that have been running their lives for so long.[253]

To this point, the entire discussion in this book has been based on research. This section on humor and therapy is the exception to that rule. The use of humor among therapists remains an art or skill whose impact is difficult to assess in research. Some therapists are comfortable and confident in using humor with patients, but others are not. Individual therapists have strong convictions about the usefulness of humor because they see its impact on patients. By definition, every patient condition and use of humor by a therapist is unique. This makes the kind of systematic comparison that is essential for research impossible. So we are left with the conclusion that many therapists *claim* that humor is a valuable ally in treating a broad range of emotional/mental conditions.

Humor and Spirituality

Many people look to religious or spiritual sources to regain the strength to carry on in the midst of crises. And there is some evidence that the active use of humor and laughter serves as a source of spiritual strength among breast cancer patients.[254] When another group of women with breast cancer were interviewed regarding their use of humor and its influence on their spirituality, however, widespread differences were found. While some saw no relationship between humor and their Christian beliefs, others said that their humor and spirituality both influenced each other. Some felt that God had to have a sense of humor to set up some of the things they had to deal with.

E-MAIL FROM GOD

One day God looked down at Earth and was dismayed at the behavior of His divine creation. So he asked one of His angels to go down to Earth and observe for a while. Upon his return, the angel said, "Yes, it's bad on Earth; 90% are behaving very badly. God reflected on this and decided to send another angel for a second opinion. That angel confirmed the findings of the first. Only 10% were behaving as God would like.

God was not pleased, so He decided to send the 10% who were being good an e-mail to offer them hope and encouragement in the midst of a world heading in a bad direction. Do you know what that e-mail said? (Turn the page for the answer.)

Children who more often use prayer to cope also tend to use humor as a coping strategy.[255] This is an especially interesting (and surprising to me) finding, although it is not clear just how this might relate to the possible link between humor/laughter and one's level of spirituality. The one study I know of which specifically related a measure of sense of humor to spiritual well-being found no significant relationship between the two.[256]

Holy Laughter

Certain religious groups began in the 1990s to use laughter as a vehicle for generating a sense of communion with God. The best-known church promoting holy laughter was (and may still be) the Toronto (Canada) Airport Christian Church. The pastor of this church would use Christian humor to get the laughter started, but also had an infectious laugh himself. People would come prepared to laugh, and once it started within the congregation, individuals would allow themselves to totally "let go" to the urge to laugh. They sometimes found themselves involuntarily falling on the floor laughing, often sobbing or shaking in the process. The experience appears to be one of religious ecstasy, as those in the church described themselves as being "moved by the Holy Spirit" to laugh. Given the contagiousness of laughter, convulsive laughter quickly spread through the congregation.

"God is a comedian playing to an audience that is afraid to laugh."

(Voltaire)

When interviewed after such experiences of holy laughter, church members reported that they were totally filled with the Holy Spirit; some said that they'd never felt as close to God as during the laughter episodes. Just as speaking in tongues is considered to be under divine control, so is this laughter considered to be under God's control. When these individuals left the church, they felt spiritually uplifted and ready to confront the challenges of the day.

While it was only two decades ago that the Toronto Airport Church and other churches in North America began their "laughter revivals," the practice is clearly not a new one. Certain U. S. Pentecostal churches in earlier centuries had a similar practice. For example, the well-known Cane Ridge (Kentucky) Revival of 1801 had a "laughing exercise."[257]

Humor and Happiness/Life Satisfaction

From its inception, a major focus of Positive Psychology has been the identification of effective paths which support the pursuit of a happy and satisfying life. The evidence we've seen documenting humor's effectiveness in boosting resilience and coping with stress suggests that it should make a major contribution to the achievement of increased levels of happiness and life satisfaction.

Within the context of the notion of emotional intelligence, we have seen that humor is a most useful tool for "managing your mood" or emotional state throughout the day. Happiness should be elevated to the extent that one is able to "let go" of negative emotions instead of carrying them around for lengthy periods of time, substituting a more positive, joyful frame of mind (and emotion) in the process.

E-MAIL FROM GOD

You don't? OK, just checking. I didn't get one either.

Barbara Fredrickson's widely-accepted "broaden-and-build" theory of positive emotion (see Introduction and beginning of this chapter for a discussion) further clarifies the mechanisms by which humor should contribute to happiness and life satisfaction. For example, positive emotion contributes to the building of creativity and other problem-solving skills, important social skills (including a general sense of interpersonal competence), more satisfying marital and other personal relationships, and a more positive sense of self. These skills contribute to more effective functioning in everyday life, generating the kind of feedback that should further contribute to happiness and satisfaction with one's life.

Many different character strengths and virtues can boost our happiness.[258] New evidence suggests that the key character strengths that lead to the happiest lives are those that generate meaning and engagement in life, along with pleasure.[259] These qualities are essential to what constitutes a "full" life in happy people. Love and gratitude are also key elements of a happy life. Evidence from both the USA and Switzerland suggests that humor plays a significant role in all of these components. In both countries, humor is associated with a life that is more engaged, more meaningful, and experienced as having more pleasure in it. It is also associated with greater life satisfaction. Together, these create a happier life.[260] Other evidence similarly shows that more frequent use of humor is associated with increased happiness.[261] Even the act of sustaining a mental image of yourself laughing is enough to increase your level of happiness.[262]

In his book, *Happiness: The Science Behind Your Smile*, Daniel Nettle distinguishes between three different kinds or levels of happiness.[263] Events that trigger specific experiences of joy and pleasure generate momentary boosts in happiness. A particular funny event clearly falls into this category. (See Chapter 3 for evidence that specific funny events activate pleasure centers in the brain.) His second level of happiness reflects a sense of satisfaction (based upon some reflection) with one's life in a general sense. (The evidence documenting a positive link between humor and life satisfaction is discussed next.) His third level of happiness centers around the experience of "flourishing" in life as a result of fulfilling a held ideal about the "good life."

This concept of flourishing is the same notion adopted by Barbara Fredrickson and her colleagues (discussed above and in the Introduction). No data are available yet specifically documenting humor's contribution to the achievement of a sense of flourishing in one's life, but to the extent that humor boosts one's daily resilience and generates daily inputs of positive emotion over the years of one's life, there is every reason to believe that the possession of a good sense of humor does support flourishing. As already noted, Fredrickson's research suggests that we generally need about a 3:1 ratio of positive to negative events in our day on an ongoing basis to flourish as a person. Obviously, there are a couple of ways of going about this. We can minimize the occurrence of negative emotions or generate positive emotion more often. An ideal tool for sustaining this ratio would involve both. Humor provides such a tool.

Sonja Lyubomirsky and her associates have noted that although that are numerous popular books available discussing how to achieve happiness, there is actually little research on techniques that have been shown to boost happiness levels—not to mention how long such increases in happiness actually last.[264] She defines happiness in terms of "frequent positive affect, high life satisfaction, and infrequent negative affect." The first question, she notes, is whether any permanent change in happiness is possible at all. There is evidence that genetic factors produce a kind of "set point" for happiness, accounting for around 50% of differences in happiness levels among people.[265] This presumably provides the basis for the close link commonly found between certain personality traits (e.g., extraversion) and happiness.[266] This genetic set point for happiness is presumably minimally changeable—if it is changeable at all. (Although Ed Diener and his colleagues have recently argued that radical life-changing events do alter this set point.[267] Of the remaining 50% of influences on our "chronic" happiness level, Lyubomirsky argues that 40% can be altered by "intentional activity" we engage in, while 10% is a reflection of circumstances we find ourselves in at the moment. It has already been shown that intentional engagement in activities known to produce positive emotion can generate lasting increases in happiness.[268]

Humor is an ideal candidate for an intervention activity to boost happiness levels within this 40% considered changeable. Research already discussed shows that all three of Lyubomirsky's three prerequisites of happiness are met by humor: increased positive emotion, reduced negative emotion and higher life satisfaction (discussed next). While having a good sense of humor and building high amounts of humor into one's life may not guarantee happiness, it certainly helps provide the emotional conditions which many researchers consider essential for happiness to occur.

Three studies of the effectiveness of my Humor Skills Training Program (discussed above) suggest that humor skills training can also be viewed as an effective happiness-promoting intervention within Lyubomirsky's model. In combination, these studies show that this humor intervention provides a significant boost in positive mood,[269] trait cheerfulness,[270] and optimism[271] and a decrease in bad mood[272] and depression and general negative affect[273]—and increased life satisfaction.[274] These changes were still present one to three months after completion of the program (the follow-up data were collected either one, two or three months later).

One of the most difficult challenges to sustaining a high level of happiness is the death of one's spouse. It has long been known that the surviving spouse is especially vulnerable to depression—and even death—in the two years following the partner's death. But a broad range of positive and negative emotions are experienced by most people in this situation.[275] The experience of positive emotion during the bereavement process appears to make an important contribution to one's adjustment and coping during this period.[276] Again, humor provides a very helpful tool in building some positive emotion into one's life during the difficult period of bereavement. Consistent with this idea, among a group of recently widowed women, those who used or experienced humor more often experienced less bereavement stress, anxiety and depression.[277] Among another group of bereaved men and women, experiencing greater amounts of humor and laughter was associated with more favorable adjustment during bereavement—and greater happiness.[278]

One group of researchers, in discussing the psychobiology of resilience, has suggested recently that the dopamine-based reward or pleasure center in the brain may serve to predispose some individuals toward greater or lesser happiness, depending on the extent of genetically-based sensitivity of their dopamine receptors.[279] Highly sensitive dopamine receptors would lead to more frequent experience of pleasure and positive affect from a wide variety of sources; humor would be just one of these sources. People with less sensitive systems would be more vulnerable to stress-induced depression. They discuss the use of drugs as one means of increasing dopamine function in key areas of this reward system (like the nucleus accumbens).

As noted in Chapter 3, humor and laughter activate this same dopamine-based pleasure or reward system—including the nucleus accumbens. It is unlikely that humor can be used as an effective technique for boosting the effectiveness of the operation of this reward system (by increasing the sensitivity of one's dopamine receptors) among individuals who have a genetic basis for less sensitive dopamine receptors, but there is now no doubt about humor's ability to generate pleasure and positive affect via this system. It may be, then, that the impact of humor upon this system helps account for its resilience-boosting power.

Other investigators have also begun to speculate about the neural circuitry involved in the experience of happiness.[280] Mirth, laughter and humor are viewed as playing an important role within this new model of happiness, based on their activation of the pleasure centers in the brain just mentioned. This model suggests that we can boost our happiness level by using humor to generate positive emotion and trigger activation of this ancient pleasure-based reward system.

So there is every reason to expect humor and laughter to make a valuable contribution to happiness—both on a daily basis and in the long run. But can this increased happiness also generate increased life satisfaction? The available evidence shows that the extent to which individuals possess humor as a character strength is positively related to life satisfaction.[281] Older adults who use humor as a coping style have also been shown to experience higher levels of life satisfaction.[282] And the strength of this relationship among seniors has been found to be mediated by individuals' effectiveness in coping with life stress.[283]

Consistent with these finding, it was noted above that a systematic humor skills training program generated increased life satisfaction (which was still present two months following completion of the program). There is even some evidence that even passive exposure to humor may boost life satisfaction. Among a group of older adults, weekly exposure to humor (with no focus on developing humor skills) as part of a therapeutic recreation program in an urban senior center over a 10-week period significantly improved measured levels of life satisfaction.[284]

Finally, coping with a physical illness generally has a negative impact on life satisfaction. However, having a physical illness was shown to have less impact on life satisfaction among individuals who have humor as a character strength than among those who lacked this character strength.[285] This is consistent with the general thrust of findings throughout this chapter. It was noted in the Introduction that it is the boost in resilience associated with positive emotion that accounts for the connection between positive emotion and increased life satisfaction. Given humor's clear effectiveness in generating positive emotion, regular doses of humor can be used to help sustain resilience on an ongoing basis.

Considering the research as a whole, then, building more humor into your life deserves your serious consideration as a path that can help generate a happier and more satisfying life—even in the midst of the stress you're sure to encounter while on that path.

CHAPTER 2
HUMOR AND PHYSICAL HEALTH

"Over the years, I have encountered a surprising number of instances in which, to all appearances, patients have laughed themselves back to health, or at least have used their sense of humor as a very positive and adaptive response to their illness."

(Raymond A. Moody, M.D.)

"Laughter is the most inexpensive and most effective wonder drug. Laughter is a universal medicine." (Bertrand Russell)

MOST PEOPLE HAVE NOTICED THAT it feels good to have a real belly laugh. They sense intuitively that it must be good for you, since they feel good/better after hearty laughter. The familiar phrase, "Laughter is the best medicine"—repeatedly emphasized by *Readers Digest* through most of the 20th century—reflects the folk wisdom that humor and laughter are healthy daily habits. And yet the prevailing attitude toward humor was a negative one until the late 19th century.[1] Until that point, laughter was commonly considered detrimental to both physical and spiritual well-being—not to mention impolite and sinful. A notable exception to this prevailing view was Henri de Mondeville, a 13th century surgeon, who argued that laughter facilitates recovery from surgery, while negative emotions slow recovery. Also, Immanuel Kant, in his *Critique of Reason*, suggested that laughter improves health by restoring equilibrium to the body.

Until the early 1980s, there was no solid research that could be used to convince the alien mentioned at the beginning of Chapter 1 (or you, if you've long been one of the skeptics) that humor and laughter are important for good health. After a slow beginning at that point, we are now witnessing an explosion of research interest in the benefits of humor and laughter. The bulk of this research has provided a rapidly-growing amount of evidence for the view that laughter really is good medicine. Since this research is discussed in more detail than you may be expecting, use this general summary to help guide you through the details provided below.

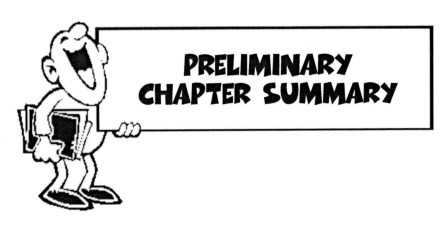

PRELIMINARY CHAPTER SUMMARY

The emergence of the new field of medical research called psychoneuroimmunology in the 1980s has stimulated an enormous amount of research (hundreds of studies) over the past quarter century on the impact of your mind on the body's basic health and healing systems. This work has focused on the influence of thoughts, attitudes, beliefs and (especially) emotions on health and well being. While we have long known that chronic negative emotion has a negative impact on health, there is now strong evidence that positive emotion supports good health. The suddenly popular research on humor's contribution to good health reflects—in part—the growing interest in the much broader role of positive emotion in general in sustaining good health. Humor and laughter are simply one means (albeit an especially effective one) of generating the positive emotions of joy and exhilaration—and of sustaining a positive daily mood.

While some studies have failed to demonstrate a positive impact of humor and laughter on health, the general picture emerging from the bulk of existing research suggests that that humor and laughter promote health by 1) strengthening the immune system, 2) reducing pain, 3) lowering blood pressure (in the long run), 4) triggering muscle relaxation, 5) reducing blood levels of stress-related hormones (like cortisol), 6) supporting the healthy structure and function of blood vessels (especially important in connection with coronary heart disease and diabetes, 7) helping manage both asthma and diabetes, and 8) reducing certain kinds of allergic response.

Researchers have only recently started looking at the impact of humor on specific diseases. The work that has been done, however, suggests that humor and laughter make significant contributions to health in connection with coronary heart disease, asthma, certain allergies and even diabetes. While many cancer patients swear that they are alive today because of their sense of humor—and many oncology units of hospitals have adopted "therapeutic humor programs" (see discussion in this chapter)—researchers have not yet made much effort to determine whether humor is capable of boosting cancer survival rates. The first large study to examine this question did find—amazingly—that among a group of people diagnosed with cancer, those with a stronger sense of humor had a 70% higher survival rate over the following seven-years than those who possessed a poor sense of humor.

The available research certainly does not suggest that a regular dose of humor and laughter can overcome any disease, or that it can serve as a substitute for the care and recommendations of your physician. It does, however, mean that doing things to maintain a more positive emotional state in your day-to-day living through the use of your sense of humor helps sustain conditions in your body which get your body's basic health and healing mechanisms working *for* you—not *against* you. You cannot use your mind and emotional state to take full control over your health and well being, but you can certainly use them as an effective ally in boosting your chances of remaining healthy.

Other exciting new findings are not yet well established (they need to be replicated), but point to possible additional key contributions of humor to health. These include preliminary evidence that humor and laughter support the destruction of damaging free radicals—long known to have a detrimental effect on many different aspects of health. And a very recent dramatic finding has shown that humor and laughter are even capable of directly influencing the level of expression of a gene that is crucial in the regulation of a key enzyme (rennin) known to be crucial in managing diabetes. This suggests that humor could become a valuable resource in helping diabetics learn to manage their disease, aiding in the prevention of some of the common damaging effects resulting from failure to keep blood sugar levels under control.

The Popular and Academic Humor and Health Movements Origins and Influences

You've probably noticed (if you're over 30) that an increasing amount of attention has been given over the past 15 years in magazine and newspaper articles (as well as on television and radio) to the idea that humor is good for you—physically, mentally and emotionally. Some people make outlandish claims about humor's power to cure what ails you, while others just say that they know they feel better when they have a good belly laugh or find a light side of their tough days—so it must somehow be good for you. I've even heard physicians say things about the health benefits of humor that have no foundation in research.

All of this media attention is a reflection of what has come to be referred to as the "humor and health movement." The movement has grown steadily over the past 25 years and is now very evident in hospitals, certain corporations, senior residential communities and the daily lives of people across the country. After 15 years or so of endless popular claims about humor and health, scientists have finally decided that it is time to see if there is a valid foundation for the claims being made. Before we look at this evidence of humor's power to support a healthy body (Chapter 1 showed its importance for resilience and mental/emotional health), we'll first look at the major events that stimulated both the popular humor and health movement and the research designed to determine whether the movement has a firm scientific foundation or is just another fun fad.

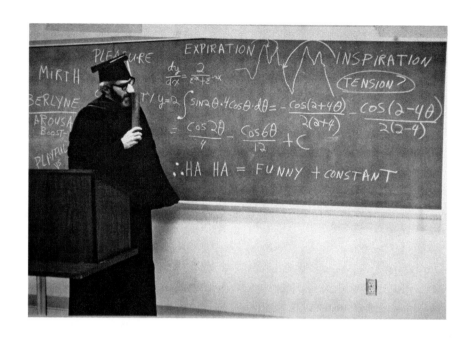

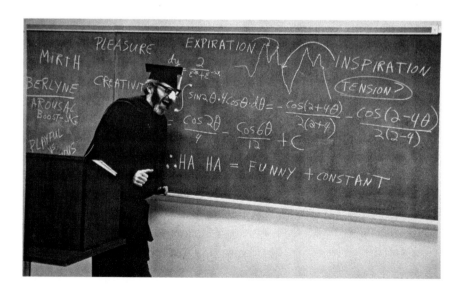

Early Academic Resistance to Humor Research

When I finished graduate school (with a PhD in psychology) and made a commitment in the early 1970s to use the same scientific rigor in studying humor that one would use in studying cancer (or any other serious topic), it was difficult to get other researchers to take the topic seriously. It was OK to study humor in a university setting, but to get tenure, you also had to do something "important." Humor was seen by academia as a frivolous and superficial topic, so that even if you did get a good study completed and published, very few other researchers paid much attention to it.

A good demonstration of the scientific community's reaction to the idea of conducting research on humor can be found in my first (and only) experience with the prestigious American Association for the Advancement of Science in 1971. The AAAS had decided to devote one day-long symposium to humor, with the morning session taking a serious look at research on humor while the afternoon session invited scientists of all persuasions (chemists, biologists, psychologists, etc.) to poke fun at themselves and the work they do. The afternoon session was basically a spoof session. I was a new PhD and one of three "serious" presenters. To my amazement, few among the 200+ scientists in the morning session wanted to hear about scientific investigations of humor. They just wanted to laugh and have fun. There was little interest in discussing the nature of humor or its importance in our everyday lives. While I no longer remember the funny stories shared that day, these scientists wanted to hear something like the following story told to me by a nurse.

One evening a family brings their frail, elderly mother to a nursing home, hoping she will be well cared for. The next morning, the nurses bathe her, feed her a tasty breakfast and set her in a chair at a window overlooking a lovely flower garden. She seems OK, but after a while she slowly starts to lean over sideways in her chair. Two attentive nurses immediately rush up to catch her and straighten her up. Again she seems OK, but after a while she starts

to tilt to the other side. The nurses rush back and once more bring her back upright. This goes on all morning. Later the family arrives to see how mom is adjusting to her new home. "So Ma, how is it here? Are they treating you OK?" they ask.

"It's pretty nice," she replies. "Except they won't let me pass gas."

Newspaper reporters in the 1970s also fell into this camp. I used to have a collection of AP and UPI articles which had been written following a meeting of the American Psychological Association (the academic conference I regularly attended). These reporters generally looked for a presentation they thought would be of interest to the average reader, and they often chose a humor symposium because they knew readers found the topic interesting. Among other things they would write about in their article, they often emphasized the idea that "These are hard times; we've got the threat of nuclear war, pollution, cancer, etc. . . . and now they're trying to take that away from us." The essence of the idea expressed was that if a bunch of scientists start studying humor, this will somehow rob us of our sense of humor. Like the prevailing attitude toward research on sex and love in an earlier era, they felt that the great mystery of humor and laughter is best left alone. Some painted a picture of a friendly round of sharing of jokes and funny anecdotes being replaced with deadly serious people sitting around analyzing why this or that is funny—a set-up for boring anyone.

I talked to a lot of non-academic people in the 1970s, however, about what they thought about the importance of humor in our everyday lives and they generally had a quite different view. They loved to share funny stories, but they were very interested in the idea that humor might be important for your general health and well being. Many said they'd have a hard time getting through a lot of their days if it weren't for their sense of humor. Their own experience told them that humor had to somehow be good for you.

The other reaction of news reporters to scholars and scientists studying humor in that decade was to simply poke fun at them. The idea of a bunch of researchers studying humor was considered funny in its own right. Often, it was the titles of scientific presentations that led to great guffaws by reporters and the reading public alike. I'll never forget being lampooned myself on the front page of one section of the *Manchester Guardian* (in England) following my presentation at the first-ever international academic conference on humor and laughter in Cardiff, Wales in 1976. The title of my talk was "Phylogenetic and ontogenetic considerations for a theory of the origins of humor" (OK, I know . . . I deserved the ribbing).

> **A nurse was leaving the hospital one day when she found the doctor standing by the shredder with a piece of paper in his hand. "Listen", said the doctor, "this is important and my assistant has left. Can you make this thing work?"**
>
> **"Certainly", said the nurse, flattered that the doctor had asked her for help. She turned the machine on, inserted the paper and pressed the start button.**
>
> **"Excellent! Excellent!" said the doctor as his paper disappeared inside the machine. "I need two copies of that."**

Over the past 20 years, the number of published research articles relating to humor and health has progressively increased. What was once a slow back burner of research interest is now an exciting area for new PhDs. And this research has become truly international in recent years. Studies of humor and health are now being done in Europe, as well as the USA, and the biggest surge of new areas of research (on specific disease conditions) is occurring in Japan.

In the United States, the growing emphasis in recent years on preventive medicine and doing things to sustain one's own health and wellness has served to simulate new research interest in humor. In the 1990s, the National Institutes of Health, in Washington D. C., even created a new department of research funding designed to sort out which "alternative" or "complementary" health-related therapies do and do not work. Studies of humor have ridden the coattails of this much broader interest in new ways of promoting health. However, researchers who have eagerly participated in the recent explosion of interest in Positive

Psychology (and positive emotion generally) have, surprisingly, not yet extended their interest to humor as a source of positive emotion. This is very reminiscent of the disinterest among psychologists generally in the field of humor research over most of the past 30 years.

The Impact of Normal Cousins: The Sputnik of Mind-Body Research

The frequent negative media reactions to the idea of doing research on humor abruptly changed after 1979. I never saw another newspaper article poking fun at researchers studying humor or laughter after 1979. Even researchers in universities began to become more open to the importance of studying humor. Agencies that granted money for research even got into the act and began to fund a few studies on humor. People also began talking about health benefits offered by humor.

I attribute this sudden shift in the popular culture's attitude to the importance of humor to the publication of a single book in 1979 by Norman Cousins; that book was *Anatomy of an Illness*. Cousins, the former editor of *Saturday Review* magazine, was in constant pain as a result of a degenerative spinal condition called ankylosing spondylitis. He could not turn over in bed without pain. A friend of Alan Funt, of *Candid Camera* fame, he invited friends over and watched a lot of *Candid Camera* videos and other comedy programs. He laughed a lot while watching these programs and discovered that he had less pain (and increased mobility) after the laughter. He reported in his last book, *Head First: The Biology of Hope*, that 10 minutes of laughter (someone kept track of the actual amount of time spent laughing) would give him two hours of pain relief. While Cousins' experience was just an anecdote, and certainly didn't prove that laughter reduces pain, his story convinced many that laughter somehow has a natural analgesic effect. As you will see later in this chapter, subsequent research his shown that they were right.

Cousins' book was translated into many languages and was read around the world by untold millions of people. This one book had an amazing impact on our collective view of the healing power of humor. For many years, it seemed that everyone had heard about Cousins' idea that you can laugh your pain away. The idea turned up in conversations over coffee, among spouses, at the workplace, etc. The media nurtured this awareness by reporting regularly on Cousins' talks around the country in which he would emphasize the importance of humor, and positive emotion generally, in sustaining good health. It was a very small step from accepting the idea that humor and laughter can reduce pain to a willingness to consider that they may contribute to health and wellness in other ways, as well.

Norman Cousins' sense of humor is evident in an incident that occurred while he was still in the hospital. A specimen bottle had been left on his breakfast tray for Cousins to provide a urine sample. On the same tray was a small bottle of apple juice. Cousins put some of the apple juice in the specimen bottle. When the nurse came to pick it up, she looked at it and said, "Hmm, it looks a little cloudy this morning Mr. Cousins." Cousins picked it up, examined it, and said: "You're right; we'd better run it through again." He then promptly drank it!

Since this story is widely shared, other patients have been known to try the same trick. If you try it, be sure to keep track of which specimen bottle is yours!

Emergence of Psychoneuroimmunology

Another major development which opened the minds of both researchers and the general public to the idea that humor and laughter might support health and healing was the emergence of the new medical field called psychoneuroimmunology—referred to as PNI. This impossibly long term refers to the combination of your mind (psycho) nervous system (neuro) and immune system (immunology). While we have long known that the mind is a product of the (central) nervous system—i.e., the brain—we had always assumed that there was no direct connection between the brain and the immune system. Even neurologists and physiologists were confident that there was no way these two parts of your body could talk to each other.

In the late 1970s and early 1980s, it became evident that this was not the case. A large body of evidence emerged making it clear that thoughts, beliefs, attitudes and (especially) emotions can play an important role in either boosting or suppressing the immune system. There is now an enormous amount of research supporting this idea. Most of it has nothing to do with humor, but it does clearly demonstrate the impact of both positive and negative emotion on health. PNI research further opened the door to acceptance of the notion that humor—as one potent source of positive emotion—might be especially supportive of health and wellness.

Rethinking the Placebo Effect: Early Clues Regarding the Impact of Mind and Emotion on Health. Drug researchers had strong evidence of the mind's influence on the body for decades without realizing it. This evidence had long been a source of annoyance in studies designed to demonstrate the effectiveness of drugs. Even people with no scientific training are now aware of the so-called "placebo effect." This is the idea that a biologically neutral substance or "sugar pill" can have a dramatic effect on physiological processes simply because it was expected to have the effect. The term comes from the Latin term for "I shall please." The key to placebo effects is a patient's or research subject's knowledge or expectation of what a drug or treatment is supposed to do.

Drugs that go through rigorous clinical trials have to demonstrate a significant effect over and above this placebo effect in order to be proven effective. Amazingly, research over the last half century has—on average—demonstrated that about 1/3 of the subjects tested with a placebo treatment show the same kind of effect as subjects getting the real drug. How is this possible? How can a belief in a certain outcome—i.e., a genuine expectation that something is going to happen in your body—trigger real physical change? For example, how can treatment with a neutral substance cause your hair to fall out in a study of a new cancer drug? (Virtually all cancer patients know that hair loss is one of the side effects of chemotherapy.)

There are many well known examples of the power of the placebo effect. One of the most dramatic was the classic case of the 1950s drug Krebiozen. One patient's experience with this drug has long been part of medical folklore.

The Krebiozen Miracle

"The patient had an advanced case of cancer of the lymph nodes. His abdomen, groin and neck were riddled with tumors—some the size of an orange, and he was bed-ridden and gasped for air. His doctors had given him about two weeks to live. But the man had heard about a promising new 'miracle cancer drug' called Krebiozen and insisted that he be admitted to clinical trials. (Luckily, the clinic where his doctor worked was involved in the testing of the drug.) His doctor finally consented to giving him the drug, giving him the first injection on a Friday (subsequent doses would be administered, Monday, Wednesday and Friday). To the doctor's amazement, when he saw the patient again on Monday, he was up and walking around—joking with the nurses. His tumors were only about half their size from three days earlier. Within 10 days, he seemed to his doctors to be disease free, and he was released from the hospital.

After two months of good health, newspaper reports appeared documenting that Krebiozen appeared to be of no value as a cancer treatment. Soon after these reports, the patient had to be readmitted to the hospital—the tumors were back again. The doctor—being a good researcher—decided to use the patient as his own control. He told the patient that those earlier batches of Krebiozen were actually faulty, but that the doctor would give him a new double dose of the 'new' and stronger Krebiozen. But this time, he was not given Krebiozen at all; he was given only injections of sterile water. Just as the first time, the patient's tumors disappeared in a matter of days. His doctors were stunned in disbelief. Again, he lived a symptom-free life for another two months.

This all changed when another news report appeared declaring that 'Nationwide AMA tests show Krebiozen to be worthless as a cancer treatment.' Within a few days of these reports, the man was back at the hospital, his body again riddled with tumors. Two days later, he was dead. As his doctor put it at the time, 'His faith was now gone, his last hope vanished, and he succumbed in less than two days.'"[2]

This sequence of tumor reversals has long been used to provide anecdotal support for the idea that one's belief system has a powerful effect on the body's ability to rally its own healing resources. While the case is clearly an extreme one, countless similar cases support the power of one's belief system to reduce symptoms. Among doctors who have accepted the notion that one's beliefs and emotions can have an impact on health and wellness, the most common approach to acting on this knowledge involves using positive emotions and beliefs to *get patients' own healing mechanisms working for, and not against them—thereby optimizing treatment outcomes.*

BUILD YOUR HUMOR SKILLS

[Work on both jokes before checking the answers.]

1. A young woman with severe PMS asked a friend to recommend a gynecologist. "I know a great one," said the friend, "but he's very expensive. He charges $500 for the first visit and $150 for every visit after that." So the woman decided to give him a try. Trying to save money, she greeted the doctor with a loud "I'm back!" When the doctor finished his exam, he said, "Everything looks OK. Just continue _____."

1st clue: The doctor knows what she's up to.
2nd clue: How can the doctor play just as good a joke on her?

2. A man walked into a doctor's office and the receptionist asked why he'd come. The man said "shingles." After a while the doctor asked him what he had, and the man again answered "shingles." The doctor examined him thoroughly and finally said, "I'm sorry I just can't find them." The man said, "They're _____.

Clue: He's not there as a patient; he's a delivery man.

Early Research Showing the Impact of Emotion on Health. A great deal of non–humor research conducted in the 1980s and 1990s laid a clear foundation for the notion that your sense of humor might have a tremendous impact on your health and general well being. Generally speaking, this research showed that the body's own healing system responds favorably to positive attitudes, thoughts, moods and especially to emotions (e.g., love, hope, optimism, caring, intimacy, joy, laughter and humor) and negatively to negative ones (hate, hopelessness, pessimism, indifference, anxiety, depression, loneliness, etc.).

So early PNI studies made it clear that it is important to organize your life in a way that maintains as positive a focus as possible. (Recall the Chapter 1 conclusion that positive emotion plays the key role in generating personal resilience.) This does not mean you should avoid negative emotion; anger, anxiety or feeling down may well be appropriate emotions in a difficult life circumstance. The key, however, is to avoid carrying these negative emotions around with you day after day. You need techniques that keep you from wallowing in resistance–lowering negativity. The longer negative states persist in your mind/body, the greater the likelihood that they will lead to some negative health outcome. Love is probably the most powerful tool we have to overcome negativity, but humor, in my view, comes a close second. The power of humor to promote wellness appears to lie in its ability to manage your daily emotional state, helping to sustain a more positive daily mood instead of a negative one (which accompanies ongoing stress).

The new hospital CEO was determined to rid the institution of all slackers and bring real fiscal discipline to the hospital. On his first tour of the facility, he notices a guy leaning on a wall near the staff lounge. The room is full of doctors, nurses and aides and he wants to let them know he means business! He walks up to the guy and asks, "And how much money do you make a week?"

A little surprised, the young fellow looks at him and replies, "$300 a week. Why?"

The CEO hands him $1,200 in cash and screams, "Here's four weeks pay, now GET OUT and don't come back!"

Feeling pretty good about his first firing, the CEO stands a little taller, looks around the room and asks, "Does anyone want to tell me what that goof-off did here?"

A nurse grins and says, "He's the pizza delivery guy."

Candace Pert noted in her book, *The Molecules of Emotion*, that emotions—registered and stored in the body in the form of chemical messages—are the best candidates for the key to the health connection between mind and body. It is through the emotions you experience in connection with your thoughts and daily attitudes—actually, through the neurochemical changes that accompany these emotions—that your mind acquires the power to influence whether you get sick or remain well.

ANSWERS TO JOKES

1. with the prescription I gave you last time. (Other similar answers will work just as well.)

2. in the truck. Where should I unload them? (Or any other answer making reference to the shingles you use on your roof.)

We learned in the 1980s that there is a hard-wire connection between the brain and the immune system. Neural connections between the brain and the lymph nodes, bone marrow, thymus and spleen develop in early childhood and diminish with old age (this partly explains why our immune system works less well in our senior years).[3] The key to the operation of these interconnected systems is found in complex molecules called neuropeptides. "A peptide is made up of amino acids, which are the building blocks of protein. There are twenty-three different amino acids. Peptides are amino acids strung together very much like pearls strung along in a necklace."[4] Peptides are found throughout the body, including the brain and immune system. The brain contains many different neuropeptides, including endorphins. These neuropeptides are the means by which all cells in the body communicate with each other. This includes brain-to-brain messages, brain-to-body messages, body-to-body messages and body-to-brain messages.

So individual cells, including brain cells, immune cells, and other body cells, have receptor sites that receive neuropeptides. The kinds of neuropeptides available to cells are constantly changing, reflecting changes in your emotions throughout the day. The exact combinations of neuropeptides released during different emotional states have not yet been determined.

The kind and number of emotion-linked neuropeptides available at receptor sites of cells influence your probability of staying well or getting sick. "Viruses use these same receptors to enter into a cell, and depending on how much of the . . . natural peptide for that receptor is around, the virus will have an easier or harder time getting into the cell. *So our emotional state will affect whether we'll get sick from the same loading dose of a virus.*"[5] (Italics are McGhee's.) As this book shows, building more humor and laughter in your life helps assure that these chemical messages are working for you, not against you.

"The chemicals that are running our body and our brain are the same chemicals that are involved in emotion. And that says to me that . . . we'd better pay more attention to emotions with respect to health." (Candace Pert)

1) Negative Emotion

Early PNI research showed that negative emotion has a strong impact on both survival rates and severity of symptoms. Among older people, for example, the death rate for both men and women increases sharply following the death of their spouse.[6] The greater the level of depression experienced, the greater the impact on the surviving spouse's health.

All of us have down days where we feel blue or depressed. But this does not become a risk factor until it begins to persist. Among adults given a test for depression, those who died from cancer 17 years later were twice as likely to have had high depression scores (when the study started) than those who developed no cancer at all.[7] Among patients with AIDS Related Complex in the 1980s, those who had weaker beliefs that they could do things to influence the course of the disease were less successful in fighting off AIDS.[8] These studies suggest that, at least in some circumstances, persistent negative emotion can put you at greater risk of death.

Among patients with heart disease, those with a pessimistic outlook about their ability to recover enough to eventually resume their daily routine were more than twice as likely as optimists to have died one year later, even when severity of condition was taken into account.[9] In a group of patients recovering from heart attacks, those who scored high on tests of sadness and depression were eight times as likely as more optimistic patients to die within the next 18 months.[10] Risk of death was tripled both among those who tended to hold in their anger and those judged to be very anxious.

"We're all in this together—by ourselves."   (Lily Tomlin)

It is not surprising that the grief you feel after the death of a loved one can damage your health. But even the commonplace bad moods and negative attitudes that we all suffer can set you up for increased symptoms of illness—if they occur day after day, month after month. This is difficult to document in research, but the herpes simplex virus (responsible for small ulcers, fever blisters and cold sores around the mouth) provides a good way to demonstrate it. This virus, carried by about 1/3 of the U.S. population, normally remains latent, but persistent negative emotions often trigger an outbreak.[11] Pessimistic students, who can be expected to generally have more frequent negative moods than optimistic students, have been shown to develop more symptoms than optimistic students around exam time.[12]

157

PAUL McGHEE, PhD

In 1991, an article in the *New England Journal of Medicine* finally established that stress makes you more vulnerable to the common cold. Your daily mood and coping skills also influence susceptibility to colds and the flu.[13] In fact, people with low morale, and who cope less well with stress, are three times more likely to catch the flu during a flu epidemic.[14] Among more severe illnesses, increased stress among heart disease patients has been shown to increase the level of angina pectoris experienced.[15]

Multiple Sclerosis is a good example of a disease known to incur exacerbations (worsening symptoms) in the presence of negative emotional states. Anything MS patients can do to sustain a positive frame of mind helps keep these exacerbations from occurring. One man who had difficulty controlling his shaking hand demonstrated his ability to stay positive when he told me, "MS also has its good points; I never have to worry about stirring my coffee anymore."

2) Positive Emotion

Numerous studies have examined the link between longevity and the tendency to show positive affect or emotion on a daily basis (psychologists call this "trait positive affect"). The best studies along these lines measure one's level of positive affect at one point in time and then follow up with these same individuals years later to see who is living and who is not. This is called a "prospective" study. Such studies are generally done with older (over 60—and often including subjects into their 90s) populations, so that the follow-up data can be collected in a shorter time frame. Some studies only use people documented to be in good health, while others statistically control for health status at the start of the study.

"This I believe to be the chemical function of humor: to change the character of our thought." (Lin Yutang)

The great majority of these studies found that a greater amount of positive affect at the first measurement time among people aged 60+ (all living in the community, not in institutional settings) was associated with greater longevity.[16] Other studies have shown this same longevity advantage associated with positive emotion for other groups of people.[17]

THINGS YOU DON'T WANT TO HEAR DURING SURGERY

Ya' know . . . there's big money in kidneys . . . and this guy's got two of 'em.

Oops! Hey, has anyone ever survived 500 ml. of this stuff?

This patient has already had some kids, am I correct?

Bo! Bo! Come back with that! Bad Dog!

Better save that. We'll need it for the autopsy.

Wait a minute, if this is his spleen, then what's that?

Hand me that . . . uh . . . that uh . . . thingie.

Everybody stand back! I lost my contact lens!

What's this doing here?

That's cool! Now can you make his leg twitch?!

Sterile, shcmerile. The floor's clean, right?

What do you mean he wasn't in for a sex change?

Don't worry. I think it's sharp enough.

FIRE! FIRE! Everyone get out!

Isn't this the guy with the really lousy insurance?

A few prospective studies have looked at the impact of positive affect among individuals who are already sick. In this kind of study, the key is getting good information on the severity of the illness at the start of the study so that this can be controlled for statistically. These studies show that positive affect does not extend one's survival for individuals who have diseases generally accompanied by short periods of survival or who are in the "end stages" of their disease. *Any underlying physiological processes occurring in response to positive emotion, then, are clearly not strong enough to overcome severe disease conditions.*[18]

The picture is quite different, however, for individuals with diseases (or disease stages) accompanied by a greater period of expected survival—including cancer and AIDS. In this case, greater positive affect is associated with longer survival.[19] Among HIV+ men, those showing greater amounts of positive affect survived longer—even when various factors associated with disease progression were controlled for.[20] It seems clear, then, that there is something about a habitual positive emotional state that promotes a longer (and healthier) life.

> *"Our doctor would never really operate unless it was necessary. He was just that way. If he didn't need the money, he wouldn't lay a hand on you."* (Herb Schriner, 1950s comedian)

Among patients with metastatic (spreading) cancers, those who expressed greater hope at the time of their diagnosis survived longer.[21] When over 400 reports of spontaneous remission of cancer were reviewed and analyzed, the patients themselves attributed their cure to a broad range of causes, but only one factor was common to all cases—a shift toward greater hope and a more positive attitude.[22]

Striking evidence of the impact of optimism was obtained when it was showed that among a group of individuals 65 and older, those who were optimistic about their health—in spite of lab tests that showed them to be in poor health—had lower death rates over the next six years than those who were pessimistic about their health—in spite of health records which documented that they were in good health.[23] Optimism, in this case, became a self-fulfilling prophecy, leading individuals in relatively poor health to fare better than their healthier, but pessimistic, peers.

BUILD YOUR HUMOR SKILLS

[Work on both before checking the answers.]

1. The proctologists considered the financial condition of the hospital and refused to go along with the decision, saying "We are currently in _____."
Clue: They are behind in their payments for medical equipment.

2. The osteopathic doctors did not like the decision; felt they were being _____.
Clue: Osteopaths sometimes do the same thing chiropractors are known for.

"If I'd known I was going to live this long, I'd have taken better care of myself."

In terms of symptoms, positive emotion has been found to contribute to protecting you against the common cold. When cold viruses were directly introduced to individuals' noses (followed by three days of being quarantined), those who had a more positive "emotional style" (i.e., tended to experience more daily positive emotions) subsequently developed fewer colds than those who had a more negative emotional style.[24]

With respect to health in general, one team of researchers reviewed all the existing research along these lines in 2005 and concluded that

". . . the studies virtually unanimously support an association between higher PA [positive affect] and health. The more critical (in regard to the hypothesis that PA is the causal factor) prospective morbidity [the state of being diseased] studies found benefits of trait PA in conditions as diverse as stroke, rehospitalization for coronary problems, the common cold, and accidents. . . . the near unanimity of results supporting a beneficial association of PA and morbidity is impressive."[25]

Attitudinal and emotional factors have even been linked to wound healing. For example, more optimistic patients showed the most rapid healing following an operation for a detached retina.[26] Consistent with this finding, one investigator concluded, following a thorough review of research in psychoneuroimmunology, that positive emotions do facilitate the healing of wounds.[27] He felt that they did this by disrupting the production of neurotransmitters, hormones, and other substances which interfere with certain steps of the healing process.

> **A patient walks into a doctor's office with a cucumber crammed into one ear, a bouquet of parsley jammed into his mouth and two large carrots hanging from his nostrils. He manages to mumble, "Doc, you gotta help me. I feel awful. What's wrong with me?"**
>
> **The doctor replied, "You're not eating properly."**

Evidence is also emerging to show that hope—like optimism—contributes to symptom improvement. For example, among spinal injury patients with comparable injuries, those who expressed greater hope for improvement became more mobile and coped better emotionally than those who saw their situation as hopeless.[28]

The Role of Feeling a Sense of Control. We have known for decades that a major obstacle to sustaining a positive outlook in the midst of a serious disease (or any other major stressor) is a feeling of helplessness—the sense that you just have no control in the matter. If you know of a way to handle a problem, you generally do it and the stress disappears (or is, at least, reduced). The damaging effect on health occurs when the stressful event seems out of your control to deal with—and when this feeling persists over time.

ANSWERS TO JOKES

1. arrears   2. manipulated

While this link is now well established with people, it was first demonstrated in rats decades ago. Pairs of rats were put in individual cages in which a mild electric shock could be administered. One animal could avoid the shocks by turning a wheel in its cage. The other also had a wheel, but turning it had no influence on whether a shock was received. The apparatus was set up so that whenever one rat received a shock, the other also received it. So there was no difference in the number of shocks received, but only one rat could take control over whether a shock did or did not occur. The importance of control was evident in the fact that the "helpless" rats developed significantly more ulcers than the rats that had control of the occurrence of the shocks.[29] A great deal of evidence similarly points to negative health effects of perceived helplessness among people.

> *"If you think you have caught a cold, call a doctor . . . Call in three doctors and play bridge."*   (Robert Benchley)

We all know people who seem to take no active steps to manage a problem when it seems like the easiest thing in the world to do. They strike us as pitiful people who wallow in their depression or upset for days instead of just doing what needs to be done. This phenomenon is generally referred to as "learned helplessness." Marty Seligman used dogs to demonstrate how this works. Two groups of dogs were placed in a harness and raised in the air so that their feet did not touch the ground. Both groups were given a mild electric shock following a warning tone, but only one group could avoid the shocks (by pressing a plate with their nose).

After a period of this kind of training, they were then placed in a box where a shock (again preceded by a tone) could be applied to their feet. Both groups could avoid the shock by simply jumping over a small barrier out of the box. Animals with no prior shock experience, as well as the animals who had already learned to avoid a shock by pressing the plate with their nose, quickly jumped out of the box—the obvious thing to do. The dogs that had no control over the shock in their previous experience in a completely different situation just cowered in the box and endured the mild shock.[30] Their prior experience had taught them to become helpless even though it was the very easy to avoid the shock. They had learned to be helpless. Seligman has emphasized that people who have extensive prior experience with having to endure stressful life experiences often develop a generalized learned helplessness—a habit of not even making the effort to cope, even when they have the opportunity to do so.

When you have access to your sense of humor in a stressful situation, it reduces your sense of helplessness in two ways. First, it gives you some degree of control over your emotional state in the situation. Both this chapter and Chapter 1 document humor's power to pull you out of a negative mood, substituting a positive one in its place. Second, once in this more positive emotional state, it is easier to plan effective strategies for dealing with the cause of the stress of the moment. As Chapter 1 also shows, however, you can use humor to simply hide from your problems if you're not committed to dealing with them. This just temporarily eases your stress by blocking it from your mind. The choice of actively coping with it is up to you. Humor at least gives you the choice.

Dr Bernie Siegel's "Exceptional Cancer Patients"

In the 1980s and 1990s, Dr. Bernie Siegel wrote a series of very popular books (including *Love Medicine and Miracles* and *Peace, Love and Healing*) related to the mind's role in maintaining good health. Especially noteworthy was his Exceptional Cancer Patient Program (ECAP). He documented many examples of cancer patients who beat the survival odds given them by their doctors. He noted a pattern in the characteristics these unlikely survivors had in common. They were upbeat, optimistic and determined—one way or another—to overcome their cancer. They were not going to let it be a death sentence. They also tended to be "difficult" patients—patients who insisted on having all the information they could get from their doctors, even when their persistence became annoying to the doctors. They were clearly not passive individuals who just got depressed and waited for the cancer to take them. They were determined to somehow take control. Some patients had a specific future event they wanted to stay alive for. For example, one woman just wanted to live to see her daughter graduate from college. After far outliving the life sentence given by her doctors, she died within days following the graduation.

Millions of people read Dr. Siegel's books, and many more attended his frequent lectures on mind-body issues given all over North America for 25 years. His popularity made a major contribution to general public awareness of the importance of using your own emotions, attitudes and beliefs to support good health.

Steadily Mounting Job Stress

At some point in the 1980s, concerns about rising stress levels on the job began showing up more and more often. Phrases like "doing more with less", "downsizing" and "rightsizing" became part of our everyday vocabulary. The dreaded metaphor "raising the bar," initiated in the 1990s and commonly heard ever since, meant that employees were asked to do just a bit more each year than in the previous year. This approach worked fine for a while, but as the trend continued through the 1990s and into the new century, stress levels began 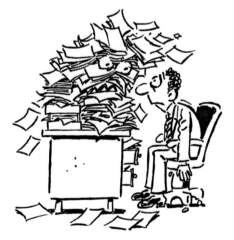 to get so high that they interfered with job performance. Even people who were lucky enough to still have jobs they loved soon began to burn out and hate their work. The predictable result of all this is that job performance began to suffer.

A man comes into the ER and yells, "My wife's having her baby in the cab!" The ER physician grabs his stuff, rushes out to the cab, lifts the lady's dress, and begins to take off her underwear. Suddenly he notices that there are several cabs, and he's in the wrong one.

While most employers continue this trend of expecting more from their employees each year, a growing number over the past decade have come to realize that they have a responsibility to provide employees with tools that help manage the increased job stress that goes with raising the bar. One common approach (among those that are pertinent to this book) to achieving this goal has been to find innovative ways to make work "fun." While the primary goal here is to boost job performance by providing an effective tool for managing work-related stress, this approach has—in the process—elevated both employers' and employees' awareness of humor's contribution to health and well-being.

The Emergence of "Laughter Clubs"

In the 1990s, Dr. Madan Kataria, a physician in Bombay (now Mumbai), India began searching for some means to help the average (generally poor) Indian cope with the daily stress that goes with trying to eek out a living with limited resources in an exceedingly overpopulated city and country. He decided to use humor. At the beginning (March, 1995), small groups of men and women got together to share funny jokes at the start of their day. He soon discovered, however, that it was hard to keep coming up with new jokes every day; also the women were often offended by the jokes that were told (mainly) by the men.

Kataria's solution to this problem was to forget the humor and focus entirely on laughter. He devised a series of laughter exercises (some of which are quite funny looking) and groups of people used the exercises to "laugh for no reason." Each laughter exercise typically lasted 30-45 seconds. This caught on quickly in India, so that thousands of people were soon getting together in small groups (generally at the start of their day) to spend 15 minutes or so just laughing together. I have seen photographs of more than 10,000 people at a race track in Mumbai going through these laughter exercises together. I participated in them with Dr. Kataria a decade ago, and I could see that even though we started laughing in the absence of anything funny, things got very funny pretty quickly as I saw the exaggerated and distorted laughing faces around me. (My favorite was the lion laugh, in which you stick your tongue out as far as you can while laughing hard.)

The quick acceptance in India of this approach to laughter for "good health" and stress reduction, and starting one's day on a positive note, was probably due to longstanding yoga traditions in India that include a form of laughter as a breathing exercise. And yet, even countries that lack this yoga tradition have taken a strong interest in getting together in small groups to start their day with laughter (comparable to the earlier Chinese approach of starting the day with tai chi in public parks—which 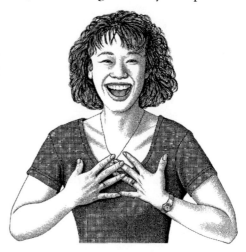 we first began to witness following Richard Nixon's breakthrough visit to China in the early 1970s). Hundreds of laughter groups now get together in the United States, Canada and Europe in their workplaces, parks, senior communities and other settings to share laughter "for no reason." The success of these laughter groups is partly due to the growing conviction that laughter is good for you— even if there is no humor involved. Some support has already been obtained for this idea. It was noted in Chapter 1 that even forced, non-humorous laughter generates a more positive mood.

The First Wave
General Health-Promoting Effects
of Humor and Laughter

There have been two distinct waves of research linking humor and laughter to good health. The first wave began in the early 1980s and focused mainly on pain reduction (in response to Norman Cousins' well-known claim of reduced pain in response to humor), strengthening of the immune system and the reduction of stress. In more recent years, this first wave has been extended to muscle relaxation and the lowering of both stress hormones and blood pressure. What the different parts of this first wave have in common is a concern with general health-promoting systems—not specific disease conditions.

> *"I was caesarian born. You can't really tell, although whenever I leave a house, I go out through a window."* (Steven Wright)

It was only after humor's power to boost these general health-promoting mechanisms was demonstrated that the second wave of research began. This second wave has focused on specific disease conditions and remains in its infancy.

Pain Reduction

I lived in Paris for three years in the 1980s. During two of those years, I spent a lot of time in a little neighborhood cafe, and almosts every time I stopped by for my daily expresso, there was an old man at his usual corner table laughing with friends. He rarely went more than 10 minutes without laughing. I was amazed at this and asked him how he managed to stay in such a wonderful mood all the time. To my surprise, he said his laughter didn't always mean he was in a good mood. He laughed for two reasons. One was in order to get into a good mood. He lived alone and didn't like it. He knew that laughter would lift his spirits, so he forced himself to laugh until he really was feeling good.

The other reason was that he had arthritis and had a lot of aches and pains. One day (several years prior to my conversation with him) he and his friends were doubling up with laughter about pranks they had played when they were kids. He noticed that his arthritis pain had disappeared during the laughter and didn't show up again until an hour or so later. From that day on, he was a laugher. It was his way of managing pain. He took control of his pain in a way that also improved his mood and the quality of his life. About 40 studies completed since the early 1980s have supported the effectiveness of his approach to pain management. This pain-reduction effect of humor and laughter is now a well-established effect. Only a sample of this research is discussed here in order to give you a good sense of the breadth of the supporting data.

Doctor to patient: "You have nothing to worry about. You'll live to be 80.
Patient: "I am 80!"
Doctor: "See, what did I tell you?"

Back pain, along with other areas of musculoskeletal pain, has become very common among adults—both in the USA and other countries.[31] It has become clear that psychological factors make an important contribution to the experience of this kind of pain.[32] In work environments, the extent to which it is experienced is increased by negative emotional states and reduced by positive ones.[33]

Pain, of course, is a totally subjective experience. You can only measure it by asking people how much pain they feel. But the level of pain experienced—both among individuals suffering from chronic pain and when it is experimentally induced in some way—is easily influenced by your emotional state of the moment. An enormous body of research covering a broad range of medical conditions shows that pain is worsened by negative emotion.[34] This is a long-established finding. But it is only in the past couple of decades that investigators have studied the impact of positive emotion on pain.

As noted above, Norman Cousins drew the attention of the medical community to humor's power to reduce pain in his book *Anatomy of an Illness.* His spinal disease left him in almost constant pain. But he quickly discovered while watching comedy films that belly laughter eased his pain. Dr. James Walsh, an American physician, had noted a half century earlier in his 1928 book *Laughter and Health,* that laughter often reduced the pain experienced following surgery and appeared to promote wound healing, but the medical field seems to have been unaware of Walsh's observation until Cousins sparked new interest in humor and pain reduction.

Cousins' "apple juice/urine" prank (noted earlier in this chapter) is well known. On another occasion, Cousins was about to take a bath in a tub filled with an oily substance designed to ease some of his joint problems. He described it as "a cross between stale oatmeal and used crankcase oil." When the nurse left for a moment, leaving the bottle containing the oily stuff near the tub, Cousins poured most of it down the drain. When the nurse returned, he held up the bottle and said, "I'm terribly sorry, but I can't get the rest of this down."

Humor and Experimentally-Induced Pain. Most experimental studies of humor and pain have adopted either of two approaches to inducing pain. In one, subjects are asked to leave their hands in ice water (at one degree centigrade) for as long as possible before it becomes too uncomfortable/painful, and then remove it. A baseline is established before having subjects watch either a comedy or some other kind of video. The ice water procedure is then repeated. The other approach involves the use of a standard blood pressure cuff on the arm. Pressure is steadily increased until the subject asks to have it stopped—because it becomes too uncomfortable/painful. The question tested is whether humor and laughter increase an individual's pain threshold (i.e., the length of time the hand is in water or the level of pressure reached with the blood pressure cuff).

Research using these approaches has demonstrated humor's power to both increase the time individuals are able to leave their hand in the ice water[35] and withstand higher levels of pressure on the arm using the blood pressure cuff.[36] Similar findings have been obtained with children using the ice water approach.[37] Although there is widespread support for these findings, it is still not clear whether humor just raises the threshold at which pain begins to be experienced or increases the capacity to withstand pain.

We also don't know just how long this pain reduction effect of humor and laughter lasts, but you will recall Norman Cousins' observation that 10 minutes of actual belly laughter would give him two hours of pain relief. The limited available experimental evidence suggests that the effect lasts at least as long as 20 minutes.[38] And it may last longer.

Given the compelling evidence that humor does increase pain thresholds (or reduce pain), it makes sense that those who get the greatest enjoyment from the humor presented would show the greatest pain reduction effect. We have little evidence one way or the other about this, but it was recently found that pain reduction was greatest among individuals whose faces reflected greater degrees of enjoyment.[39] Surprisingly, increased laughter was not associated with greater pain reduction. So this supports the idea that it is the mental enjoyment of humor (perhaps due to humor's distraction power) that is the key, not the laughter itself. This issue is discussed below.

BUILD YOUR HUMOR SKILLS

[Work on both before checking the answers.]

1. Gastroenterologists just have a _____ feeling about which is the right decision.
Clue: Anotherr word for intestines.

2. Microsurgeons have no trouble agreeing because they're always thinking along the same _____.
Clue: A blood vessel.

Although it was noted above that there is a great deal of evidence documenting the worsening effect of negative emotion on pain, there is also—amazingly—evidence that the specific negative emotions associated with both repulsion and tragedy (as experienced from watching a video) have an effect similar to that of humor. That is, they both increase the threshold for experiencing experimentally-induced pain.[40] It is not clear how to make sense out of this, although researchers have concluded from these findings that anything that is physically and emotionally arousing may raise pain thresholds (making the experience of pain less likely).[41] This is consistent with the frequent observation that individuals suffering terrible injuries in accidents often fail to notice pain if they are mainly concerned about doing something to insure the safety of a young child or other loved one also involved in the accident.

The apparent discrepancy between the conclusion (above) that negative emotion commonly worsens pain and these studies showing comparable pain-reduction findings for humor and repulsion or tragedy may also be explained by the fact that most of the literature documenting a worsening of pain as a result of negative emotion concerns chronic sources of pain—not acute pain generated in a laboratory setting.

> **A man returns from Africa and is feeling very ill. He goes to see his doctor and is immediately rushed to the Hospital to undergo a barrage of tests. He wakes up after the tests in a private room at the hospital and the phone by his bed rings.**
>
> **"This is your doctor. We've had the results back from your tests and we've found you have an extremely nasty virus, which is extremely contagious!"**
>
> **"Oh my gosh," cried the man, "What are you going to do, doctor?"**
>
> **"Well, we're putting you on a diet of pizzas, pancakes and pita bread."**
>
> **"Will that cure me?" asked the man.**
>
> **The doctor replied, "Well no, but . . . it's the only food we can get under the door."**

If watching a comedy video in a research laboratory reduces pain thresholds, should we expect the same result for people who have a good sense of humor (as evidenced by higher scores on a sense of humor test)? There is some evidence that individuals who score higher on sense of humor tests show reduced pain sensitivity,[42] but there are just as many studies showing the opposite.[43] The reason for this inconsistency may lie in the fact that any pain reduction (or increase in threshold for experiencing pain) that results from humor presumably occurs for only a limited period of time. We have some evidence that it lasts up to 20 minutes (and Cousins' personal observation of a two-hour reduction in pain), but we still just don't know much about this issue. The duration of pain reduction may well depend on both the intensity and length of laughter, as well as the level of enjoyment or amusement experienced. Since some people who express great amusement at funny events laugh very little, the latter factor could contribute independently to the pain reduction experienced.

ANSWERS TO JOKES

1. gut   2. vein

Humor and Chronic Pain. While negative emotion tends to worsen pain among individuals suffering from chronic pain, positive emotion is associated with pain reduction in these individuals. Of course, when people with any serious illness or injury are in a lot of pain, we don't expect them to show much positive emotion. Pain puts us all in a bad mood. But some people have an enduring trait of being more upbeat and positive than others, regardless of their circumstance at the moment. Individuals who have this kind of "trait positive affect" report less pain in coping with such conditions as cancer,[44] rheumatoid arthritis[45] and fibromyalgia.[46] This also holds for hospital inpatients suffering from a broad range of pain-inducing conditions.[47]

"Humor is the instinct for taking pain playfully." (Max Eastman)

For people who don't have an enduring positive mood as a general personality trait which can help manage their pain, humor offers an effective means of putting oneself in a good mood. Using humor to generate positive emotion has been shown to be an effective means of reducing pain in connection with a broad range of medical conditions. For example, listening to an hour of traditional Japanese comic stories (Rakugo) reduced the pain experienced by Japanese rheumatoid arthritis patients.[48] This is an important finding, since the symptoms experienced by these patients (as well as by patients with multiple sclerosis and numerous other medical conditions) generally worsen in the presence of negative emotional states.

Laughing when you're in pain helps substitute a more positive mood for the negative one you're likely to be in and lifts your spirits at the same time that it reduces the pain. This may explain why rheumatoid arthritis patients who report more chronic pain also say they look for humor more often in everyday life.[49] Like the old man in Paris who learned to laugh to ease his pain, they've learned that humor helps manage their pain.

Among patients in a rehabilitation hospital, 74% agreed with the statement, "Sometimes laughing works as well as a pain pill."[50] The patients had such conditions as traumatic brain injury, spinal cord injury, arthritis, limb amputations, and a range of other neurological or musculoskeletal disorders. When elderly residents suffering pain in a long-term care facility watched funny movies, the level of pain they experienced was reduced.[51]

A man went to his doctor complaining of painful headaches. After concluding his tests, the doctor said, "There's only one solution, but it's extreme: castration." The patient said he could never do that and he walked out.

As the weeks went on, his headaches got so bad that he couldn't take it any longer. He went back to the doctor and agreed to the castration. The operation was a success and the patient couldn't believe that his headaches were finally gone. He felt like a new man. He was so excited about his new life that he went to a tailor and bought a whole new set of clothes—suits, shirts, socks, coats . . . even underwear.

In jotting down all the appropriate information, the tailor finally asked, "What size underwear do you wear?"

"Forty," replied the man.

"Oh no," said the tailor. "You're a 44. If you wear underwear that tight, you'll get terrible headaches!"

Pain management is an important consideration for many patients following surgery. So it is worth noting that watching a funny video reduced the level of minor pain medication requested by patients following surgery.[52] Given the power of humor and laughter to reduce pain, it is not surprising that humor has been applied as a "treatment" in managing pain associated with burns and dental work[53] and as a component of general nursing care.[54]

There is also widespread anecdotal evidence that laughter can help manage pain. Norman Cousins once described in a speech how he, Dr. Carl Simonton and Jose Jimenez (a comedian from the old *Steve Allen Show* in the 1950s) went to talk to a group of patients at a VA Hospital. Jimenez had them falling off their chairs laughing. The doctors later told Cousins that 85% of the patients had been experiencing pain when they entered the room. But the laughter reduced or eliminated the pain for most of them.

Nurses often tell me they know a patient who tried Cousins' idea of laughing a lot while watching funny videos and found that it also reduced their pain. But not all who try it experience pain reduction. The reason for this inconsistency remains unclear.

"A clown is like an aspirin, only he works twice as fast."

(Groucho Marx)

If you're someone who is not very good at using your own sense of humor to help cope with pain or any other source of stress, is it possible to learn to use humor to manage pain? The answer appears to be "yes." A Swedish physician reported that six women suffering from painful muscle disorders got significant pain relief during a 13-week course on humor therapy.[55] Throughout this period, they read funny books, listened to or watched funny tapes and worked at "giving higher priority to humor in their everyday lives." They also attended lectures on humor research. Those patients who laughed the most in group sessions showed the greatest symptom reduction.

My book *Humor as Survival Training for a Stressed-Out World* (also published by Author House) provides you with a ready-made humor skills training program, so that you can—over a period of two to four months—progressively build the skills needed to use humor as an ally in managing your daily pain, regardless of whether it is physical or emotional pain.

Using Humor to Ease Painful Medical Procedures with Children. Many medical procedures cause pain. Such procedures are difficult for all of us to get through, but they can be an especially big source of distress for children. To take just one condition—cancer—as an example, many painful procedures must be endured, including inserting and removing catheters and drug delivery systems, injections, bone marrow aspirations and lumbar punctures. Children who go through these procedures experience a great deal of distress and pain; and the distress generally increases over time with the need to repeat the procedures.[56]

Given the strong evidence that humor helps manage many forms of pain, some hospitals have looked at ways of using humor to help manage this pain. The use of clowns in pediatric units of hospitals (discussed below) is—at this point—the most common approach to helping kids cope. The clowns are used to boost the children's spirits and take their minds off their pain or discomfort. Some hospitals have also explored other approaches to bringing humor to pediatric patients.[57]

An exciting study has now been underway for several years at the Mattel Children's Hospital at the University of California at Los Angeles. This ongoing project—called Rx Laughter—is studying the power of humor to help children manage painful medical procedures and to support patients' wellness in general. One of the researchers, Dr. Lonnie Zeltzer, noted that she could recall many children finding their own ways to use humor to cope with medical procedures over the years before Rx Laughter was begun.

"It is interesting that many years ago, in the early 1980s, when I was studying the impact of children using their imagination to control severe medical procedure pain, many children would spontaneously imagine themselves watching a TV program, and almost invariably these imaginary programs were funny. Many of these children would be smiling or even giggling during the procedure, and when asked they would describe the funny things they were seeing on their imaginary program. *Children who did this had significantly less pain and discomfort during the medical procedure.*"[58] (Italics are McGhee's.)

Consistent with Dr. Zeltzer's observation, research has shown that some children do learn to use humor to manage pain on their own. These children also tend to initiate other adaptive ways to distract themselves from the pain.[59] One test was developed which specifically measures the extent to which children use humor to cope with pain. Among pre-adolescent children going through various painful procedures while hospitalized, those scoring higher on the humor measure rated the procedures gone through to be less "unpleasant" than children with lower humor scores.[60] So their own humor coping style served them well in reducing the unpleasantness of their hospital experience.

Dr. Zeltzer's Rx Laughter Project has shown that children are able to leave their hands in painful ice water longer while watching comedy videos.[61] Interestingly, children who watched the comedy video with their hands in the ice water did not rate the procedure as being less painful. But the fact that they left their hand in longer suggests that they were distracted enough by the video to not notice the painfulness of the ice water until it became more intense.

Dr. Zeltzer shared an observation from Rx Laughter which captures the way in which humor can transform a child's experience in a pediatric unit.

"Yesterday we went . . . on a tour of the children's hospital at UCLA with some of the members of the board of advisors for Rx Laughter, and I was really struck by a young boy in the dialysis unit, and he was just sitting there quietly. Two of the former writers from *I Love Lucy* had come up to him and asked him if he ever watched the show. He said he loved the show . . . [and that his favorite episode was] where she was going on an airplane and was trying to hide a huge cheese she was bringing on board, so she put it under her blouse and pretended she was pregnant. He was laughing as he described the story. The writers began to tell him how they got the idea for that episode, and the child was laughing. Watching this boy, who was in his teens, and these writers, who were probably in their late 70s or early 80s, laughing hysterically while he was in the middle of hemomdialysis made me think of the power of laughter."[62]

What Causes the Pain Reduction Associated with Humor and Laughter? For those who do experience pain reduction following humor and laughter, why does it occur? We have known for a long time that emotional stress makes pain worse for many conditions, so part of the pain-reducing impact of humor may be due to humor's amazing ability to help cope with stress and reduce negative emotion (this is discussed in Chapter 1). But what is the physiological mechanism that is responsible for humor's pain-reducing power? There has been no definitive answer to this question, but the four most likely candidates are discussed below.

1) Mental Distraction

One possibility is distraction. Humor—especially the kind that is fully engaging and really cracks you up—is an effective means of drawing attention away from the source of pain or discomfort, and there is every reason to think that this influences the brain's pain channeling mechanisms.[63] There is some evidence that humor, music and a mentally-engaging arithmetic task result in comparable levels of increased tolerance of painful stimulation; this is consistent with the view that the key to humor's pain reducing power may be distraction.[64]

"When you're hungry, sing. When you're hurt, laugh."

(Jewish proverb)

2) Release of Endorphins?

It has long been speculated that humor—or the act of laughter itself—causes the release of endorphins or other endogenous opioids (natural pain killers) in the body, and that this provides an analgesic effect for some period of time. The net effect of this would be reduced pain. This explanation makes good sense, and the mass media have been reporting for the past 25 years that humor and laughter produce endorphins. Until recently, however, there have been no published data to support this view. Two early studies failed to show the endorphin-humor connection[65] but a 2007 study did find that both the anticipation and watching of a humorous film led to increased endorphin production.[66] Since two of three studies have shown no endorphin effect, the jury remains out on whether the well-established pain reduction effect associated with humor and laughter is even partly due to the body's production of endorphins.

3) Muscle Relaxation

Regardless of whether laughter/humor does or does not trigger the release of endorphins into the blood stream, its ability to reduce pain is undoubtedly partly due to its reduction of muscle tension (see discussion below and in Chapter 1). Even brief relaxation procedures (in the absence of humor) have been shown to reduce pain—both in laboratory and clinical settings.[67] Many pain centers around the country now use meditation and other relaxation techniques to reduce the level of pain medication needed by patients. Laughter is just one additional technique for achieving the same effect. There is some evidence that genuinely mirthful laughter (i.e., laughter associated with the experience of humor) triggers a stronger muscle relaxation effect than laughter without mirth.[68]

This muscle relaxation effect has its practical side in hospitals. Some nurses tell patients jokes before giving them shots, because they know it keeps them from tightening up their muscles in anticipation of the shot.

4) Activation of Pleasure Centers in the Brain

Recent research (discussed in Chapters 1 and 3) has documented that humor activates known pleasure or reward centers in the brain. The elevation of dopamine levels by humor in connection with these pleasure centers may either directly or indirectly reduce the level of pain experienced. This view is strengthened by recent findings that pleasurable and painful (or otherwise aversive) stimuli appear to share some of the same neural circuitry.[69]

Strengthening of the Immune System

Your immune system is crucial to sustaining good health. We are all constantly bombarded by viruses, bacteria and other antigens that could seriously harm or even kill us. This threat is present every day of our lives, so anything we do to bolster the effectiveness of this system is clearly important. But can humor really make your immune system stronger?

It has long been recognized that chronic stress weakens the immune system, leaving you more vulnerable to illness—although short-term, acute stress may boost the immune system.[70] If you find yourself constantly stressed out by your job, a financial crisis, deteriorating health, an unsatisfactory marriage or any other persisting personal problem, your odds of coming down with some kind of health problem increase.

One of the first hints of a solution to the puzzle of how one's mental or emotional state might influence health came from studies of animals showing that the immune system could actually be conditioned to respond to something that would normally have no impact at all on its functioning. In a now classic study, rats were given a drug known to suppress the functioning of the immune system. The (at the time) commonly used sweetener saccharine was put in the animals' drinking water and presented simultaneously with the drug, leading to the expected suppression of the immune system. After a period of time following the cessation of drug-plus-saccharine, the animals' immune systems fully recovered. At that point, the saccharine alone was presented. Amazingly, the immune system was again suppressed, just as it had been by the drug.[71] A clear conditioning effect had occurred. After simply being paired with the drug in the animals' experience, the saccharine acquired the ability to suppress the immune system—an effect that never occurs in the absence of such prior pairing. This and other similar findings clearly established that the functioning of a basic health-sustaining mechanism like the immune system can be influenced by our experience and expectations—including, perhaps, our emotions.

By the early 1980s, researchers finally began to study the impact of humor and laughter on the immune system. The best evidence that humor boosts the immune system comes from studies where immune system measures are taken before and after a particular humorous event—usually a comedy video.

Immunoglobulin A. The greatest amount of research to date has focused on immunoglobulin A, which protects you against upper respiratory problems, like colds and the flu. Secretory IgA (or SIgA) is a kind of antibody found in the mucosal areas of the body—including saliva. It is the first line of defense against antigens in these areas. There are now more than a dozen studies showing that watching as little as 30 or 60 minutes of a comedy video is enough to increase both salivary[72] and blood levels of IgA.[73] This has been shown for children, as well as adults.[74] (It should be noted that a few studies have failed to show this increase, but the general thrust of the data clearly favors the immunoenhancement effect.) It should also be noted that films that are exciting, but not funny, also boost salivary IgA.[75] These findings do not mean that you won't get a cold or the flu if you have a good sense of humor. Rather, they suggest that humor and laughter reduce your odds of catching a cold or the flu—or reduce their severity if you do get sick.

Humor, of course, is just one tool for generating positive emotion. Other approaches to creating a positive emotional state have similarly produced increased SIgA.[76] So anything you do to keep yourself in an upbeat, positive mood helps keep this part of your immune system functioning well.

Natural Killer Cells. While most of the early research on humor and the immune system focused on salivary IgA (because it is convenient and inexpensive), several researchers have argued that there are problems with this measure, and that it may not reliably reflect immune function.[77] It was argued 20 years ago that a natural killer (NK) cell immunoassay would be a better tool for assessing immune function.[78] As a result, researchers have more recently focused on NK cell activity in determining the effect of humor on the immune system.

Natural killer cells seek out tumor cells and destroy them by releasing a toxic substance. They also battle the latest cold- and flu-generating viruses and other foreign organisms. They are another part of the body's first line of defense and can attack foreign organisms even if they've never seen them before. Several studies have shown that watching a humorous video increases the activity—or number—of natural killer cells.[79] In one case, this increased NK cell activity occurred only for those individuals who laughed out loud during the comedy video.[80] Just watching a comedy video did not, in itself, increase NK cell activity. (Presumably, this means that it only occurred for those who found the video funny.) Amazingly, the correlation between amount of laughter subjects showed and the extent of increase in NK cell activity was .74. Other studies have not shown this strong link between laughter and NK cell activity, so it remains unclear whether it is laugher or the mental enjoyment of humor that is the key to generating the immune boost.

Most studies of NK cell activity have not assessed subjects' sense of humor, but two that did measure it found a positive relationship between sense of humor and NK cell activity among cardiac patients[81] and cancer patients.[82] Watching a comedy video, however, did not boost NK cell activity in these patients. (It should be noted that NK activity is generally suppressed in cancer patients.)

It appears that a number of factors can influence the extent of this positive impact of humor on NK cells. For example, the immunoenhancement effect may occur only for individuals whose NK cell activity is lower than average.[83] But the extent of increase in NK cell activity seems to be reduced if one is depressed or angry prior to watching the funny video.[84] A recent Japanese study focusing on the impact of laughter on gene expression among diabetes patients unexpectedly shed some important light on how humor and laughter influence NK cell activity. The analyzed some 41,000 genes and found that 39 were "up-regulated" 90 minutes following the viewing of a comedy video. After four hours, 27 of these genes were still up-regulated. Of the 27, 14 were specifically related to NK cell activity. They concluded that ". . . laughter influences the expression of many genes classified into immune responses . . ."[85]

Among cancer patients, reduced natural killer cell activity is associated with an increased rate of spread of tumors.[86] So the significance of laughter's ability to increase the activity of these cells among those with cancer is clear. The just-mentioned finding that humor's ability to boost NK cell activity is greatest among those with lower starting levels of NK cell activity is especially important for cancer patients and oncologists to keep in mind. This may be one reason oncology units of hospitals have become so interested in humor as a form of therapy.[87] If you work in oncology, and your hospital or center has never had a program on the importance of humor as part of its National Cancer Survivors Day celebration, you now have a good foundation for suggesting such a program.

A country doctor went out to the boondocks to deliver a baby. It was so far out, there was no electricity. When he arrived, no one was home except for the laboring mother and her five-year-old son. The doctor instructed the child to hold a lantern high so he could see while delivering the baby.

The child did so, and the mother pushed. After a little while, the doctor lifted the newborn by the feet and spanked him on the bottom to get him to take his first breath.

The doctor asked the boy what he thought of the baby.

"Hit him again," the boy said. "He shouldn't have crawled up there in the first place!"

The functioning of one's immune system is sensitive to shifting moods or emotional states throughout the day. Method actors were asked to generate the emotion of joy within themselves. Amazingly, an increase in the number of NK cells circulating in the blood stream occurred within 20 minutes. Once they got themselves out of this positive state, their levels of NK cells quickly dropped again.[88] This kind of finding makes it very clear just *how important it is to have tools for sustaining a positive emotional state as much as possible throughout the day.*

This is consistent with findings discussed below indicating that a positive mood is associated with increased NK cell activity, while a heightened negative mood is associated with reduced NK cell activity. Since humor and laughter provide a quick and effective means of generating the experience of joy, they give you a means of taking at least a bit of control over your immune system by helping to sustain a positive mood throughout the day.

A very new approach to treating cancer involves activation of the patient's own immune system to get it to battle the cancer more effectively. It is called immunotherapy and uses a drug to bolster the immune system. For example, at the time of writing of this book, researchers at the Roswell Park Cancer Institute in Buffalo, New York were giving certain cancer patients high doses of a drug called Interleukin2 to stimulate the immune system. Unfortunately, these high doses are often difficult to tolerate, and the drug only seems to work with certain patients. But when it does work, the effect is dramatic. According to one of the researchers testing the drug, "In those patients where we really get a response out of IL2 therapy, it is nothing short of extraordinary. You can have a situation where a patient with metastatic disease will have their tumors melt away."[89] The language used to describe the drug's impact (the observation that the tumors just seem melt away) is very reminiscent of the doctors' description of the effect of Krebiozen (discussed earlier) a half century ago.

Investigators studying the impact of immunotherapy are excited about its potential, but there is no definitive research documenting its effectiveness at this point. It is brought into the discussion here to emphasize that *immunotherapy does the very same thing that humor does*—although much more intensely. That is, it provides a boost to the immune system, helping the body to fight disease on its own. Presumably (if it does prove to be effective in battling cancer), Interleukin2 would provide a much more potent immune system boost than that provided by humor, but this in no way devalues the importance of humor as an ally in the battle.

Other Immunoenhancement Effects. Little research has been completed on the impact of humor on other parts of the immune system. There is some evidence that both IgG[90] and IgM are also enhanced as a result of humor/laughter.[91] IgM is the antibody that arrives first as part of the humoral immune response. IgG antibodies are present in the greatest amount in the body and are responsible for producing long-term immunity. When you are immunized for a particular illness, it is the IgG antibodies that are tested to see if the procedure has worked.

This same study showed that watching a comedy video produced increased levels of complement 3, which helps antibodies pierce through defective or infected cells in order to destroy them.

In terms of other parts of the cellular immune system, again only limited research has been completed, although what has been done supports the findings for NK cells. B cells are produced in the bone marrow and are responsible for making the immunoglobulins. The one study that has looked at B cells found that simply watching a comedy video was enough to increase the number of these cells circulating in the blood.[92] This is not surprising, of course, given the evidence of increased levels of immunoglobulins following humor.

Humor may even have a place in the battle against AIDS. T-cells are immune cells produced by the thymus gland. The AIDS virus attacks "helper T-cells." Humor and laughter have been shown to increase the number and level of activation of helper T-cells; they also increase the ratio of helper to suppresser T-cells.[93]

The humor/T-cell findings are supported by evidence that relaxation techniques increase levels of helper T-cells. For example, medical students' levels of helper T-cells are reduced on the day of exams.[94] But learning a relaxation technique increased their level of helper T-cells. And the degree of increase was directly related to the extent to which they practiced the techniques learned. So the increased helper T-cell production found for humor and laughter may have been due to their ability to produce relaxation. Relaxation techniques also increase antibody production, natural killer cell activity, and the effectiveness of cytotoxic T-cells.[95]

"The art of medicine consists of keeping the patient amused while nature heals the disease." (Voltaire)

While we wait for researchers to settle this issue, I fully agree with the advice given by an early long-term AIDS survivor, Michael Callen (who died in 1993): "It simply makes sense to try to mobilize whatever immune-system enhancing effects might flow from marshaling the mind. After all, even if your T-cells don't increase, how can having a cheerful, frisky, life-affirming attitude possibly hurt? . . . I highly recommend daily doses of laughter."[96]

Finally, one study has also shown that humor increases levels of gamma interferon, a complex substance that plays an important role in the maturation of B cells, the growth of cytotoxic T cells and the activation of NK cells.[97] It also tells different components of the immune system when to become more active and regulates the level of cooperation between cells of the immune system. Given the specific types of immunoenhancement resulting from humor discussed above, this effect on gamma interferon is to be expected.

Taken as a whole, it's clear that there is something about humor and laughter that "turns on" the immune system metabolically and causes it to do more effectively the very thing it is designed to do—promote health and wellness in the face of internal or external threats. *But your sense of humor is not some kind of magic bullet which will cure cancer or other illnesses. Rather, it creates internal conditions which support the body's own basic healing and health-maintaining mechanisms.* It helps assure that these mechanisms are working *for* you, *not against* you.

Free Radical Scavenging Capacity. The level of free radicals in the body has received a great deal of attention in recent years, since they have been implicated in faster aging, inflammation, cancer and other pathological conditions. Antioxidant vitamins have become very popular because of their presumed ability to reduce the level of free radicals in the body. It is generally believed that anything which helps reduce free radicals in the body is important when it comes to sustaining health in the long run.

Japanese researchers have shown that watching a comedy video increases the free radical scavenging capacity in human saliva.[98] (This new research is really part of the second wave of health-related humor research, not the first wave—even though it deals with a general health-promoting mechanism.) Just as importantly, those who reported higher levels of "pleasant feeling" while watching the video showed higher levels of free radical scavenging. This is an exciting finding in support of a key general health-promoting mechanism and is consistent with the bulk of evidence showing that humor boosts the immune system.

BUILD YOUR HUMOR SKILLS

[Work on both jokes before checking the answers.]

1. How is a hospital gown like health insurance? You're never _____ as much as you think you are.
Clue: You should not need a clue for this one.

2. Two podiatrists opened up offices on the same street. As you might expect, they soon became _____ enemies.
Clue: Part of the bottom of your foot.

Sense of Humor and Immunity. Given all the evidence that watching a humorous video strengthens the immune system, individuals who have a better-developed sense of humor—meaning that they find more humor in their everyday life, seek out humor more often, laugh more, etc.—should have a stronger immune system, since they presumably get more of the same benefits that result from watching a comedy video by exercising their sense of humor more often. Consistent with this expectation, there is some evidence that people with higher scores on a sense of humor test have higher "baseline levels" of IgA.[99] But there are also several studies which failed to find this expected relationship, so the picture for the relationship between sense of humor and the immune system is not as clear as that obtained for watching a funny video.

> **John was a clerk in a small drugstore, but he wasn't much of a salesman. He could never find the item the customer wanted. Bob, the owner, had had enough and warned John that the next sale he missed would be his last.**
>
> **Just then a man came in coughing and asked John for their best cough syrup. Try as he might, John could not find the cough syrup. Remembering Bob's warning, he sold the man a box of Ex-Lax and told him to take it all at once. The customer did as John said and then walked outside and suddenly stopped and leaned against a lamp post.**
>
> **Bob had seen the whole thing and came over to ask John what had transpired. "He wanted something for his cough but I couldn't find the cough syrup. So I substituted Ex-Lax and told him to take it all at once," John explained.**
>
> **"Ex-Lax won't cure a cough!" Bob shouted angrily.**
>
> **"Sure it will," John said, pointing at the man leaning on the lamp post. "Look at him. He's afraid to cough!"**

The reason for the inconsistent findings for sense of humor may lie in the finding noted above that one's immune system fluctuates throughout the day as a function of shifts in mood. While a good sense of humor increases the likelihood that you will have more frequent occasions for mood-elevating laughs throughout the day, it is no guarantee. Even people with a great sense of humor may go hours without laughing.

It was noted in Chapter 1 that a distinction between positive and negative humor styles is crucial to psychological benefits associated with humor; only positive styles of humor were positively linked to psychological well-being when this distinction was made. It may be that the failure to distinguish positive from negative styles of humor is similarly responsible for the inconsistency in research linking sense of humor to immunoenhancement effects. It may be that only positive styles of humor boost the immune system. Researchers have not yet attempted to resolve this issue.

It was also noted earlier that many researchers have doubts about the use of IgA as an index of humor's ability to boost the immune system. Greater confidence has been shown in NK cell activity as an indicator of immune effects. As discussed above, a positive relationship was obtained between sense of humor scores and NK cell activity among both cardiac and cancer patients.[100]

If people with a better sense of humor do have a stronger immune system than their humor-impaired friends, those with a less-developed sense of humor might be expected to show a stronger immune boost from watching a comedy video. But the opposite is true. People with higher sense of humor scores show the greatest increase in IgA after watching a funny video.[101] This suggests that those with a better sense of humor may have appreciated the videos more or laughed more.

ANSWERS TO JOKES

1. covered   2. arch

"The simple truth is that happy people generally don't get sick."
(Bernie Siegel, M.D.)

Humor's ability to protect against immunosuppression during stress was evident when people with a well-developed sense of humor (they found a lot of humor in everyday life or frequently used humor to cope with stress) were compared to people with a poor sense of humor. Among the latter, a greater number of everyday hassles and negative life events was associated with greater suppression of their immune system (IgA). Among those with a well-developed sense of humor, on the other hand, everyday hassles and problems did not weaken the immune system.[102] Their sense of humor helped keep them from becoming more vulnerable to illness when under stress.

The Role of Mood. Your immune system is very sensitive to your mood, being stronger on your "up" days, and weaker on "down" days. This has been shown for both IgA and natural killer cell activity.[103] It appears to be the negative emotion or mood that accompanies stress that is responsible for the reduced level of antibody response that occurs when the immune system is asked to fight a virus or other antigen. This has been documented with reduced levels of NK cell activity,[104] lymphocyte proliferation,[105] serum antibody response to Hepatitis B vaccine,[106] and salivary IgA response to a novel antigen,[107] to name a few.

Part of the health-promoting power of humor, then, lies in its ability to help keep negative events from disturbing your mood.[108] Experiencing humor makes it easier to keep an upbeat, optimistic outlook, even in the face of stress. Dr. Bernie Siegel has long emphasized the importance of a positive, optimistic mood in fighting cancer and sustaining wellness,[109] and your sense of humor is one of the best ways you have to maintain this mood on high-stress days.

Which is More Important, Laughter or Humor? A key question concerns the relative importance of laughter versus the mental/emotional experience of humor. Only two studies have addressed this issue. In one, half the participants were encouraged to laugh while watching a comedy video, while the other half were asked to suppress laughter while watching. Comparable levels of increased salivary IgA were found for the two groups.[110] Since laughter did not add to the amount of IgA increase, this suggests that the experience of humor may be more important than how much you laugh. This is consistent with other evidence that the act of laughter itself is less important in accounting for observed increases in the threshold for experiencing pain than the level of enjoyment (as indicated by facial expression) of the humor presented.[111]

Another study, however, showed no relationship between the funniness of a video and the amount of IgA increase shown.[112] The way in which one's sense of humor provides immunoenhancement benefits is clearly complicated and not yet well understood. So we cannot answer the question of which is more important for health. As long as you're someone who is comfortable having a good belly laugh when you find something funny, it makes no difference which is really responsible for the immune strengthening benefit (or any other health benefit) you receive in your daily life. Your body gets the benefit, even if your mind doesn't know why.

Lower Sedimentation Rate

Sedimentation rate is a measure of inflammation in the body. Norman Cousins' illness—ankylosing spondylitis—involved severe inflammation of the joints and spine, making it very painful for him to even turn over in bed. So his sedimentation rate was very high. But his doctor (William Hitzig) measured Cousins' sedimentation rate before and after bouts of laughter at comedy films with his friends. The laughter sharply lowered his sedimentation rate.[113] Dr. Hitzig noted that "just a few moments of robust laughter . . . knocked a significant number of units off the sedimentation rate. What to him was most interesting of all was that the reduction held and was cumulative."[114]

This was an important observation, but its possible significance for health went unnoticed for more than a quarter of a century. It is only recently that humor's impact on inflammation has been studied. As noted later in this chapter (see discussion of Arthritis and "How humor promotes cardiac health"), two studies have now shown that a daily diet of humor videos over a lengthy period of time reduces levels of inflammatory cytokines and C-reactive proteins (an additional marker of inflammation).[115] Other evidence shows that even short-term exposure to a comedy video is sufficient to reduce levels of inflammatory cytokines in arthritis patients.[116]

Reduction of the Health-Damaging Effects of Stress

Stress has long been known to cause or worsen health problems. It can even cause brain cells to atrophy and die.[117] It also damages artery walls, causing them to lose their elasticity; this, in turn, leads to reduced blood flow and increased blood pressure, speeding up the risk of coronary heart disease .

Stress even speeds up normal aging processes. We all inherit a certain limit in the number of cell divisions that the cells of our body are capable of. Stress increases the rate at which these cell divisions occur. So chronic stress actually accelerates the aging process at the cellular level.[118]

As a result of mounting job-related stress over the past quarter century, stress management has become a multi-million dollar business in the United States; it is rapidly growing in other countries, as well. In addition to the direct positive influences of humor and laughter on health already discussed, humor also helps sustain health by reducing or eliminating the negative effects that persistent stress has on health and well being. Chapter 1 documents the many ways in which humor helps to cope with life stress. The discussion here is restricted to how humor counters some of the effects of stress known to have a negative influence on health.

Muscle Relaxation. Many stress management techniques have been developed, including physical exercise, progressive relaxation, biofeedback, deep breathing, meditation, massage, etc. The main goal of all of these techniques is muscle relaxation and the easing of psychological tensions that goes with it. But you don't have to spend a lot of time, effort and money learning special relaxation techniques. You just have to find more humor in your life—and laugh more! Belly laughter naturally produces muscle relaxation.[119] And genuinely mirthful laughter (i.e., laughter associated with the experience of humor) appears to trigger a stronger muscle relaxation effect than laughter without the experience of mirth.[120] The recent research documenting this relaxation effect of laughter supports the observation made by researchers over 75 years ago that laughter produces a loss of muscle tone (known as hypotonia).[121]

This relaxation effect is easily noticeable when you have a good laugh. In my keynote addresses, I have a funny routine which culminates in getting everyone in the room doing belly laughter for half a minute or so. Afterwards, I ask them to describe any changes they notice in their bodies or in how they feel. The first comment is usually, "I feel more relaxed." The next time you have a good long laugh, look for this feeling of relaxation and reduced tension.

We've all at some point heard someone say, "I laughed so hard I couldn't stand up." If you've ever watched preschoolers laughing hard, you're sure to have seen some of them fall down and roll around on the floor laughing. Most of us have learned not to fall down when we're laughing hard, but little kids just go with the flow. If those muscles relax, they go down. In your own experience, you'll notice that if you're sitting down when you're laughing hard, you generally fall back in your chair, rather than sit up straight. This is the adult equivalent of falling down from laughter.

> **An elderly lady came in for her annual eye exam. When asked to cover her left eye and read the 3rd line of the eye chart, she replied, "I can't dear."**
> **"Okay, cover your other eye and read the chart.**
> **"I can't dear," was the reply again.**
> **The doctor then asked if she could read.**
> **"Oh yes dear," came the reply.**
> **"Well read the chart for me then."**
> **"I can't dear," came the reply again.**
> **The puzzled doctor asked if she could see the chart.**
> **"Oh yes dear," came the reply.**
> **Finally, he asked why she could not read the chart.**
> **The answer came, "Because I can't pronounce it!"**

Two separate mechanisms cause this relaxation effect. Muscles not directly participating in the act of laughter relax while you're laughing. That's why little kids fall down during fits of laughter. It's also why you seem to lose your strength when you're laughing (try carrying something heavy across the room while laughing hard). When you stop laughing, the muscles that had been contracting relax. This is no different from what happens with any other physical activity. When you stop working muscles, their natural tendency is to relax. In combination, these two mechanisms produce a general pattern of muscle relaxation throughout your body.

> "There ain't much fun in medicine, but there's a heck of a lot of medicine in fun."   (Josh Billings)

Biofeedback is one popular approach used by many to learn to relax. People using a biofeedback apparatus are able to relax muscles more quickly after watching funny cartoons than after looking at beautiful scenery.[122] The importance of this relaxation effect may be seen in the fact that relaxation not only reduces stress; it also helps alleviate heart disease,[123] headaches,[124] chronic anxiety,[125] and other problems. For patients with rheumatism, neuralgia, or other conditions characterized by a spasm-pain-spasm cycle, the reduced muscle tension that results from laughter disrupts this cycle and reduces the pain experienced.

Reduced Stress Hormones. When you're under stress, your body undergoes a series of hormonal and other changes which make up the "fight or flight" response. Even though there's no physical threat to your life, your body reacts as if there were. One byproduct of stress is the release of cortisol and other stress hormones into the blood stream. These hormones are crucial to assuring survival; they prepare your body to meet the challenge of the moment.

The problem, as we have long known, is that modern threats are generally to our psychological survival—not our physical survival. And psychological stressors have a nagging tendency to persist over time. We have ongoing work-overload on the job, financial or relationship problems, health crises, and so on. As I write this in 2009, we are in the midst of the greatest financial crisis this country has seen since the Great Depression of the 1930s. The health risk comes when cortisol and other stress hormones associated with this crisis continue to circulate throughout our bodies day after day.[126] For example, heightened cortisol levels contribute to inflammatory diseases.[127] Anything which reduces the level of stress hormones in the blood on a regular basis helps reduce this health threat.

"Stress-related disease emerges, predominantly, out of the fact that we so often activate a physiological system that has evolved for responding to acute physical emergencies, but we turn it on for months on end, worrying about mortgages, relationships, and promotions."[128]

The importance of learning to manage negative emotion is evident in the fact that high levels of it are associated with increased levels of stress hormones—throughout the day and in specific times of stress.[129] So it is no surprise that people showing high levels of negative emotion as a general personality trait have higher levels of circulating cortisol in their bodies.[130] This link is made all the more clear by evidence that inducing negative emotion in a laboratory setting increases circulating stress hormones.[131]

The impact of humor and laughter on cortisol and other stress hormones is a new area of study, but five studies have documented that humor significantly reduces cortisol levels in the blood.[132] In fact, the mere anticipation of watching a funny film may be enough to reduce cortisol levels.[133] This is consistent with evidence that other relaxation procedures[134] and other approaches[135] to inducing positive emotion also reduce cortisol levels. And people who habitually show more positive affect on a daily basis tend to have lower cortisol levels. Similarly, a steady daily diet of (at least 30 minutes of) humor on TV or DVD/videos for 12 months among diabetic patients reduces levels of epinephrine and norepinephrine (suggesting lower stress levels).[136]

Another hormone—growth hormone—is associated with joint pain and swelling. These symptoms are a common complaint in rheumatoid arthritis (RA) patients. Consistent with the cortisol data, humor and laughter reduce the level of circulating growth hormone in RA patients.[137] Before exposure to humor, the growth hormone level of the RA patients was significantly higher than the level of a comparable group without the disease. This difference between the groups disappeared after the exposure to humor, with the level for the RA patients closely approaching that of the non-RA individuals.

Lower Blood Pressure. Another clear byproduct of stress is elevated blood pressure. While the evidence for blood pressure is limited at this point, humor and laughter over an extended period of time appear to lower blood pressure. Of course, as your heart beats more rapidly during laughter, it pumps more blood through your system, producing the familiar flushed cheeks. Not surprisingly, blood pressure increases during laughter, with larger increases corresponding to more intense and longer-lasting laughs.[138] If this were a lasting increase, it might point to a harmful effect of laughter, but blood pressure soon returns to its base line once the laughter stops. In fact, it may briefly drop below the pre-laughter baseline, although this drop is short-lived.[139] And we certainly would not expect any long-range blood pressure effect from a single episode of laughter. The best test of their ability to generate a lasting drop in blood pressure would come from studying the effect of increased amounts of humor and laughter over a more extended period of time.

In an especially important finding along these lines, watching a comedy video three times a week while participating in a one-year cardiac rehab program significantly lowered blood pressure in people who had suffered heart attacks.[140] This long-term outcome is important for everyone, but it is especially important for those suffering from coronary heart disease. On the other hand, a six-week laughter exercise intervention did not lower blood pressure.[141] This may mean that a period longer than six weeks is required to show the reduction effect. But since the former study emphasized humor, while the latter focused on laughter exercises, this may point to the relatively greater importance of humor than laughter alone in managing one's blood pressure. Again, the limited current research in this area makes it impossible to tell.

In another important study, a better sense of humor among a group of middle-aged police chiefs was associated with lower blood pressure—in spite of the fact that those with a better sense of humor also smoked more and consumed more alcohol.[142] Presumably, their better sense of humor provided them daily doses of muscle relaxation and reduced stress hormones, setting up in their bodies the conditions we expect to help lower blood pressure.

Consistent with this finding, women who more often used humor to cope had lower (systolic) blood pressure than women who used coping humor less often.[143] Surprisingly, high-coping-humor men showed the opposite pattern, having higher blood pressure. So having a better sense of humor in coping with stress did nothing to lower these men's blood pressure. When these same men were exposed to a series of stress-inducing tasks, however, their better sense of humor did help keep their blood pressure from elevating (it did increase for low sense of humor subjects). When women were confronted with the same set of tasks, having a stronger coping sense of humor did not protect them from increasing blood pressure; their blood pressure went up just as it did for low sense of humor women.

So the picture of the relationship between humor and blood pressure remains one of confusion. It seems likely that if a blood pressure lowering effect of humor is to be found, it will be found for ongoing regular exposure to humor. It was noted in Chapter 1 that it is crucial to distinguish between positive and negative aspects of one's sense of humor when considering any physical or mental health benefits. It may well be that a strong positive sense of humor (or "humor style") contributes to lower blood pressure, while having a hostile, sarcastic or otherwise negative sense of humor provides no blood pressure lowering benefit at all—it may even elevate it. The authors of this study suggested that higher amounts of humor among these men may have reflected their greater competitiveness and aggressiveness, leading to increased blood pressure.

Better Health Practices?

Better diet, sleep and exercise habits are all associated with a reduced risk of illness and death.[144] And people who habitually show more positive affect do exercise more[145] and have a better quality of nightly sleep.[146] (On a personal note, my wife is a firm believer in the sleep-inducing power of humor. She has an endless supply of videotapes of *I Love Lucy* and other classic comedy shows. These gentle forms of humor are essential tools in relaxing her, helping her let go of the problems and hassles of the day and ease into a sound, healthy night's sleep.) There is no evidence, however, that people with a stronger sense of humor have better health habits in general. In fact, the opposite may be true. Individuals scoring higher on sense of humor tests are less focused on health concerns and engage more often in smoking and drinking alcohol. (See the section on "Does humor increase longevity?" below.)

Better Social Network

Having a sense of humor is a quality that most of us admire and seek out in others. From childhood on, those who have a good sense of humor tend to be more popular and are sought out more often by others as friends. So a sense of humor should help build a good social network at any age. The importance of this lies in the fact that a stronger social network reduces the risk of illness and death.[147] And people who have higher trait positive affect have a higher quality of social ties with others and also socialize more often.[148]

The Second Wave Impact of Humor and Laughter on Specific Diseases

The first 15-20 years of research on the health benefits of humor and laughter focused on the general health promoting mechanisms just discussed. By the beginning of the new century, these promising health-promoting findings stimulated interest in humor's impact on specific disease conditions.

Coronary Heart Disease

Coronary heart disease is the number one cause of death in the United States (for women and men), as well as in most other industrialized nations; it is responsible for about 20% of deaths.[149] In 2009, well over one and a quarter million Americans were expected to experience a new or recurrent coronary event. We have long known about such risk factors as a poor diet, lack of exercise, smoking, and family history, but the fact that these factors only account for half the incidents of CHD[150] has led researchers to cast their net more widely in recent years to find additional things that start some individuals down the path toward CHD. One of these additional risk factors is your daily emotional state. Learning to manage your emotions, so that you do not wallow in depression, anxiety or anger (along with doing the right thing in terms of diet, exercise, smoking, etc.) is important for maximizing your chances of sustaining a healthy heart well into your senior years.

Temporary increases in heart rate and blood pressure do not pose a health risk. This is a normal and natural response to any perceived threat. It is part of the "fight or flight" response. The risk to health comes when this condition is present day after day over a prolonged period of time;[151] and this risk is greatest for coronary heart disease and stroke.[152] There is exciting new evidence, however, that humor and laughter can support good cardiac health—both for individuals who have already suffered a heart attack and those who have not. Since this research specifically focusing on the cardiac benefits offered by humor is just starting, we'll first take a brief look at the broader field of research on the impact of negative and other forms of positive emotion (excluding humor) on heart health. This will help put the heart-healing benefits of humor in better perspective.

Impact of Negative Emotion. A very large body of research now shows that persistent negative emotions and thoughts contribute to both the onset and progression of CHD.[153] Chronic anger, especially, has been closely linked to heart disease for many years. Individuals with the classic "Type A" personality have long been considered to be on the fast track to a heart attack. These are people who are competitive, have a sense of time-urgency and can't relax, and generally carry around a lot of anger and hostility.[154] These qualities sharply increase the risk of CHD, independent of one's age, systolic blood pressure, smoking and cholesterol level.[155] Among men who have already had a heart attack (myocardial infarction), Type A men are also more likely than Type B men to have additional subsequent heart attacks.[156] This elevated hostility even shows up as greater enjoyment of hostile than non-hostile humor.[157] Chronic depression, anxiety, a sense of hopelessness and the bottling up or suppression of one's emotions are also CHD risk factors.[158]

In the case of chronic hostility and anger, the problem is that these emotions generate frequent and prolonged elevation in both heart rate and blood pressure (increased "cardiovascular reactivity"), which progressively takes you down the path toward hypertension and atherosclerosis.[159] Even among persons who do not have coronary heart disease, their current level of hostility predicts the subsequent severity and progression of atherosclerosis.[160]

A single episode of extreme anger or stress is sometimes sufficient to trigger a heart attack. In fact, the likelihood of a heart attack is twice as great in the two hours following an episode of anger.[161] About 30% of the "attributable risk of acute myocardial infarction" can be accounted for by stress. "Psychosocial stress appears to adversely affect autonomic and hormonal homeostasis, resulting in metabolic abnormalities, insulin resistance, and *endothelial dysfunction*."[162] (Italics are McGhee's.)

Sharply elevated stress in an entire community can similarly boost the incidence of heart attacks. In the 1991 war with Iraq (in which Iraq initiated attacks on Israel), death rates from heart attacks in Israeli cities targeted by Scud missiles were twice what they would normally be.[163] Similarly, on the day of the Los Angeles earthquake in 1994, deaths from sudden heart attacks were five times what would normally be expected for the day.[164] Depression, anxiety and hopelessness have also been shown to increase the risk of both the development and progression of CHD.[165]

In an especially important study, Amy Ferketich and her colleagues studied the health records of over 2800 men and 5,000 women over a 10-year period. No one had heart disease when the study began, although 10% of the men and 17% of the women were clinically depressed. Both men and women who were depressed at the start of the study showed more than a 70% greater incidence of heart disease than the non-depressed participants 10 years later. The depressed men were twice as likely as the non-depressed men to die in that 10-year period, while depressed women were (surprisingly) not at greater risk of dying.[166] Other evidence similarly shows that depressed mood predicts mortality among patients with congestive heart failure.[167]

KEY HEART-RELATED DEFINITIONS

Sclerosis: Hardening of tissues.

Arteriosclerosis: Thickening, hardening and loss of elasticity of arterial walls, leading to impaired blood circulation (sometimes referred to as hardening of the arteries).

Atherosclerosis: A form of arteriosclerosis characterized by the depositing of plaques (containing cholesterol and lipids) on the inner wall of arteries.

Coronary heart disease: A condition that reduces blood flow through the coronary arteries to the heart muscle (e.g., because of artery blockage or sclerosis).

Heart attack: An acute episode of heart disease (a myocardial infarction) due to an insufficient blood supply to the heart muscle—especially when caused by a coronary blood clot or occlusion.

Infarction: A process leading to the death of living tissue.

Cardiovascular reactivity: Extent of elevated heart rate and blood pressure.

Endothelium: Inner lining of arteries.

1) Damage to the Inner Lining of Arteries Resulting from Negative Emotion Starts You Down the Path to CHD

The integrity of the endothelium or inner lining of artery walls has long been known to be crucial to good heart health. The progressive build-up of plaque (containing cholesterol and lipids) in artery walls is called atherosclerosis, and it generates the path that sets you up for CHD as the years go by. As this process continues, it becomes increasingly difficult for artery walls to expand and contract normally. This—in combination with the plaque-induced reduction in the inner diameter of the vessels—leads to high blood pressure and sharply increased risk of CHD.

A healthy endothelium is able to effectively expand and contract to meet the demands placed on the body at any given moment. But, as arteriosclerosis proceeds, arteries become stiff and lose their capacity to expand and contract as needed. The extent of loss (dysfunction) of this expansion/contraction capacity of coronary arteries has been shown to be directly related to the extent and severity of coronary artery disease,[168] and is an independent predictor of cardiovascular "events" (including heart attacks, unstable angina and other coronary difficulties).[169] "Endothelial dysfunction precedes overt vascular disease by years and may itself be a potentially modifiable CVD risk factor."[170]

A doctor explained to a woman that her husband had died of a massive myocardial infarction. A little later, she was heard explaining to other family members that he had died of a massive internal fart.

While we have long known about the role of diet in determining how far one goes down this path, there is growing evidence that your daily emotional state makes a contribution, as well. The *key issue here is whether one's (negative or positive) emotional state can influence the endothelium's ability to expand or contract in a normal or healthy fashion.* In the case of negative emotion, both short- and long-term negative emotion interfere with this process. Among healthy middle-aged men who were exposed to a stress-inducing circumstance in which they had to defend themselves against a charge of theft, the capacity of the inner wall of arteries in the arm to dilate (in response to use of a blood pressure cuff) was reduced (in comparison to a baseline of artery dilation capacity established prior to the stressor) both 30 and 90 minutes after the stressor.[171] While the mechanism for this effect is not clear at this point, it shows that the negative emotion accompanying a specific stressful experience does reduce the capacity of arteries to expand and contract in a healthy or normal fashion.

Personality measures which assess one's habitual proneness to negative emotion similarly predict reduced capacity for vasodilation. For example, women found to show high levels of anger (and Type A behavior), anxiety or depression during their middle adult years showed significantly lower capacity for dilation of an arm artery 13 years later.[172] Depression may play an even more important role than anxiety in the development of vasodilation dysfunction.[173] (As noted above, this dysfunction of the endothelium is an accepted early marker of atherosclerosis and cardiovascular disease).[174]

Learning to manage one's emotions more effectively, then, can be added to the classic dietary advice (reducing intake of bad forms of cholesterol, fats and oils) when it comes to minimizing one's risk of heart disease. As was noted in Chapter 1, humor is an effective tool for substituting a positive for a negative emotional state.

BUILD YOUR HUMOR SKILLS

[Work on both jokes before checking the answers.]

1. How do doctors know that diarrhea is hereditary? Researchers clearly showed that it runs in your _____.
Clue: It's genetic.

2. A man was rushing his pregnant wife to the hospital, but didn't quite make it, and his wife gave birth right on the hospital lawn. The couple later received a bill of $600 labeled "delivery room fee." He wrote the hospital and reminded them that the baby had been delivered on the hospital lawn. Ten days later, he received a revised bill labeled "_____ $300."
Clue: A term sometimes used for what you pay to play golf.

Impact of Positive Emotion (excluding humor). With the recent explosion of interest in positive emotion, evidence is quickly accumulating to make the case that any source of habitual positive emotion contributes to good cardiac health. Humor is simply the most fun way to use positive emotion to help maintain heart health.

There are two key questions to answer here in connection with cardiac health. First, does positive emotion help prevent CHD or heart attacks? Second, can it help promote recovery among individuals already suffering from CHD? We will shortly ask the same questions in connection with humor.

> **An 82-year-old man went to the doctor to get a physical. A few days later, the doctor spotted him walking down the street with a woman half his age on his arm. The doctor said, "You're really doing great aren't you?"**
>
> **The man answered, "Just doin' what you said, Doc: 'Get a hot momma and be cheerful.'"**
>
> **The doctor said, "No! No! I said, 'You've got a heart murmur. Be careful!'"**

1) Preventing Heart Disease

Different forms of positive emotion have been shown to be associated with reduced risk of heart disease or heart attacks. Optimism, of course, is one source of habitual positive emotion. An optimist is a person who has a general disposition to be positive about future outcomes.[175] This does not mean that s/he is always positive or never experiences negative emotion or doubt. S/he simply has a chronic tendency to see the bright side and expect a good outcome in life. In a study of older male war veterans, optimists were less than half as likely as pessimists to suffer from angina or heart attacks over a 10-year follow-up period.[176]

2) Facilitating Recovery from Heart Disease

As noted above, Dr. Bernie Siegel noted in the 1980s that certain patients suffering from cancer outlived their doctors' prognosis for their life expectancy, while others either died more quickly than expected. He referred to the former as "exceptional cancer patients" and noted that they tended to have an upbeat, hopeful, optimistic attitude and a sense of determination to beat the disease. There was no research to confirm the significance of these observations at the time, but with the coming of age of psychoneuroimmunology and related fields over the past 25 years, we now know that his patients were quite typical of people who manage to sustain an optimistic outlook in spite of their illness. The same observation applies in connection with heart disease. Just a sample of the research relating positive emotion to heart disease is discussed here.

> *"The witch doctor succeeds for the same reason all the rest of us [doctors] succeed. Each patient carries his own doctor inside him. They come to us not knowing that truth. We are best when we give the doctor who resides within each patient a chance to go to work."*
> (Albert Schweitzer, M.D.)

Optimists have faster recovery than pessimists after coronary artery bypass surgery—both immediately after the surgery and six months later.[177] They are also less likely to be rehospitalized (for cardiac or other issues) following their surgery.[178] Similarly, among elderly patients hospitalized with cardiovascular disease, those who reported greater happiness over a 90-day period following their release from the hospital had lower readmission rates than patients with lower happiness levels.[179] In fact, the self-reported positive emotions of these patients during this period predicted their (lower) readmission rates even when their length of initial hospital stay and health status at initial release were taken into consideration.

ANSWERS TO JOKES

1. jeans (genes)   2. greens fee

Impact of Humor. While the research specifically looking at the impact of humor on heart health has only recently begun, what has been done is consistent with the findings discussed above for other sources of positive emotion and suggests that humor can play an important role in promoting cardiac health in both healthy individuals and those who have already suffered a heart attack.

1) Preventing Heart Disease

The first study to deal with this question matched (by age) 150 people who had already had a heart attack or had undergone coronary artery bypass surgery with 150 individuals with no prior history of heart disease. The group which had had a heart attack was found (using a self-report questionnaire) to be 40% less likely than the heart-healthy individuals to laugh in a variety of different situations.[180] An example of one of the situations is as follows: "If you were eating in a restaurant with some friends and the waiter accidentally spilled a drink on you, would you a) not find it particularly amusing, b) be amused but not show it outwardly, c) smile, d) laugh, or e) laugh heartily?"

Mahatma Ghandi always walked barefoot, so his feet became hard and callused. He was also a frail and spiritual person. Hunger strikes and a poor diet caused him to be thin and have constant bad breath. This is why he came to be known as a super callused fragile mystic plagued with halitosis.

The heart-attack group also reported feeling more anger and hostility. Their reduced laughter is not surprising in view of this, since most people laugh less when they're angry. It is tempting to conclude that the group with no heart-disease suffered fewer heart attacks *because* they found more humor in life and laughed more. But, as with any correlational study, we can't draw this conclusion. The study just establishes a significant association between laughter and heart attacks. It could also be that people were more angry and laughed less because they had had a heart attack in the past.

In addition to showing less laughter, individuals with CHD scored significantly lower on a measure of sense of humor. In fact, a weaker sense of humor predicted CHD even when the data were adjusted for other factors known to contribute to good/poor cardiac health, including hypertension, cholesterol level, cigarette smoking and family history of CHD. So this initial research supported the idea that humor and laughter may help sustain a healthy heart.

In an especially promising recent study, high risk diabetic patients suffering from hypertension and hyperlipidemia (elevated level of blood lipids) viewed a 30-minute humor video daily (each person chose the video they wanted to watch) for a year as an addition to their standard diabetes, hypertension and hyperlipidemia therapies. In comparison with a similar group who did not receive a daily diet of humor, the humor group suffered a lower incidence of myocardial infarction during the year.[181]

2) Facilitating Recovery from Heart Disease

Keeping your sense of humor is also important for heart health when you've already suffered a heart attack. This is a real challenge, since such life-threatening events generally rob people of their sense of humor and fun in life. People who had already suffered a myocardial infarction (heart attack) were randomly assigned to two groups before going through a standard cardiac rehab program for an entire year. Some patients just went through the regular rehab program, going to the hospital three times a week. Others also watched a comedy video while they were there for their rehab procedure. Each patient got to choose the video watched, so they presumably selected one that was funny to them.

At the end of one year, the comedy-watching group had suffered significantly fewer additional heart attacks during the 12-month period, along with fewer episodes of cardiac arrhythmia.[182] As noted earlier, the patients who watched comedy videos also had significantly lower blood pressure (there were no blood pressure differences between the groups at the beginning of the study). So humor plays an important role in promoting cardiac health even if you've already had a heart attack.

How Does Humor Promote Cardiac Health? Several different explanations have been offered for how humor supports a healthy heart.

1) By Reducing Stress-Linked Cardiovascular Reactivity

As noted above, we have known for years that the anger, tension and anxiety that generally go along with high stress have a negative impact on the heart, making a significant contribution to both CHD and hypertension.[183] Barbara Fredrickson and her colleagues have done a series of studies suggesting that humor and other sources of positive emotion have the power to overcome this link. They showed, for example, that after negative emotion (accompanied by increased cardiovascular reactivity) was induced by watching a film, watching a subsequent humorous film produced a quicker recovery to the baseline of cardiovascular reactivity than did either a negative or neutral film.[184] They concluded that *positive emotions (humor being only one path to positive emotion) restore one to a state of physiological equilibrium following negative emotion or stress.* This finding is of special importance, given the generally accepted view that chronic activation of the sympathetic nervous system (e.g., due to anger or feeling constantly "driven" to achieve, as discussed above in connection with the "Type A personality") contributes to the development of cardiovascular disease.[185]

A physician was on her way to preschool to pick up her four-year-old daughter. The doctor had left her stethoscope on the car seat, and her little girl picked it up and began playing with it. The doctor was thrilled, thinking her daughter wanted to follow in her own footsteps!

Then the child spoke into the instrument: "Welcome to McDonald's. May I take your order?"

Fredrickson has argued, based on a series of studies along these lines, that *humor—and positive emotion in general—undoes the lingering physiological reactivity that goes along with negative emotion.* She has completed several experiments which support this view. In each case, a high-arousal negative emotion was first produced (activating the sympathetic nervous system). Subjects then watched a film that induced joy (high-activation positive emotion), contentment (low-activation positive emotion), neutral feelings, or sadness. In three different samples, subjects in both the high- and low-activation positive emotion conditions showed more rapid cardiovascular recovery from negative emotional arousal than subjects in the other two groups.[186]

In one of these studies, a humor video was used as the high-activation source of positive emotion. Subjects who watched the funny video showed faster cardiovascular recovery than those who watched either a neutral or sadness-inducing video.[187] So, as these researchers noted, the positive emotion associated with humor does have "the ability to regulate lingering negative emotional arousal."

2) By Supporting a Healthy Inner Lining of Arteries

What else is there about humor and laughter that would reduce your risk of a heart attack? We saw earlier that stress and negative emotion cause arterial dysfunction, in which the endothelium (inner lining) of blood vessels shows reduced capacity to dilate/enlarge when called upon to do so. Dr. Michael Miller speculated that positive emotion might have just the opposite effect, increasing the ability of an artery to dilate when conditions call for it to do so. He noted in 2000 that "We don't yet know why laughing protects the heart, but we know that mental stress is associated with impairment of the endothelium, the protective barrier lining our blood vessels. This can cause a series of inflammatory reactions that lead to fat and cholesterol build-up in the coronary arteries and ultimately to a heart attack."[188] Humor and laughter might reverse these effects.

To check out this possibility, he completed a follow-up study in which he examined the effect of humor and laughter on the endothelium itself. Subjects watched both a stress-inducing and funny video (with a two-day time lapse between videos). Some watched the former first, while others watched the latter first. He used the same blood pressure cuff procedure described above. That is, a standard arm blood pressure cuff was used to restrict blood flow for a period of time. When the cuff is removed, there is a sudden increase in blood flow in the brachial artery of the arm. Another device measured how well the artery dilated to accommodate the increased surge of blood.

Watching the comedy movie segment led to a 22% increase (average across subjects) in blood flow in comparison to a preestablished baseline for each subject. This endothelium-relaxation effect occurred in 19 of the 20 participating subjects. Watching a stressful movie segment (the opening scene of the movie *Saving Private Ryan*) had the opposite effect, leading to vasoconstriction and a 35% (average) decrease in blood flow.[189] This amounts to a 57% difference in the extent of artery dilation in response to the stressful and funny films. Dr. Miller noted that the magnitude of changes observed in the endothelium in response to humor is similar to those associated with aerobic exercise[190] and statin therapy.[191]

Miller speculated in 2006 that the vasodilation effect might be due to the lowering of such neuroendocrine hormones as cortisol. He subsequently argued that humor and laughter (as well as other positive emotions) lead to the direct release of nitric oxide (not nitrous oxide, or laughing gas) by the endothelium, and that this is responsible for the relaxation effect that occurs.[192] Nitric oxide reduces clotting and inflammation—a clear benefit in sustaining healthy arteries—while emotion-induced contraction of the endothelium is associated with increased cortisol, which may cause clotting. They specifically hypothesized that beta-endorphins play the key role in this process by activating opiate receptors, which trigger the production of nitric oxide.

Consistent with this finding, watching a brief (30-minute) comedy film has also been shown to reduce arterial "stiffness," a known cardiovascular risk.[193]

If this dilation of blood vessels occurs in response to humor in a laboratory setting, it must also be occurring in everyday life among individuals with a good sense of humor—people who find more humor and laugh more at the office, with their family, etc. In both cases, the relaxation effect counters the ongoing artery constriction and associated elevation of blood pressure that accompanies stress.

Words noticed on a trash bag on Virgin Airlines: "Virgin Recycling."

Relaxation of the inner lining of arteries, then, (and the increased blood flow that results from this) may be the means by which humor and laughter help sustain a healthy heart. This is consistent with the finding that humor and laughter cause muscle relaxation, and the easing of psychological tension in the process (see discussion of relaxation above and in Chapter 3). A direct result of this increased blood flow (associated with blood vessel dilation), of course, is lower blood pressure. The health risks associated with high blood pressure are well-established.

An individual who has a better developed sense of humor, and is able to use humor to both minimize the level of stress experienced and more quickly reduce stress when it does occur, has blood vessels which go through fewer of the endless cycles of vasoconstriction and dilation which occur when we are frequently stressed through the day. Every rise in blood pressure puts extra stress on the inner walls of your arteries and may eventually lead to small tears in the walls. While your body does initiate actions to repair the walls when such tears occur, there is every reason to think that in the long run this process leads to the eventual development of atherosclerotic plaque. If enough plaque builds up within coronary arteries, a heart attack may occur. Humor and laughter, then, can play a crucial role in slowing down this process.

3) By Reducing Catecholamines and Inflammatory Cytokines

Lee Berk and his colleagues at Loma Linda University found that a daily diet of humor videos led to reduced levels of catecholamines (long known to have an effect on the cardiovascular system) and inflammatory cytokines, along with reduced incidence of myocardial infarction.[194] They argued that the lower level of catecholamines and cytokines played a key role in reducing the occurrence of myocardial infarction among their high-risk diabetes patients.

A second study by the same research team found that watching at least 30 minutes a day of comedy TV shows or comedy videos for 12 months reduced levels of inflammatory cytokines and C-reactive proteins (another marker of inflammation and cardiovascular disease) by 66% among diabetic patients (who were taking standard medications for diabetes, high blood pressure and high cholesterol) after four months of comedy viewing.[195] A control group receiving similar medications, but not watching comedy programs, showed only 26% decrease over the same time period. A reduced level of cytokines in response to humor has also been shown to occur among rheumatoid arthritis patients.[196]

These findings documenting reductions in markers of inflammation in response to humor and laughter are consistent with the finding of a lower sedimentation rate by Norman Cousins' doctors after he and his friends engaged in bouts of hearty laughter. (See discussion above.) But the impact of humor and laughter on sedimentation rate has never been studied systematically.

4) By increasing HDL Cholesterol

One study has—amazingly—also demonstrated that humor and laughter increase high density lipoprotein (HDL)—the good kind of cholesterol.[197] High-risk type-2 diabetes patients who also had high blood pressure and high cholesterol levels were asked to watch a comedy video or TV show at least 30 minutes a day (they chose a video on their own that they thought would be funny). A separate control group of comparable diabetic patients was not asked to watch comedy videos or TV shows. Both groups received standard medications for diabetes, high blood pressure and high cholesterol. By the second month, the humor group's HDL levels were lower than those of the control group (no differences were present at the beginning of the study). After 12 months of daily humor exposure, the humor group's HDL levels had risen 26%, in contrast to 3% for the control group.

5) By Pulling You Out of a Negative Mood and Substituting a Positive Mood in its Place

Depression and emotional distress were shown above to be significant predictors of mortality due to heart-related problems among both individuals in good and poor cardiac health. Chapter 1 documents humor's power to sustain a positive mood and substitute a positive for an already-existing negative mood. Given the ability of positive emotion to reduce cardiovascular reactivity, this mood-altering power of humor undoubtedly contributes to its ability to support a healthy heart.

Cancer

Virtually no research (to my knowledge) has yet been undertaken to determine the importance of humor and laughter in either preventing cancer or helping battle the disease among individuals already diagnosed with cancer. This is in spite of the fact that several studies have now demonstrated that humor does boost the activity of natural killer cells (which seek out and destroy tumor cells). Similarly, immunotherapy has in recent years shown promise as a tool in battling certain cancers. Immunotherapy typically uses drugs like Interleukin2 to stimulate the immune system—boosting the body's own ability to battle the cancer.

My own conversations with oncologists and oncology nurses following some of my Cancer Survivors Day programs has made it clear that many of them are unaware of the evidence pointing to humor's impact on NK cells. Others are aware, but (perhaps correctly) assume that any potential effect of humor in boosting the immune system's ability to battle cancer would be negligible.

The one exception to this void in research is the recent study of a very large group of individuals followed over a seven-year period in Norway. Among individuals diagnosed with cancer during this period, those scoring higher on a sense of humor test at the beginning of the study had a 70% higher survival rate than those with a poorer sense of humor.[198] This research is discussed below in the section on humor and longevity.

Many cancer patients have taken it upon themselves to use their sense of humor to at least help them cope—if not to directly battle the cancer. An increasing number of hospitals also now make an active effort to bring humor to their cancer patients. Over the past 15 years, I have done many programs for cancer patients (generally for National Cancer Survivors Day, in early June). More than half the time, someone comes up to me and says, "You know, you're right! If it weren't for my sense of humor, I wouldn't have survived the treatments—let alone the disease." Increasingly over the past 20 years, cancer patients have gotten the message that it is important to keep your spirits up and laugh whenever the opportunity arises.

The number of cancer patients who strongly believe in the importance of humor was evident in a study of patients in the rural Midwest, with 50% indicating that they used humor to cope with the stress of cancer.[199] Among another large group of breast cancer patients, 21% said they used humor to cope with their cancer.[200]

Over 25 years ago, Allen Funt was filming a segment for his *Candid Camera* TV show at a meeting of The Wellness Community, attended by many cancer patients. He asked those present if anyone really believed that laughter made a difference in their health. One person said,

> "I know laughter is good for me. I don't know if it is helping me get better, but *it makes me feel better—not only mentally but physically as well*—and it takes my mind off my situation. Life and its pleasures have become very real to me and I know just how important it is to enjoy each minute. *So when something strikes me as laughable, I laugh. I want to be conscious of every joyful part of life.*
>
> Before cancer, I only paid attention to the problems of life . . . and I took the pleasant and joyful parts of life as routine and as my due.
>
> That's all different now. Now I accentuate the positive and eliminate the negative. . . Most importantly, I make sure that I am aware of the good times when they come along. *So when something is funny, I laugh; and that reinforces my certainty that life is good.*"[201] (Italics are McGhee's throughout.)

Pulmonary Health

Researchers have recently begun to study the pulmonary benefits of humor and laughter. If you are already in good health, their contribution to pulmonary health is probably negligible. For individuals with a respiratory illness (or who are confined to a bed), however, the picture may be quite different. Such individuals are more likely to have a shallow breathing pattern, which leaves a larger (than desired) volume of "residual air" (the air remaining in the lungs when your outward breath is replaced by the next inhalation) in the lungs. More active individuals breathe out more of the residual air and replace it on a regular basis with new oxygen-enriched air.

The risk associated with excess residual air in the lungs on an ongoing basis lies in the fact that there is a progressive buildup in this air of both water vapor and carbon dioxide. This leaves shallow breathers and chronically inactive people at greater risk of pulmonary infection. As this residual air stays in the lungs for longer periods of time, its oxygen content drops, and the levels of water vapor and carbon dioxide increase.[202] Again, the health risk here arises for individuals already prone to respiratory difficulties, since the increased water vapor creates a more favorable environment for bacterial growth and pulmonary infection.[203]

You know from your own experience, however, that there is a dramatic change in your breathing pattern when you have a good belly laugh. When you laugh, you repeatedly push air out of your lungs (with each "ha") until you can't push out any more. Then you take a deep breath and start the same process all over again. This is repeated over and over until the exhilarating feeling of amusement has passed. Each time you laugh, you get rid of the excess carbon dioxide and water vapor that's built up and replace it with oxygen-rich air. So frequent belly laughter reduces the risk of pulmonary infection by emptying your lungs of more of the air that's taken in.

Hospitalized patients with respiratory problems are often encouraged to breathe deeply and exhale fully, but nurses generally have difficulty getting them to do so. Most patients enjoy a good laugh, though, so many nurses have learned to tell them a joke from time to time or give them a comedy tape to view. This automatically achieves the respiratory goals the nurse has for the patient. This is also one reason why many nursing homes now provide comedy programs to their residents on a regular basis (especially humor from their early adult years that still makes seniors laugh).

A 90-year-old woman went to see a new doctor. He asked her how she was doing, so she gave him the full list of complaints—this hurts, that's stiff, I'm tired and slower, etc.

He responded with, "Mrs. Weiss, you have to expect things to start deteriorating at this point in life. After all, who wants to live to 100?"

She looked him in the eye and said, "Anyone who's 99."

If you've ever had a good belly laugh in the midst of a cold, you're sure to have noticed that the laughing quickly turns into coughing. The laughing and coughing reflexes are very similar, so the laughter is quickly overtaken by persistent coughing. This laughing-coughing link is normally just an annoyance, since coughing is not nearly as enjoyable as laughing (as noted in Chapter 3, humor and laughter activate known pleasure or reward centers in the brain; while no one has yet studied the impact of coughing on these reward centers, I would bet my retirement fund that they are not activated by a hacking cough).

There are some conditions, however, in which the laugh-cough connection is a good thing. For example, nurses and respiratory therapists often encourage certain patients to cough to help discharge mucous plugs accumulating in the respiratory tract. The problem is that even well-motivated patients have a difficult time following through on the advice to cough periodically. But if you can get patients laughing from time to time, this problem takes care of itself. The laughter triggers coughing and automatically achieves the goal of clearing mucous from the respiratory system—and the patients have a good time in the process.

A pulmonary researcher has emphasized to me, however, that there are good coughs and bad coughs when it comes to many pulmonary conditions.[204] A good cough is one that clears out mucous plugs; a bad one is irritating and actually causes more inflammation. In cases where the lungs are already inflamed, repetitive coughing (which is likely to be triggered by laughter) just worsens the irritation and inflammation.

COPD. Intuitively, you would assume that laughter would not be a good idea for patients with chronic obstructive pulmonary disease, or COPD—a condition (which may result from emphysema or chronic bronchitis) characterized by generally irreversible airway obstruction (air trapping), resulting in a slowed rate of exhalation. In COPD, the bronchial passages are seriously impaired in their ability to rid the lungs of air, leading to hyperinflation. "Pursed lip" breathing is often recommended to help patients get a good exchange of air in the lungs. Bronchodilators are also used to help empty air and reduce the level of hyperinflation.

On the one hand, you might expect the forcefulness of hearty laughter to help force more air through the bronchi and reduce the level of trapped air. We know that laughter does reduce residual air in the lungs of healthy individuals.[205] But if the laughter does not successfully push out trapped air in COPD patients, it could actually cause more air to get trapped in the lungs. When a healthy person laughs hard, a series of expiratory pushes (the "ha ha's") rapidly forces air out until we run out of air. We then take a quick deep breath and continue pushing air out until the hilarity settles down. For a COPD patient, if the lungs do not permit this rapid expulsion of air, the deep inspirations could actually increase the level of trapped air. This is why slow and steady breathing is generally seen as the way to go for these patients.

One very recent study has taken the first step toward determining the possible value or harm of laughter for COPD patients.[206] Lung volume was measured in patients with severe COPD and healthy controls both before and after a performance by a clown within the hospital. (COPD patients have greater lung volume in their residual air, as well as immediately after a full inspiration—defined as "total lung capacity" or TLC—in comparison to healthy individuals). This was a very funny clown who worked well with adults, and a lot of laughter occurred among both patients and the control adults. Total lung capacity was significantly reduced among the COPD patients, but not in the control group. (This reduction in TLC was relatively short-lived, however; it was no longer present two hours later.) Among those patients showing the greatest reduction of TLC (10% or more), there was a sharp drop in residual air volume. This suggests that a reduction in air-trapping did occur for them.

Since one concern prior to this study was whether laughter would even be safe for COPD patients, it should be noted that the researchers concluded that mild laughter is safe for this patient group—even for patients with severe COPD. But they also found that patients showing the most intense laughter did show increased hyperinflation. It was "gentle" laughter that was associated with reduced lung volume. This suggests that *COPD patients should be cautioned to restrict their laughter to more moderate levels.*

Of special interest is the finding that those patients who showed the greatest reduction in trapped residual air smiled more than patients showing minimal reduction in trapped residual air. So smiling may actually be more beneficial than laughter in helping COPD patients get rid of trapped air and breathe more easily. These researchers specifically recommended that smiling-while-breathing be considered as an additional breathing technique, along with the traditional pursed-lip breathing. To be most effective, this should be encouraged in the context of comedy videos, friendly banter, or any other approach to generating amusement in patients.

Asthma. Another pulmonary condition for which a health-promoting benefit from humor has been demonstrated is asthma. Asthma is a chronic respiratory condition in which breathing is impaired because of muscle spasms, mucous and inflammation of the airways. The airway inflammation makes the paths through the lungs smaller, resulting in coughing or chest tightness and difficulty moving air in and out. In the year 2000, asthma affected over 17 million Americans, resulting in 5400 deaths and half a million hospitalizations annually.[207]

The new interest in humor's impact on asthma sufferers lies in the fact that we have long known that stress and negative emotion lead to constriction of the airways among individuals with bronchial asthma.[208] One's emotional state, of course, is just one trigger (among others) for asthmatic attacks. But given humor's power to quickly pull you out of a negative emotional state and substitute a positive one in its place, it is an ideal tool to help asthmatics gain some control over this particular cause of airway constriction.

The best demonstration of humor's potential in preventing (or reducing the severity of) attacks of bronchial asthma was provided by a Japanese researcher. Hajime Kimata administered a substance (metacholine) known to cause bronchoconstriction (resulting in increased airway resistance and greater difficulty breathing) to both healthy individuals and people suffering from asthma.[209] All subjects in the study then watched both a humorous and a control (nonhumorous) video. The funny video reduced the level of both healthy and asthmatic subjects' negative mood and increased their positive mood (the two mood measures were obtained separately). While the funny video had no impact on healthy subjects' airways, it reduced the level of bronchial constriction among asthmatics. *So humor enabled them to breathe more easily.*

These are exciting findings for asthma suffers, but it may be premature to conclude that humor is a key tool in managing attacks for everyone suffering from asthma, since the act of laughter itself triggers asthmatic attacks in some people—about 1/3 of asthma patients, according to one study[210] and 56% in another.[211] The key here may again be how hard you laugh, with extended belly laughter bringing on the attack. The research is not yet clear on this point. In the Kimata study, all participants laughed during the funny video, but the laughter was certainly not the kind of extreme laughter we have all experienced at times—where something is just so funny you can't stop laughing. It has been suggested that asthmatic children may be especially vulnerable to this kind of laughter.[212] If this is the case, then humor obviously becomes a health risk for these individuals—not a source of healing and wellness.

Humor (in the absence of extreme laughter) is not alone in its capacity to alleviate asthmatic symptoms. Other positive emotional states also relieve airway constriction in individuals with bronchial asthma.[213] On the other hand, non-humorous forms of positive emotion can sometimes increase airway resistance (making it more difficult to breathe).[214] When this restriction of airway passages does occur in response to positive emotion, however, it is generally less severe than that which occurs in response to negative emotion.

A man went to see his doctor because he was feeling miserable. His doctor spent weeks trying to diagnose the source of his problems, with no success. Over the weeks, he prescribed a series of pills, shots, exercises . . . even dietary changes, but nothing helped.

On his last visit, the doctor told the man to go home and take a hot bath. As soon as he was finished bathing he was to throw open all the windows and stand in the draft.

"But Doc, if I do that, I'll get pneumonia."

"I know," said the doctor, "but I can cure pneumonia!"

The key to making sense out of these apparent inconsistencies in asthma research is not whether the emotion experienced is positive or negative; rather, it is the level of "emotional arousal" experienced in connection with either kind of emotion.[215] It appears to be events that are highly emotionally arousing that create breathing problems for asthmatics. In the case of humor, then, *moderately funny humor accompanied by mild laughter should support good pulmonary function among asthmatics, while extreme funniness accompanied by extended hearty laughter should interfere with it.*

The unique nature of laughter also contributes to the confusion about its role in triggering or relieving asthma attacks. Laughter is a vigorous muscular activity, but—as discussed earlier—also causes muscle relaxation (some muscles relax while you're laughing; others relax after you stop). In the case of asthma, it used to be assumed (two decades ago) that any form of behavioral relaxation would improve lung function—that it would relax the bronchi, leading to easier breathing.[216] There is no evidence, though, to support the view that muscle relaxation elsewhere in the body relaxes the bronchi.[217] In fact, the opposite turns out to be the case. For both healthy and asthmatic individuals, muscle activity or exercise causes dilation of the airways.

The key here is that *brief* muscle activation should occur to get the dilation effect. For example, simply briefly activating the facial muscles facilitates breathing among asthmatics, leading one expert in the field to suggest that "...*brief dynamic exercise of the facial muscles should be practiced to induce bronchodilation.*" [218] (Italics are McGhee's.) *Mild laughter, and its accompanying exercise of several facial muscles, then, is just what the doctor ordered.* However, if you have asthma and notice that other forms of moderate exercise trigger asthma attacks in you,

you should probably make a special effort to stifle your laughter since this form of exercise is likely to trigger an attack in you, as well.[219]

BUILD YOUR HUMOR SKILLS

[Work on both jokes before checking the answers.]

1. A man felt his way into an optometrist's office, stumbling as he went. He said, "I sat on my glasses and broke them. Will the doctor have to examine me all over again?" The receptionist said, "No, just _____."
Clue: This is really more like a kid's joke. Focus on the words "all over."

2. A new nurse noticed that Dr. Tinsley would periodically shout out "tetanus!," "flu!," "measles!" or "typhoid!". She finally asked another nurse, "Why does he do that?" "Oh," said the other nurse, "he just likes to _____ around here."
Clue: He likes to be (or sound) in charge.

The chances of laughter causing an asthmatic attack may depend on how well a patient's asthma is under control at the time. Patients have reported that they can laugh longer without symptoms when their asthma is well controlled. This means that laughter-induced asthma (especially when the laughter is mild) may be used as a signal that the patient needs to get the asthma under better control.

As noted above, strong negative emotion is a common trigger for asthma attacks. While the role of emotion in asthma is complicated (in that the intensity of the emotion may be more important than whether it is positive or negative), it becomes even more confusing in view of evidence that suppressing negative emotions can worsen breathing problems for asthmatics. One researcher concluded after an extensive review of the evidence that "suppression or inadequate expression of emotions were far more important in the precipitation of attacks of asthma than the type of emotion experienced."[220] This puts asthmatics in somewhat of a "can't win" situation. Both expressing and holding in anxiety or anger can cause an attack. But this really does make sense, since holding in negative emotions just keeps us stewing in our emotional juices—sustaining or even increasing the level of emotion experienced.

The key for asthmatics, then, is to find a way to manage their emotions on a regular basis—a way that helps prevent negative emotions from occurring and pulls them out of negative moods when they do occur. As discussed in Chapter 1, humor is ideally suited to achieving this goal.

Arthritis

Rheumatoid arthritis (RA) is an autoimmune disease which is characterized by progressive destruction of joints. Its cause is not yet understood, but certain inflammation-inducing cytokines play a major role in triggering the inflammation and tissue destruction.[221] Three Japanese studies have now shown that listening to an hour-long traditional Japanese comic story ("Rakugo") told by a professional story teller significantly reduced the level of the pro-inflammatory cytokine interleukin 6 (IL-6) in RA patients.[222] When the RA patients were split into those whose disease symptoms were easily managed or difficult to manage, this effect was strongest for those whose disease conditions were difficult to manage.[223] Since stressful life events worsen the joint symptoms associated with RA,[224] using humor or other effective tools to manage daily stress is especially important for people whose RA is difficult to manage.

Growth hormone (GH) has also been shown to be associated with joint swelling and pain in RA patients. But, again, exposure to a traditional Rakugo story resulted in reduced levels of serum GH in RA patients, but not in healthy individuals.[225] In fact, the humor—in this case—reduced the RA patients' GH levels to a level similar to that of the healthy subjects.

Allergies

The role of humor and laughter in managing allergic reactions has also been studied, and the early evidence suggests that laughter (or the humor that triggers it) helps counteract certain allergies. (It should be noted that stress often increases allergic response.)[226] Again, it is the Japanese researcher Hajime Kimata who has completed several breakthrough studies along these lines. For example, laughter while watching a comedy video reduced an allergic skin response in patients with dermatitis,[227] as well as an allergen-specific (a particular kind of Japanese cedar tree) immunoglobulin E response among patients with dermatitis.[228]

ANSWERS TO JOKES

1. your eyes
2. call the shots

Dr. Kimata has also shown in more than one study that watching a tear-producing movie similarly reduces the level of allergic response.[229] This is reminiscent of the finding (discussed above) that certain types of negative emotion reduce pain, just as humor and laughter do. It is not clear how to interpret these findings when it comes to the role of emotion in supporting wellness. But if sadness-inducing and joy-inducing experiences eventually prove to be equally effective in reducing the level of one's allergic response, I—for one—will always go for the funny approach.

Atopic (meaning that it's probably hereditary) eczema (AE) is a common form of chronic allergy-linked dermatitis (inflammation of the skin). Patients who have AE tend to suffer frequent bacteria-induced infections, including infections from *Staphylococcus aureus* bacteria.[230] The use of antibiotics does help battle this disease, but there are concerns that the prolonged use of antibiotics may produce drug-resistant strains of *Staphylococcus aureus*. Given the evidence documenting the positive impact of humor and laughter upon certain types of allergic response, along with the evidence showing a generalized immunoenhancement effect of humor and laughter (including increased scavenging for free radicals), Dr. Kimata speculated that humor and laughter might enhance antimicrobial immunity in other body fluids, as well—including sweat.

He has shown that this is, indeed, the case. AE patients have deficient levels of a peptide called dermcidin, and low levels of dermcidin from sweat glands have been linked to increased colonization of skin bacteria.[231] Antimicrobial peptides appear to be derived from dermcidin. Watching a 90-minute comedy film (Charlie Chaplin) significantly increased the levels of dermcidin from these patients' sweat glands.[232] Given this promising finding for a single comedy movie, Dr. Kimata had 14 patients with AE watch funny videos daily for one week—with no medication. Patients' dermcidin levels increased and—most importantly—"the number of patients colonized by *S. aureus* [bacteria] decreased from 14 (before viewing) to 4 (after viewing)." So humor and laughter are helpful in battling yet another disease condition—apparently as a result of a strengthened or more aroused immune system.

As a side note, atopic dermatitis patients often have difficulty sleeping through the night. Children with this condition were found to have less night-time awakening following viewing of a humorous film (a non-humorous film had no effect).[233]

The health benefits of breast feeding for babies have long been known. Dr. Kimata has shown that humor and laughter among breast feeding mothers also help their babies battle at least one kind of allergy. Mothers again watched a 90-minute Charlie Chaplin film (or a non-humorous control film). Breastfed babies with atopic eczema showed reduced levels of allergic skin response (to latex and house dust mite) following viewing of the comedy film (but not the control film).[234] The reason for this effect is not clear, but Dr. Kimata did note that the laughter increased levels of melatonin in mothers' breast milk. Melatonin is a hormone that has been associated with relaxation, and people with eczema generally have low levels of it. His guess at this point is that the relaxation effect resulting from laughter is responsible for the increased melatonin levels following the funny film, and that the increase in melatonin reduces allergic responses by "inhibiting mast cell responses." (Mast cells are large cells in connective tissue that contain substances that mediate allergic reactions.) As with the new asthma-humor research, these initial findings hold exciting promise for yet another wellness-promoting benefit of humor and laughter. More research along these lines is sure to follow in the near future.

Diabetes

The rapidly increasing prevalence of diabetes in the U. S. is well documented. The health risk of diabetes, of course, occurs when blood glucose levels get dangerously high. People with diabetes are unable to naturally produce the appropriate levels of insulin required for the body to use the glucose present in the blood, causing blood sugar to get too high. If not managed well, persistent high glucose levels can lead to circulatory problems (sometimes resulting in amputation), heart disease, stroke, kidney failure or blindness.

Can humor and laughter help keep blood glucose levels under control—or even reduce the risk of developing diabetes to begin with? *While there is no reason to expect humor to be helpful in preventing diabetes, it is helpful in managing it.* A different team of Japanese researchers, led by Dr. Takashi Hayashi, recently plunged into this totally unexplored area by having both healthy individuals and diabetics first listen to a monotonous 40-minute college lecture and then (on a different day) sit in on a 40-minute comedy show (as part of an audience of 1000 people). The healthy and diabetic groups had identical meals prior to attending these events. Among the healthy subjects, there was no difference between blood glucose levels following the comedy and serious lecture. But among diabetics, glucose levels were significantly lower following the comedy show (most subjects in both groups rated themselves as laughing a lot during the comedy presentation).

So the *laughter (or humor) served to reduce the level of blood glucose increase "in the presence of insufficient insulin action."*[235] It was concluded that "This favorable effect of laughter may include the acceleration of glucose utilization by the muscle action [of laughter] during the comedy show. However, it is possible that positive emotions such as laughter acted on the neuroendocrine system and suppressed the elevation of blood glucose level."

In any case, the researchers suggested that these findings point to *"the importance of daily opportunities for laughter in patients with diabetes."* (Italics are McGhee's.) This glucose-reducing effect of humor and laughter was subsequently replicated by the same research team in three additional studies,[236] so this is now a well-established finding. It was not determined whether the key to lowering glucose levels was the experience of humor or the laughter that followed. But this finding is especially noteworthy in view of evidence that negative emotion tends to increase blood glucose level among diabetics.[237] A similar follow-up study showed that humor and laughter help counter the neuropathy (any disease of the nerves) that often accompanies diabetes.[238]

The key question here, of course, is what is responsible for this important glucose-lowering effect of humor/laughter in diabetics. A summary of the researchers' explanation (included here because of its importance) is provided here, but the answer is a highly technical one. There is evidence that what is called the "renin–angiotensin system" may play an important role in diabetes. Renin is an enzyme produced by the kidneys that helps produce angiotensin, a protein that—among other things—causes constriction of blood vessels. This system plays an important role in the maintenance of normal blood pressure and electrolyte balance.[239] High blood sugar levels stimulate the production of renin.[240] Individuals with diabetes show elevated levels of renin in the blood, and this elevated renin appears to be associated with microvascular problems in diabetics.[241] These vascular complications often occur in the kidney, retina (e.g., diabetic retinopathy or blindness) or nervous system. So anything which reduces blood renin levels should reduce these vascular complications and support better health in diabetics.

Mr. Jones goes to the doctor's office to collect his wife's test results. The lab tech says, "I'm sorry, but there has been a mix-up and we have a problem. When we sent the samples from your wife to the lab, they got mixed up with the samples of another Mrs.

Jones, and we are now uncertain which one is your wife's. Frankly, it is either bad or terrible news!"

"What do you mean?"

"Well, one Mrs. Jones has tested positive for Alzheimer's and the other for AIDS. We can't tell which is your wife."

"That's terrible! Can we do the test over?"

"Normally, yes. But you have an HMO, and they won't pay for these expensive tests more than once."

"Well, what am I supposed to do now?"

"The HMO recommends that you drop your wife off in the middle of town. If she finds her way home, don't sleep with her."

This same Japanese research team exposed diabetic patients (all had type 2 diabetes and were not receiving insulin) to a six-month regimen of watching comedy videos once a week. At the beginning of the study, these diabetic subjects' plasma renin concentration was five times higher than that typical of non–diabetics. *By the third month of watching comedy videos, this concentration had dropped (on the average) by 2/3, and the drop was maintained into the sixth month. The drop put the renin levels into the normal range for 50% of the participating subjects.*

Parallel to these changes, angiotensin levels decreased over the first three months of the study (and were sustained through the sixth month). The researchers speculated that laughter-linked hormonal changes (see discussion of hormones above and in Chapter 1) may play a role in causing these changes. They suggested that the effect of laughter on the endocrine system might be to "suppress the secretion of renin from the kidney and stimulate the synthesis of angiotensinogen from the liver." In any case, the key benefit for diabetics is the significant drop in renin and its health-damaging potential. The researchers concluded that "*laughter therapy can be used as a non-pharmacological treatment for the prevention of diabetic microvascular complications.*"[242] (Italics are McGhee's.)

Another benefit from humor in connection with diabetes lies in the communication between patients and their physician. Medical noncompliance is common in connection with most diseases, but it is especially high among diabetics (where complex regimens involving medication, diet and exercise must be followed).[243] Many patients do not communicate their lack of compliance with eating guidelines—especially when the communication style adopted by their doctor is an authoritative or negative one.[244] Establishing a lighter style (by the doctor) of inquiring about compliance habits helps establish trust in the doctor–patient relationship and may also increase commitment to compliance with eating regimens.

Impact of Humor and Laughter upon Gene Expression. As the field of mind/body medicine has continued its explosive growth over the past 25 years, the inevitable question of whether one's emotional state (or "mind" in general) can influence the basic expression of one's genes has been raised.[245] The same Japanese research team of Takashi Hayashi and his colleagues have obtained evidence that humor and laughter can alter gene expression. (As noted in the discussion of the immune system, they also found that humor and laughter up-regulate the expression of genes related to NK cell activity.) They studied the effect of humor and laughter on prorenin, a precursor of the kidney enzyme renin. Again using diabetic patients in a design similar to the one discussed above (watching a boring lecture vs. a live comedy show), they found that prorenin levels were significantly higher in diabetic than normal individuals. (Prorenin is involved in diabetic complications.) These

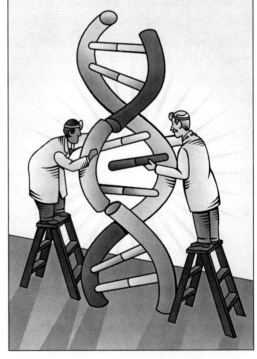

levels were not influenced by the comedy show in non–diabetics, but dropped sharply following the comedy viewing in diabetics—

including both those who had and had not already suffered some degree of nephropathy (kidney damage).[246] This supports the notion that diabetic patients would do well to build more humor and laughter into their lives.

Perhaps the most exciting finding from this study was that it demonstrated that humor and laughter influence the expression of inherited genes. Initially, ". . . the prorenin receptor gene was less expressed in the patients . . . compared with normal subjects . . . [but] This gene was up-regulated significantly . . . after watching the comedy show."[247] The comedy had no significant impact on the expression of this gene in the non-diabetic subjects. Given the suggestion that a decreased expression of this prorenin receptor gene is to some extent responsible for the increased blood prorenin concentrations that contribute to the exacerbation of diabetes-related problems,[248] this ability of humor/laughter to up-regulate expression of prorenin receptor genes (thereby reducing microvascular complications that accompany diabetes) is an exciting finding.

Similar findings were obtained in a follow-up study. Again, laughter decreased blood levels of prorenin. Laughter "normalized the expression of the prorenin receptor gene . . . this demonstrated the inhibitory effects of laughter on the onset/deterioration of diabetic complications at the gene-expression level."[249] *If humor and laughter are capable of influencing gene expression in ways that promote health and wellness in connection with diabetes, it may well be that this is one of the key (but now poorly understood) mechanisms by which humor sustains health in general.* This is an area that researchers are sure to tackle in the years ahead.

> **"Mrs. Torrence, you were supposed to lose some weight by your next visit," said the doctor. "But you've gained 20 pounds since I last saw you. What happened to your diet?"**
>
> **"Well, to tell you the truth, doctor, I've been off my diet for a month of sundaes."**

It was noted earlier that humor and laughter up-regulate genes specifically related to natural killer cell activity. The subjects used in that study all had type 2 diabetes. Given that humor and laughter do help keep blood glucose utilization under control among diabetics, the researchers speculated that it may be this up-regulation of NK cell-related genes which is responsible for the blood glucose ameliorating effect.[250] This is consistent with the finding that injecting animals with NK cells improves glucose intolerance.[251]

Humor as a Weight-Loss Technique

Another threat to health today is the rapidly growing number of Americans suffering from obesity. While humor is very effective in both preventing emotional weight-gain (think of it as a "stress-deodorant") and losing emotional weight once you've gained it, can it help you let go of those unwanted physical pounds? Your body is doing a lot of work when you have a real belly laugh. Just observe your own heart rate and loss of breath the next time you share hearty laughter with your friends if you have any doubts about this.

Amazingly, the amount of energy expended during laughter has now been determined. That expenditure is about 10-20% higher than the energy expended during inactivity or rest.[252] (Jogging can increase energy expenditure up to 100%.) As you would expect, the more intense the laughter, the greater the amount of energy expended. The researchers conducting this study concluded that a daily average of 15 minutes of laughter a day would utilize 10-40 kcal a day, depending on the person's weight and the intensity of the laughter. Other things being equal, this would result in a weight loss of 1.1 to 4.4 pounds a year. So, if you're looking for a good source of health-related motivation to build more humor into your life, focus on the emotional weight loss, not physical weight loss.

Do People with a Good Sense of Humor Get Sick Less Often?

Throughout this chapter, we have seen many pieces of evidence that humor and laughter positively influence your body in ways that promote health and wellness. This suggests that people with a better sense of humor should get sick less often. Surprisingly, very little attention has been given to this question. Some of this limited research was discussed above in connection with specific diseases. But what about common minor illnesses like colds and flu? Can humor help here? Since humor appears to boost IgA levels, and those with higher levels of salivary IgA are less likely to get colds[253] or be infected with Streptococcus,[254] a good sense of humor—or a daily diet of lots of humor from "outside" sources—should reduce the frequency of colds.

Diets are for those who are thick and tired of it.

The waist is a terrible thing to mind.

The only study to directly examine this question found that the impact of one's sense of humor upon colds depends on the kind of sense of humor you have.[255] It was only individuals whose sense of humor took the form of seeking out and appreciating humor from outside sources (not initiated by themselves) who had fewer and less severe colds/flu than their low humor counterparts. Surprisingly, those whose sense of humor took the form of initiating humor more often did not have fewer or less severe colds/flu. The researchers argued that being a person who likes to tell jokes or otherwise initiate humor takes them into more frequent contact with other people, which serves to expose them to infectious agents more often, robbing them of the advantage that a more active sense of humor otherwise offers. Obviously, more research is required to clear up this confusing picture. (Recall from Chapter 1 that, until recently, researchers failed to distinguish between positive and negative styles of humor, and that this appears to be an important factor influencing the extent of positive benefits associated with humor.)

The importance of active use of one's sense of humor in producing any health benefits was confirmed, however, in another unusual way. Among mothers of newborn infants, those who actively used humor to cope with the stress in their lives had fewer upper respiratory infections—and their infants also had fewer infections.[256] This seemed to be because these mothers had higher levels of immunoglobulin A in their breast milk. Other similar findings showed that mothers with low levels of IgA at the time of birth had babies who showed more illnesses in the first six weeks postpartum.[257] So breast-feeding mothers now have all the more reason to build plenty of laughter in their life every day. Consistent with these findings, among children battling cancer, those scoring higher on a sense of humor measure reported fewer infections than young cancer patients with low sense of humor scores.[258]

Among adults, if we look at bodily symptoms alone, independent of any diagnosed illness, higher scores on a sense of humor test are associated with better self-reported health and fewer self-reported illness symptoms.[259] Individuals who have more negative reactions to humor (finding a lot of different types of humor aversive or objectionable) report more bodily symptoms and complaints[260] and complain more often of cardiovascular symptoms.[261]

In the study of patients in a rehabilitation hospital described earlier, 94% of the patients indicated that when they laughed, they felt better.[262] Finally, sense of humor has been shown to be positively correlated with perceptions of one's own health among both college students[263] and older adults.[264]

While the bulk of evidence does support a positive link between sense of humor and health, some studies have not been supportive.[265] It is not clear why these inconsistencies exist. However, we have noted several times that the distinction between positive and negative components of one's sense of humor is important when considering the coping benefits of humor. Since the research failing to show a positive relationship between humor and general indicators of health and wellness was done before measures making this distinction were developed, this may account for their failure to show a consistent positive relationship with health.

Another clue to the failure of some studies to show the expected positive relationship between sense of humor and health may lie in the recent finding that among middle-aged police chiefs, having a stronger sense of humor was also associated with factors known to interfere with good health, including a higher body mass index (i.e., being overweight), increased alcohol consumption and increased smoking.[266] So *it may be that many people with a good sense of humor also engage more often in behaviors known to be negative influences on health.* Any such behaviors would tend to counteract the positive outcomes resulting from humor and laughter and cloud the relationship between a sense of humor and health. Researchers are only now beginning to study this issue.

Other recent evidence suggests that individuals with a good sense of humor may have fewer health-related concerns and preoccupations in general. Those scoring higher on a sense of humor measure worried less about illness and pain and were less preoccupied in general with "negative bodily sensations."[267] They also expressed less fear of death and serious diseases—including cancer and heart disease. In contrast to the police chief study, however, these high sense of humor college students did not engage in more risky health-related behavior. If the link of sense of humor to risky behavior does occur, then, it may begin to show up beyond the college years.

It is hard to imagine a greater stressor for children than a diagnosis of cancer. If a good sense of humor does have an immunoenhancement effect among children, it would be wonderful to demonstrate that it is also occurring among pediatric cancer patients. Among elementary-school aged children with cancer, those who more often used humor to cope had higher levels of (salivary) IgA and a lower frequency of different kinds of infections.[268] As the level of cancer-related stress increased for these children, the high-coping–humor kids were significantly less likely than the low-coping–humor kids to come down with infections. *This reduced infection finding is especially important, since it suggests that the immunoenhancement effect of humor is strong enough to help sustain other aspects of health and wellness as these children and their doctors battle the cancer.*

"For my sister's 50th birthday, I sent her a singing mammogram."   (Steven Wright)

As noted earlier in this chapter, coronary heart disease has long been linked to the so-called Type A personality. It was observed over 25 years ago that only type B individuals use humor as a coping tool in dealing with stress and hostile feelings.[269] Hostile humor has also been found to be the main kind of humor enjoyed by Type A patients, while Type B patients enjoy non-hostile as well as hostile humor.[270] This is consistent with the findings showing a close relationship between hostility and heart disease. While laughter at hostile humor may provide some benefits for CHD-prone individuals, those benefits are not enough to offset the negative bodily effects caused by hostility to begin with. Developing non-hostile aspects of one's sense of humor to counteract this effect is essential for Type A individuals.

Does Humor Increase Longevity?

For about 20 years, the letterhead on my stationary has included the phrase, "They who laugh, last." I love this idea, since it captures the notion that humor helps endure or cope with the most difficult of life circumstances. It could also be interpreted to mean that those with a better sense of humor live longer. This is a claim that is often made, and people generally point to famous comedians or humorous performers who lived very long lives (like George Burns, Bob Hope, Victor Borge or Red Skelton from decades past) to back up the idea.

To this point, we have seen that humor and laughter make important contributions to health. But can humor lead to a longer life? The discussion of PNI research above presented evidence showing that positive emotion from other sources *does* predict survival rates—both among healthy individuals and people who are seriously ill. So there is every reason to think that humor may add years to your life. And there is some support for this idea.

Dr. Sven Svebak, a psychologist in Norway, tracked the health status of 54,000 fellow Norwegians over a seven-year period. When he looked only at those who developed cancer during this period, *individuals scoring higher on a measure of sense of humor at the beginning of the study (2015 patients) had a 70% higher survival rate* than those with lower sense of humor scores.[271]

An elderly man hobbles into the doctor's waiting room full of a bunch of seniors and collapses into the chair next to an alert, but white-haired gentleman with sallow, wrinkled skin. The hobbling man says, "Whatcha in here for?"

"Just a general checkup," says the other.

"Well, you look pretty good to me. What's your secret?"

No secret. I drink a quart of bourbon a day, smoke a cigar, and am out late with a young woman most nights."

"That's amazing," said the first. "How old are you?"

"Twenty four."

Dr. Svebak also studied a group of patients who had been diagnosed with end-stage renal (kidney) failure. Forty-six percent of them died during the following two years. Again, *sense of humor predicted who survived longer. Those scoring above the median on a sense of humor scale increased their odds of survival by 31%.*[272] While the cause of the better survival rate of these high sense of humor individuals is not clear, Dr. Svebak concluded that the most important factor was probably the better coping skills shared by those with a better sense of humor. These superior coping skills, he argued, reduced the health-deteriorating effects of disease-related stressors typically experienced by these patients. The last 25 years of research on mind-body relationships have made it clear that better coping skills, along with other "psychological" variables are closely linked to underlying neurophysiological changes which either support or interfere with good health. In the years ahead, we can expect to better understand just how these changes contribute to improved kidney functioning/health.

Even if humor does not add years to your life, it certainly adds life to your years.

While the above findings are promising in their suggestion that humor and laughter may lead to a longer life, there is also some evidence that is inconsistent with this conclusion. Cheerfulness as a long-standing personality trait is one quality that tends to go with a better sense of humor. In an analysis of data of more than 1000 individuals from a famous long-term longitudinal study (known as the Terman Life Cycle Study, begun in 1921), individuals found to be more cheerful at an earlier point in their lives (this was assessed at age 12) actually had *higher* death rates throughout their lifetimes than less cheerful people.[273] The explanation offered for this surprising finding was that these more cheerful people actually tended to engage in more risky behaviors than their less cheerful peers. Like the high sense of humor police chiefs discussed earlier, more cheerful people smoked more, drank more alcohol and engaged more often in other behaviors known to be health risks.[274]

The specific health-promoting effects of humor and laughter discussed throughout this chapter, then, may be countered in everyday life among those with a strong sense of humor by behavior that interferes with health and wellness. *There may be on ongoing tug-of-war between health-promoting and health-weakening influences in the bodies of those with a good sense of humor throughout their lives. The outcome of this battle would obviously be unique to each individual. The overall balance of positive vs. negative health influence here would depend on the extent of daily illness-promoting behaviors. The greater the frequency and extreme to which illness-promoting behaviors occur on an ongoing basis, the greater the extent to which any health-promoting benefits of humor and laughter would be canceled out.*

The Humor-in-Hospitals Movement

You've probably never been in a hospital with a humor program. The very idea of humor in hospitals may even strike you as an oxymoron (like "giant shrimp" or "smart bombs"). If ever there were two things that don't go together, it is humor and hospitals. After all, hospitals are places for the very sick.

The last decade, however, has witnessed a (slowly building) revolution in health care, as more and more hospitals become convinced of the therapeutic power of humor. The humor-in-hospitals movement has also gained support because of the growing trend toward depersonalization in recent years, as focus has shifted away from the person and toward application of the latest technology. Many patients now crave a more personalized and human relationship with care providers, and humor helps establish it. Also, a growing number of hospitals now recognize the importance of providing care that supports patients' emotional, as well as physical needs. Humor is increasingly being viewed as a means of filling the need for such "patient-centered care."[275]

BUILD YOUR HUMOR SKILLS

[Work on both jokes before checking the answers.]

1. A man long known to be a heavy drinker hears from his doctor, "Even with all our tests, I can't find any cause for your illness; but frankly, I think it's due to drinking." "In that case," said the patient, "I'll come back when _____."
Clue: The patient thinks the doctor has been drinking.

2. A woman kept going to the eye doctor because here eye hurt all the time. The doctor finally discovered the cause of the problem and told her to stop drinking tea. The patient protested, "But I love my morning tea." "OK," said the doctor, "as long as you _____."
Clue: The problem is not the tea itself, but the way she drinks it.

Hospitals within the United States have become increasingly competitive in recent years. This has led to a greater preoccupation within upper management with levels of patient satisfaction related to their hospital stay. Humor—in combination with providing the best medical care possible—is being seen by some hospitals as a tool for boosting patient satisfaction scores.[276]

What's the difference between an oral thermometer and a rectal thermometer? The taste.

Most patients arrive at the hospital in a state of stress and anxiety. They are then placed in a strange environment, submitted to degrading and embarrassing procedures by people they don't know and have their independence and sense of control removed—and they don't always get the explanations they would like for procedures or tests. Humor provides a means of establishing a more personal relationship between patients and hospital staff, easing tensions and anxiety and helping patients cope. The nurse who maintains a high level of competence, but also has a "light touch," has an extra way of saying, "I care."

Children are especially vulnerable to anxiety upon admission to the hospital. The importance of addressing these anxieties is evident in the fact that more than three million children will require hospital care in the USA in a typical year these days. In addition to the emotional demands of struggling with the illness itself, children have little understanding of the hospital environment and the procedures they must submit to—not to mention a complete lack of control.[277] Additional stress comes from separation from their family and the pain resulting from very intrusive procedures. In fact, children report pain to be the most upsetting part of being in the hospital and that any kind of diversional activity to counter this is appreciated.[278]

Nurses and hospital administrators are often concerned that patients will perceive them as unprofessional and unconcerned about their health problems if they show a sense of humor while interacting with patients. Most patients, however, appear to welcome the opportunity for humor and a chance to laugh during their hospital stay. The figures in brackets indicate the percentage of patients in one study who *agreed* with the following statements:

"Nurses should laugh more often with patients." [80%]
"Nurses should try to get their patients to laugh." [83%]
"Laughing helps me get through difficult times." [83%]

The following statements generated strong *disagreement* by the same patients:

"Nurses who laugh with patients are unprofessional." [94%]
"Nurses who laugh are insensitive to patients who are suffering." [91%]
"Laughter does not belong in a rehabilitation hospital." [89%][279]

Humor is just as important when the patients are children. Almost half of the hospitalized children in another study said that humor and other light-hearted interactions with nurses were important in adjusting to their hospital stay.[280]

One nurse to another: "What do you give a man who has everything?" "Amoxicillin."

As a result of the steadily mounting evidence of humor's importance for both physical and mental health, physicians have finally begun discussing among themselves just what the role of humor should be in healthcare. They are finally asking questions like "When is it okay to joke with patients? When is it not okay . . . When is it okay to laugh about cancer?"[281]

ANSWERS TO JOKES

1. "you're sober"   2. take the spoon out

One problem faced by doctors and nurses who may want to use humor in healthcare settings (either for their own or for their patients' benefit) is lack of awareness of what is going on with other patients who are near. A nurse may want to share a laugh during a routine visit to the patient's room, but there is always the possibility that a patient sharing the room has just gotten some very bad news—which would make any nearby laughter inappropriate. And, of course, clinical staff must keep in mind that the "sick" or "dark" humor they share with each other is *not* to be shared with patients.

Using Humor to Promote Positive Doctor- and Nurse-Patient Interaction

In addition to adopting specific kinds of "therapeutic humor programs" (discussed below) to support health and wellness and help patients cope, a growing number of hospitals now recognize the importance of having clinical staff who are comfortable using a lighter style of interacting with patients as a means of creating a more personalized and positive interaction with them. Nurses' humor, for example, can be used to develop a sense of trust by patients.[282] One rehabilitation unit of a hospital set up a humor program that was specifically designed to stimulate a more positive, patient-centered style of interaction with patients.[283] Their view was that this focus on the patient relationship was more important than any therapeutic benefits resulting from humor.

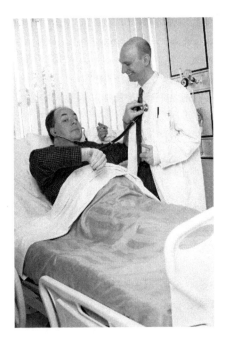 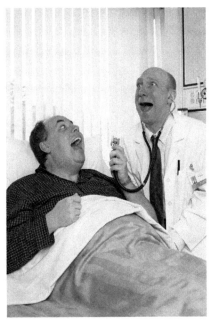

One physician has adopted the habit of helping his patients lighten up a bit by joking about the results of a brain scan. He says,

"There was nothing there whatsoever."

He then waits for a family member present to come up with a punch line. "Invariably, one of the kids will say, 'Well, mom, we knew you didn't have much up there all along.' I must have heard that 400 times; however, the family will laugh, smile, and someone will put their arm around their mom and hug her."[284] Obviously, a good personal relationship with the patient must already be established before a doctor or nurse uses this kind of humor.

Humor has long been known to be an effective ally in facilitating any kind of awkward or difficult communication. A common problem faced by physicians is how to ease patients into an understanding and acceptance of the fact that their condition is deteriorating. One doctor uses the following funny story (which you may have heard) to help communicate this bad news.

> **"Timothy is in college and he calls home to his younger brother and says, 'Jon, it's your big brother Timothy. How are you doing?' 'Oh, Timothy [pause]. Timothy, your cat died.' Dead silence. There is a bit of sobbing on the phone. Tim says, 'Jon, don't give bad news like that. You knew that cat was important to me. You should have said, 'The cat is on the roof and we've been trying, but we can't get it down; it's scared and we called the fire department.' You leave the conversation like that, knowing that I'm going to call back in a while. When I called back, you could have said that the cat fell off the roof and it's badly hurt, and it's going to the vet and everybody is concerned. Then when I called back later, you tell me that the cat died. That way, it comes in steps and it's not such a shock to me.' Jon says, 'Tim, you're right. I'm sorry. I don't know what I was thinking.' Tim says, 'You're young; you're my baby brother; you have a lot to learn.' He says, 'I learned, I learned.' Tim then says, 'Okay, what else is going on?' and Jon says, 'Mom's on the roof.'"[285]**

The chuckle that generally follows opens the door to a more open discussion of the patient's condition.

WHY DOCTORS AND NURSES MAY CHOOSE TO USE HUMOR WITH PATIENTS

1. To make the hospital seem like a more "normal" environment.
2. To established a more personalized connection with patients.
3. To help patients manage stress and anxiety related to their illness.
4. To help mobilize patients' own internal healing resources.

Consistent with this view, there is some evidence that humor is viewed by cancer patients as an effective communication strategy—especially once the perception of physician competence and trust is established.[286] But all clinical staff must always be sensitive to the patient's receptiveness to any kind of humor. Especially in the initial encounters with a patient, ". . . clinicians should be careful not to initiate humor without a clear lead from the patient."[287]

In spite of this growing conviction that humor has an important place in interactions between healthcare staff and patients, it is still not a topic that is covered in American nursing schools. Rather, nurses learn about humor on the job in clinical settings.[288] This is consistent with my own conversations with nurses following my presentations on humor and health/stress in hospital settings. I have consistently heard from them that humor was never discussed during their course work, and that they were initially put off by the (macabre or "sick") humor they saw in their hospital colleagues. That view quickly changed once they began to personally experience the emotionally draining work nurses are asked to do day after day.

Humor actually plays several important roles in healthcare settings. It not only helps humanize the healthcare experience for both the patient and care provider; it also helps reduce tension (for patients and staff), helps manage one's emotional state and helps staff work together as a team.[289]

If you are a healthcare provider, the guidelines on the following pages for using humor in healthcare settings should be followed.

CONCERNS ABOUT USING HUMOR IN HEALTHCARE SETTINGS

1. Will patients (or colleagues) consider it unprofessional?

A brief explanation of the health benefits resulting from humor, and how humor helps manage tension and anxiety, helps prevent this. This concern can also be handled by a small handout which explains why a lighter style of interaction by staff sometimes occurs. You can maintain your professionalism and still adopt a lighter style of interaction with patients and staff.

2. Will I be seen as incompetent?

Establish your competence first and then let your sense of humor emerge. Patients will generally welcome a lighter style of interaction.

3. Doesn't improving my sense of humor just increase my workload?

Learning to lighten up will not take time away from your job. Quite the opposite, you will soon find that humor lightens your workload, because it enables you to sustain a frame of mind conducive to doing your work more efficiently. You will also begin to enjoy your work more.

4. Will patients worry that I won't consider them sick, and will give them less attention if we share some laughs together?

Assure them that this is not true and that you enjoy tending to patients who are in a good mood.

5. What should I do if I really don't think the patient's humor is funny?

Don't fake laughter, but smile and acknowledge it as a joke.

6. What if the patient's humor is offensive, or somehow goes too far?

Be honest and tell them you really don't enjoy that kind of humor. Be flexible, open and supportive of their humor generally; but there are limits.

GENERAL GUIDELINES FOR USING HUMOR IN HEALTHCARE SETTINGS

1. Always establish your competence first in the eyes of a patient. The lighter style of interaction comes later. Premature use of humor may undermine the patient's confidence or trust in you.

2. Be sure other nearby patients/family members are not facing a crisis at the moment.

3. Always adopt a "toe in the water" approach. Ease into a playful interaction to gauge whether humor will be welcomed.

4. Be sensitive to whether the patient is responding positively or negatively to initial efforts at humor.

   Don't force humor upon the patient if s/he is not receptive. Think of humor as a medication. Some medications can be used with most patients, but others cannot. Two patients with the same symptoms don't always get the same medication. Some patients have allergic reactions. Be sensitive to the patient's humor allergies.

5. Remember that patients often don't feel like laughing. They may be nauseous, in pain or just not in the mood.

6. Remember that patients may not respond to humor until they have come to accept the fact of their disease.

   Do not try to use humor to overcome their depression or anger in the weeks after their diagnosis. It is important to express these emotions. The time may come, however, when humor can help them turn the corner of acceptance.

7. Avoid joking with other staff in the presence of patients who are about to undergo a test, surgery, etc.—unless you already have a good joking relationship established with them.

   Although you may need a good laugh, the patient doesn't understand that.

GENERAL GUIDELINES FOR USING HUMOR IN HEALTHCARE SETTINGS

8. Laugh together at unexpected circumstances that arise.

9. Poke fun at yourself—but not in a way that suggests lack of competence.

10. Never joke about staff incompetence.

11. Never joke at the patient's expense.

12. Never use humor when you are about to deliver bad news; compassion and empathy are called for. Consider humor later, once the bad news has been fully taken in and accepted.

13. Do not use joking to avoid discussion of sensitive issues.

14. Remember that many patients have no history of using humor under stress. It may be unrealistic to expect them to react favorably to humor in a hospital or hospice setting.

15. Remember that patients may have religious convictions which stress reverence in the midst of serious illness. This may be incompatible with any form of lighter interaction.

CONDITIONS WHERE HOSPITAL HUMOR IS INAPPROPRIATE

1. During any acute crisis. (But shared laughter can help adjust to the crisis afterwards.)

2. When the patient needs to cry.

3. When the patient needs quiet time.

4. When a patient in an adjacent bed is very ill or coping with bad news.

5. When the patient is coming to grips with any emotional crisis.

6. When the patient is communicating something important to you.

Nothing is more frustrating than having someone appear to not take seriously something that is very important to you and that you're trying to communicate. This can destroy your rapport.

7. Avoid

Ethnic jokes, sarcasm and mockery.
Humor at the expense of any other person. Laugh *with*, not *at*.
Joking about any patient or their condition.

8. If you have any doubts about the appropriateness of humor in a situation, try another approach (e.g., compassion, concern, and touch).

Types of Hospital Humor Programs

The best known approach to bringing humor to hospital settings is the use of clown volunteers. Over the past two decades, a steadily increasing number of hospitals have created programs in which clowns visit patients in their rooms to distract them from their anxieties and concerns and boost their spirits. The Big Apple Circus Clown Care Unit was initiated in New York City by Michael Christensen in 1986. It now includes about 90 "clown doctors" who provide about 250,000 bedside visits a year. The Big Apple Circus has spawned many other clown units across the U.S. and around the world (e.g., the Fondation Théodora, in France, Africa and Asia, Humour Foundation Clown Doctor Programs in Australia and Doctors of Happiness in South America, among others).

The general goal of these programs is to help children and their parents manage the stress that goes with being hospitalized. After laughing with a clown doctor with a white coat and a red nose, the child's spirits are raised and a real doctor in a white coat is not nearly so intimidating. At this point, we have no idea how many hospitals around the country (not to mention the rest of the world) have adopted some sort of clown program. [290] A growing number of nursing homes each year are also adopting clown programs.

The power of clowns is evident in the following example provided by a clown from the Big Apple Circus. An 11-year-old boy had been doused with gasoline and set on fire by an older boy.

"He was conscious, but in terrible pain with major burns over more than half of his body. I went right into emergency with him. When the surgeons began cutting away dead flesh, I began telling funny stories and promising circus tickets and making scarves appear and disappear—anything to keep his mind off the agony. Pretty soon he was rolling his eyes in amazement and finally I got him laughing behind his medical mask. It was incredible. He was staring death in the face— and he was having fun!"[291]

Like adults, children are generally very anxious prior to any surgical procedure. About 60% of children suffer anxiety in the preoperative period,[292] and since high preoperative anxiety is commonly associated with postoperative difficulties, efforts are often made to use sedatives or other tools to ease anxiety prior to surgery or other invasive procedures. The presence of clowns (along with parents) in the preoperative room does reduce the level of anxiety experienced prior to anesthesia induction.[293]

In one case, this reduced level of anxiety was still present in kids seven days after the surgery.[294] In spite of this anxiety reduction generated by the clowns, however, the operating room clinical staff in the hospital where one study was conducted still were against the idea of bringing clowns into the preoperative area.[295] They felt that the clowns 1) created a disturbance, 2) delayed clinical procedures and 3) interfered with the quality of the relationship between the medical personnel and the child. So while the movement to "bring in the clowns" continues to grow in connection with patients' rooms, hospitals may not yet be ready to let clowns near the operating room.

A few hospitals have created entire rooms devoted to fun and humor for ambulatory patients. These rooms are given names like "The Lively Room," "The Living Room," or "The Humor Room." For many years, Sunnyview Rehabilitation Hospital, in Schenectady, New York, even had a full-time humor coordinator whose job was to be sure humor was made available to all patients who wanted it.

"After two days in the hospital, I took a turn for the nurse."
(W. C. Fields)

One of the first humor rooms was established in the early 1980s at St. Joseph's Hospital in Houston. Representatives of this program have expressed to me their belief that the program leads to shorter hospital stays for many patients. The head nurse observed that *some patients are able to reduce their pain and nausea medications following a visit to the humor room.*

I know of one hospital in New Jersey which has a humor program built into its pediatrics department. At one point in the late 1990s, the hospital was short of beds for adults, so a 70-year-old cancer patient was forced to stay in pediatrics for nearly a week. Although he came in depressed, he had such a good time during his stay that when he was later re-admitted to the hospital, he specifically asked for a room in pediatrics.

A nurse caring for a woman from Kentucky asked, "So how's your breakfast this morning?" "It's very good, except for the Kentucky Jelly. I just can't get used to the taste," the patient replied. The nurse asked to see the jelly and the woman produced a foil packet labeled "KY Jelly."

Another common approach to building a lighter touch into hospitals is to create a "humor cart." This is a cart which can be wheeled into patients' rooms, and contains funny CDs, DVDs, cartoon books, games, funny props, silly nose glasses (animal noses as well as the traditional red clown nose), etc. Two hundred or more hospitals around the country now have humor carts (this is a guess; no one knows the exact number). Community volunteers often take responsibility for these programs. The patient can take anything on the cart to play with for as long as s/he wants. The basic idea here is simple—to take patients' mind off their pain or health concerns by engaging them in humor and the spirit of fun.

Some hospitals even adopt multiple approaches to keeping patients immersed in humor, including the use of satellite feeds of comedy programs (I know of one hospital that issues patients a kind of "*TV Guide*," listing when the comedy shows will occur on closed circuit TV, when they are first admitted to the hospital), a comedy cart, a humor room and even a lighter style of interaction with patients—at least with those who express interest in such interactions with staff. The latter approach is one of the most effective means of making the therapeutic benefits of humor available to patients. Nurses and other staff members can have a powerful impact on patients' mood by bringing them an occasional opportunity to laugh as they do their jobs.

The Integris Baptist Medical Center in Oklahoma City, Oklahoma created a humor program between 1996 and 2000 (funds for the program ran out after four years) in a 20-bed rehabilitation unit within the hospital. The unit was called the MIRTH unit (Medical Institute for Recovery Through Humor). The basic idea here was to use humor to create a more patient-centered environment and generate positive emotions in the midst of patients' rehab program. The main focus was on the use of humor in interaction with patients, but the unit also included cartoons, posters of clowns and classic comedians (like the Marx Brothers, The Three Stooges and Lucille Ball), puns and jokes, etc. Humor was used not just to get patients (all 65 or older, and being treated for a broad range of conditions, including cancer, heart disease, diabetes and stroke, among others) laughing, but to help them escape the role of patient for a while, bring back memories of their healthier youth, generate some positive feelings in the midst of a difficult circumstance and renew a sense of happiness and self-worth.[296]

This kind of environment was found to produce a contagious effect of humor on patients.

"When one patient appeared to be happy or amused, other patients and staff picked up on these cues and appeared to be happy or amused themselves. This was apparent when one patient would tell a story about his or her youth and chuckle, encouraging others in the room to chuckle reciprocally. Many patients in the room may have perceived a person chuckling as an environmental cue that 'allowed' them to perceive humor as well. Other environmental cues, such as quotations and posters on the walls or the 'joke of the day' also influenced the perception and contagion of humor."[297]

An observational study of the impact of this hospital humor program by a researcher not involved in the creation of the MIRTH unit led to the conclusion that using humor with patients supports more effective patient-centered care in three ways.

"First, humor provided an informal, positive environment in which providers . . . could gain valuable personal information about patients for the purpose of fulfilling their physical and psychological needs. Second, humor may have liberated patients from the 'bad patient' label by encouraging them to be open and unapologetic about their concerns and requests, leading them to take a more active part in their health care. Finally, humor may have de-emphasized some of the power disparities so often associated with patient-provider relationships."[298]

Impact on Patient Outcomes

The main goal of therapeutic humor programs in hospitals is generally to provide a positive counter-weight to the negative health circumstances that brought a patient to the hospital. But in the current climate of rising healthcare costs, it's also important to consider whether humor has any effect on recovery rate or other measures of improvement. Since more work has been done on other mind-body approaches than on humor, they are also discussed here. (The findings discussed in this first section are consistent with the broader discussion of PNI research at the beginning of this chapter.)

Humor Programs. In spite of the large number of hospitals around the world which have adopted clown visits or other types of therapeutic humor programs for patients, there has been little attempt to document their impact on such measures as speed of recovery, postoperative pain or wound healing. Hospitals have simply adopted humor programs because they can see from their own experience that these programs work in helping patients cope. (Four studies, as discussed above, have shown that clown interventions are effective in reducing children's anxiety prior to surgery or other invasive procedures.) If the program were to also save the hospital money, that would simply be icing on the cake.

As indicated earlier, Dr. James Walsh noted 80 years ago that laughter appeared to promote wound healing. PNI research has confirmed this finding for positive emotion. But one researcher suggested that *the key may be not so much what positive emotion does, but what it prevents.*[299] He feels that the positive effects found may be due to the disruption of production of neurotransmitters, hormones and other substances (associated with stress and negative emotion) which interfere with the healing process.

"I was born in 1962. True. And the room next to me was . . . 1963." (Joan Rivers)

Humor's power to speed up wound healing (observed anecdotally by some physicians) may be due to its capacity to lower blood levels of cortisol (see section on stress hormones), which can suppress natural killer cell and lymphocyte activity and suppress the production of antibodies. This possibility is supported by evidence from surgical patients who were given training in guided imagery and relaxation. These patients had more rapid wound healing than a control group and also had lower post-surgical levels of cortisol.[300]

BUILD YOUR HUMOR SKILLS

[Work on both jokes before checking the answers.]

1. A man went to his doctor because he just hadn't been feeling well for weeks. After the examination, the doctor gave him a bottle of pills and told him to take one with a full glass of water in the morning, at mid-day and in the evening. On his way out, he asked the doctor what his problem was. The doctor said, "You're not _____."
Clue: It's not what you think. The important part of the prescription is not the pills.

2. A TV commercial noted that 6 out of 10 people suffer from hemorrhoids. What comical conclusion can you draw from this? Four out of 10 _____.
Clue: Focus on the word "suffer" instead of "hemorrhoids."

Many studies (discussed above) have now documented humor's ability to reduce pain. In one case, patients were shown either comedy or serious movies (one in the morning and one in the afternoon) on two consecutive days following orthopedic surgery. In comparison with the serious movie group, those who watched the comedies requested 61% less "minor" pain medication (aspirin and mild tranquilizers) over the next two days.[301]

It is important to note that among those who watched the comedy films, the amount of major pain medication requested depended on whether they were able to choose the funny movie they watched. Patients who were allowed to choose movies that were funny to them requested less major pain medication than those who were presented a movie to watch without choosing. According to the researchers, "This unanticipated result is probably due to the fact that humor preferences are idiosyncratic, and few things are as irritating as being exposed to material that fails in its attempt to be funny. From an applied standpoint, our results suggest that care should be taken to determine a patient's humor preferences before humor is introduced into a hospital setting." While it is a bit much to expect any hospital to use precious staff time to determine humor preferences, one obvious way to handle this for those hospitals which have a humor cart program managed by volunteers is to make available to patients a broad range of comedy DVDs so that they are sure to find something that is funny to them.

> **A gynecologist who had lost interest in his medical practice decided to change careers and enrolled in auto mechanic school. He performed well in the course but was still shocked when he got an off-the-chart 200 on his final exam. He asked the instructor to explain the grade. "I gave you 50 points for taking the engine apart correctly," the teacher said, "50 points for putting it back together correctly . . . and an extra 100 points for doing it all through the muffler."**

Among a group of elderly residents who suffered chronic pain in a long-term care facility, watching a 20-minute comedy program three days a week for six weeks significantly reduced the amount of pain medication requested during this period.[302] This reduction was, not surprisingly, accompanied by a more positive mood.

The research on blood pressure suggests that humor will help many patients keep blood pressure down as they prepare for stressful medical procedures. It may even help reduce inflammation levels (see section on Sedimentation Rate).

Nurses have tremendous power to boost the spirits of their patients. And this, in turn, helps patients mobilize their own natural healing resources. If you are a nurse, you can use humor to help your patients cope. One nurse told me that her favorite line with patients following surgery is, "I was going to tell you a joke, but I can see you're in stitches already."

Patients commonly say that humor and laughter raise their spirits and take their minds off their illness and problems. (I have heard this many times following my National Cancer Survivors Day programs for cancer patients.) I know of a cancer center in Florida where the patients have such a good time during their treatments (while watching comedy videos and laughing with staff) that they often go back for visits long after their disease is in remission.

One physician reported to me that among his patients with spinal cord injuries, those who are able to laugh about their circumstances are much better at dealing with the humiliation and frustration they often feel. They also tend to have fewer complications than patients who are unable to find a light side of their condition. This doctor is convinced that humor plays an important role in their recovery.

ANSWERS TO JOKES

1. drinking enough water.   2. enjoy them.

---

1) Using Humor to Promote Hope and a Positive Outlook

Many nurses (who are generally in a primary care role with patients) make an active effort to instill a sense of hope and optimism in their patients.[303] The growing conviction that it is important to cultivate a sense of hope in patients is—at least in part—due to the large body of research documenting the health-promoting power of hope and other positive emotions. The initial impetus for this emphasis on hope came from Dr. Bernie Siegel's observation (as noted earlier) that a strong sense of hope and optimism characterized many cancer patients who beat the survival odds given to them by their doctors.

"Have you ever been treated by a doctor for this condition?"
"No, they always make me pay."

Sign in a doctor's office: "Amnesia patients must pay in advance."

Many other strategies have also been adopted by healthcare professionals to instill hope in their patients. These include prayer, discussions with other survivors of the same disease, providing a good understanding of the disease, providing care options, showing empathy, establishing a strong caring relationship, offering encouragement and cultivating good coping skills.

Key Findings from Other Types of Mind-Body Programs. Humor, of course, is just one among many approaches to bringing the known benefits of mind/body medicine to hospital patients. In one analysis of 191 different studies (involving 8600 patients), a wide range of mind/body interventions before and after surgery (e.g., guided imagery, hypnosis, relaxation procedures, biofeedback and giving information) were found to be effective in improving surgery outcomes. "These interventions have been shown to work for virtually every imaginable kind of surgery—from back surgery to coronary-bypass operations to cancer resections."[304]

Health management systems have become more concerned about length of hospital stays in recent years, so it is important to note that one analysis of 13 studies showed that "psychosocial interventions reduced hospitalization by an average of 2.4 days . . ."[305] The just-mentioned analysis of 191 studies showed that 79% of them led to a shorter hospital stay because of the mind–body procedure used.[306]

The most effective of the various mind/body procedures used over the past 25 years have been based on "psychoeducational interventions." These involve providing patients health-related information about their condition and surgical procedure, as well as *some kind of skill or exercise that helps them reduce pain or cope better.* In one analysis of 102 studies, such interventions were found to positively influence recovery rate, pain reduction, psychological well-being and satisfaction with care. This was found for thoracic, abdominal, orthopedic, gynecologic, cancer, and eye-ear-nose-throat patients.[307] An especially strong effect was found for the ability of these mind-body procedures to reduce both medical complications and the number of days following discharge before resuming normal activities.

In another review of all the research in this area, Henry Dreher concluded that in addition to providing preparatory information about the upcoming surgery, *the provision of coping and rehabilitation skills plays a key role in the gains shown.*[308] Relaxation techniques alone showed only mixed success, in spite of the fact that they are one of the most popular approaches used in healthcare settings.

Looking down at the sick man whose prognosis was very poor, the doctor decided to tell him the truth. "I feel that I should tell you. You are a very sick man, and you don't have many days left. I'm sure that you would want to know the facts. Now—is there anyone you would like to see?" Bending towards his patient, the doctor heard him feebly answer, "Yes." "Who is it?" asked the doctor. In a slightly stronger tone the man said, "Another doctor."

The positive outcomes associated with many "complementary" or "alternative" medical treatments have led to a steady increase in patient interest in such techniques over the past two decades.[309] By the late 1990s, one survey indicated that 87% of cancer patients in the rural Midwest were using some kind of complementary intervention to cope with the stress associated with cancer. Prayer was the most common approach; humor was second, with 50% of patients using humor to cope.[310] A larger follow-up study found that 21% used some form of humor or laughter therapy.[311]

So hopefully you are now convinced that you have many reasons to build more humor and laughter into your life. Lighten up! Jest for the health of it.

CHAPTER 3

HUMOR AND THE BRAIN

"Someone who makes you laugh is a comedian. Someone who makes you think and then laugh is a humorist."   George Burns

IT DOESN'T TAKE A ROCKET scientist (or any other kind of scientist studying humor!) to realize that this wonderful capacity we humans have to experience and enjoy humor is a direct consequence of our larger and more developed brain. Such a sophisticated form of mental play could only occur with the evolution of a larger cerebral cortex. It is only in recent years, however, that we have finally begun to understand just which areas of the brain are responsible for both our understanding and enjoyment of humor.

The 1990s were called the "Decade of the brain." This label was adopted at the beginning of the decade because of the development of breakthrough technologies that made possible observation of the exact areas of the brain activated during mental tasks. Researchers knew that these new methods would yield breathtaking new insights about the function of the brain. Efforts have only recently been made to study the brain's involvement during humor using these techniques, but we have already come a long way in clarifying the way in which the brain operates during the experience of humor. This chapter discusses what we've learned so far.

Two basic questions must be answered to understand the brain's role in humor. First, how is the brain involved in understanding or creating humor? Are many different areas activated, or only certain regions? Also, do the regions engaged differ for different kinds of humor? Is there any evidence for what might be called a "humor center?" That is, is there an area of the brain that is primarily devoted to humor, just as there are areas primarily devoted to vision, language, etc.? The second question is one that has always intrigued researchers studying humor; namely, why do we experience such a rush of pleasure, joy and exhilaration when we find something funny? Why do we enjoy humor so much? And why does it feel so good to laugh? We will look at each of these questions separately.

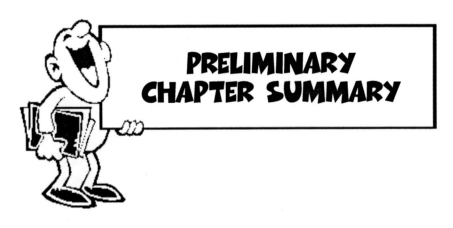

PRELIMINARY
CHAPTER SUMMARY

[Note: Some of the material in this chapter gets a bit technical. If you have difficulty following the discussion below, come back to this preliminary summary. You don't need to get bogged down in the details to get a good understanding of what we know about humor and the brain.]

There is an enormous body of research documenting the fact that the two cerebral hemispheres of the brain are in constant communication with each other and work as a team. Each side of the brain, however, appears to be specialized for certain functions— especially in connection with language-mediated thought. The issues are complex, but—put simply—in right-handed individuals (90% of the population), the left hemisphere (hereafter called the left brain or LB) is capable of mediating most basic or simple language functions while the right hemisphere (RB) increasingly comes into play for more complex and integrative uses of language. Both the LB and RB are probably engaged most of the time when we experience humor, and activation of the LB alone is often sufficient to get the point of a joke, but the RB becomes increasingly important as the challenge to comprehension increases.

Our understanding of the different ways in which the two hemispheres operate began with insights obtained from individuals who had suffered brain damage as a result of a stroke or accident. When specific types of mental or language deficits were found to be associated with damage to specific areas of the brain, it was concluded that these areas of the brain must be involved in the mental abilities found to be lacking. This early research led to the conclusion that the RB is especially important for humor in a very general sense, as well as for other forms of sophisticated thought.

By the early 1990s, new technologies were developed which allowed for the identification of specific areas of the brain activated during a particular mental task. This provided a means of testing the conclusions drawn from the early brain damage research about the role of the two hemispheres in humor. While there have been some inconsistent findings generated by these two approaches to studying the brain, they have shown remarkable agreement in many areas. Thus, both approaches suggest that while the LB plays a key role in most basic language functions and in simpler humor, the RB plays an increasingly greater role (in comparison to the LB) in a broad range of specific abilities when more sophisticated or complex thought and problem solving are required. It is too early at this point to draw conclusions about the specific areas within the RB or LB that play the key roles in humor and other complex mental activities.

The following table summarizes findings for special capacities of the RB from studies of both brain–damaged individuals and healthy persons (using neural imaging techniques). It should be noted that the fact that a given mental activity appears in one column, but not the other, does not mean that results from the two approaches disagree. Most commonly, researchers using the two techniques have simply not studied the same specific mental functions.

The first five items in the two lists are the same. Both research approaches have studied these areas, and the findings are in general agreement. Early brain damage studies used varying types of humor and generally found the RB to be important for humor, in that RB damage was associated with humor deficits. This early research failed to look at the impact of the level of complexity of the humor presented—although there was some suggestion that individuals with RB damage could understand simpler forms of humor. Investigators using new neuroimaging techniques have similarly failed to give adequate attention to the role of complexity of the cartoons and jokes used, but the findings using this approach point to the involvement of both sides of the brain in processing humor. It is suggested in this chapter that once more demanding forms of humor are presented to people using neuroimaging techniques, the RB will be shown to become increasingly important as the level of mental effort required to "get" the joke increases. This is precisely what research on other aspects of complex thought suggests.

Both approaches show the importance of the RB for understanding metaphor (although the LB alone appears sufficient for understanding some simple and familiar metaphors) and other forms of figurative or non-literal language. The RB is also critical for interpreting the influence of intonation (prosody) on meaning, along with integrating information in a meaningful way in the context of an ongoing narrative. (Most jokes and funny stories, of course, can be viewed as short narratives.)

Other types of mental abilities have also been studied using one approach, but not the other. Nonetheless, these findings form a coherent package in a very broad sense. Thus, studies of brain-damaged patients suggest that the RB is important for understanding irony and sarcasm, as well as for distinguishing between lies and jokes. The ability to appreciate irony is mentally demanding, and the ability to detect sarcasm and joking (vs. lying) requires the ability to read (often) subtle changes in intonation, facial cues, etc., something—as just noted—the LB has difficulty doing on its own.

The kinds of "indirect requests" that we use so frequently in normal discourse ("Do you think the toys should be brought in, in case it rains?") require reading behind what is literally said in order to determine what is really meant. The reduced ability along these lines among RB-damage patients is consistent with their general deficits in understanding figurative language. As with metaphors, jokes and other types of figurative language, idiomatic phrases similarly involve nonlinear uses of language—which the LB has difficulty decoding when functioning alone.

MENTAL TASKS FOR WHICH THE RB PLAYS A GREATER ROLE

BRAIN DAMAGE DATA	NEURAL IMAGING DATA
1. Humor	1. Complex humor (not puns)
2. Figurative/non-literal language	2. Figurative/non-literal language
3. Metaphor	3. Complex, unfamiliar metaphors
4. Integrating information in an ongoing narrative	4. Integrating information in an ongoing narrative
5. Changes in intonation	5. Changes in intonation
6. Distinction between lies and jokes	6. Uncommon meanings & associations
7. Irony	7. Resolving ambiguity
8. Sarcasm	8. Making inferences
9. Idiomatic phrases	9. Novelty/violation of expectation
10. Indirect requests	10. Discrepancies between input from different sources

While neural imaging studies have used individuals with healthy, intact brains and have examined other types of mental abilities, the general pattern of the data obtained is consistent with that found among patients with RB damage. Thus, the RB is more actively engaged (in comparison with the LB) in processing uncommon meanings and associations, as well as circumstances where one's expectations have been violated—as well as when confronted by something very novel. In the case of totally novel events, of course, it is not initially clear how to make sense of the situation.

The RB's increased engagement in resolving ambiguity is, again, consistent with its role in interpreting metaphor, sarcasm, violated expectancies, intonational uncertainty, etc. And the active use of the RB to process discrepancies between different sensory inputs is one more example of its general role in resolving ambiguity. Finally, the RB's special role in making inferences is consistent with its ability to integrate information in ongoing conversations or narratives and points to a special ability to go beyond the literal information given to come up with meaningful conclusions.

No attempt has yet been made to determine the relative roles of the two hemispheres in creating humor. This is clearly more mentally demanding than simply making the effort to understand a cartoon or joke that is presented to you. It is suggested here that researchers need to provide subjects with an opportunity to create humor to best demonstrate the RB's superiority in connection with humor requiring greater mental effort for comprehension.

While the RB does specialize in more sophisticated uses of language—and more sophisticated thought in general—the two hemispheres are in constant communication with each other in a healthy brain. The importance of this continuous back-and-forth communication between the two hemispheres is evident from several studies that have documented the impact of loss of this communication. A major "superhighway" of neurons connects the two-hemispheres; it is called the corpus callosum. Some individuals have a genetic defect in which they are born lacking this neural connection between the LB and RB. They typically have normal IQ levels, but show a pattern of mental deficits very similar to that of individuals with RB damage. That is, they have difficulty in understanding a broad range of "second order" meanings, including jokes, proverbs and non-literal language.

As we have seen, the RB's involvement is crucial for these more mentally demanding forms of thought. As one researcher in this area put it, the information required to makes sense out of such second order meanings is trapped in the RB, and the LB has no way of getting to it. However, it is important to note that individuals lacking a corpus callosum show no difficulty in understanding puns and other simple forms of humor—although they do show deficits in understanding complex forms of verbal humor.

Taken as a whole, findings using brain-damaged individuals, people lacking the main path (the corpus callosum) for communication between the two hemispheres, and individuals with normal brains (using neuroimaging techniques) point to the general conclusion that the relative engagement of the two hemispheres is a matter of emphasis, depending on the situation engaging our thought. The LB generally takes the lead in making sense out of new situations. Thus, it is activated first in processing humor, as well as non-humorous verbal or nonverbal inputs.

In straightforward communications and simpler forms of humor, the LB is generally able to make sense of things on its own, so the RB is minimally engaged. While some researchers suggest that the RB is not engaged at all in the processing of simpler information, a better conclusion at this point may be one of fluctuating bilateral engagement in which the RB does periodically get engaged to assess the overall coherence of thought, even when the information is not complex. When the LB encounters difficulty in making sense of the information provided, it calls on the RB for help. The RB then takes over in looking for the key pieces needed to make sense of the joke, metaphor, or other form of unexpected or puzzling information.

Several key functional differences between the two hemispheres help account for the overall pattern of differences in the contributions of the LB and RB to humor. The RB appears to have evolved to process more novel and discrepant information (i.e., information that is in some way inconsistent with the person's prior experience), while the LB has evolved to handle more familiar or routinized tasks and information. In fact, information initially processed by the RB may well eventually be transferred over to the LB for future processing as it becomes increasingly familiar.

The two hemispheres also appear to differ in the kinds of mental operations performed. The LB is better at analytical functions, while the RB is better at more holistic processing of information from diverse sources. In the case of humor, we must quickly pull together pieces of information that initially seem to have no meaningful link in order to get the joke. This clearly would be expected to utilize the holistic processing strength of the RB.

Finally, recent neuroimaging studies have now clarified the basis for the feel-good side of humor—the rush of exhilaration, joy or enjoyment we get when we find something really funny. A phylogenetically older area of the brain (the mesolimbic dopaminergic reward system) that has long been known to mediate the pleasure we experience in response to drugs (like cocaine and methamphetamine) and sex is also activated in response to humor. So while the most-recently evolved structures of the brain (the cerebral cortex) mediate our understanding of humor, very old sub cortical structures play the key role in triggering the enjoyment we experience when we get the joke.

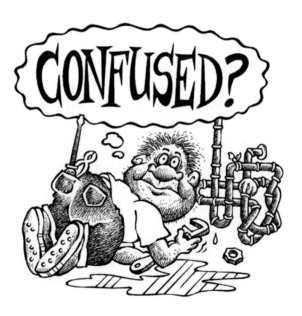

It wasn't that many decades ago that scientists were puzzled by the presence of two separate halves of the cerebral cortex. They looked similar anatomically and seemed to have the same basic shape and structure. Was one just a backup for the other in case something happened to it? Or did they have distinctive functions that had not yet been discovered?

A century and a half ago (1861), Paul Broca discovered that basic language functions were mediated by an area just above the left temporal lobe of the brain (located a bit above and forward of your left ear). Studies over the decades have supported this initial observation for right-handed individuals (who constitute 90% of the population). Despite their similar appearance, the two sides of the brain have different functions—especially in connection with the comprehension and production of language. The two halves of the cerebral cortex process semantic (semantic refers to "meaning") information in different—but complementary—ways. The left brain

> *"A very special custom occurs after a Navajo baby is born: a celebration of the baby's first laugh. The soul (also called 'the wind') enters the body soon after birth. A baby's laugh is a sign that the soul has become attached to the body."*[1]

is specialized for basic language functions, while the right becomes more active in the handling of more subtle and complex language functions—including more complex forms of humor.[2]

Understanding Humor
Will the Funny Hemisphere Please Light Up?

Two approaches have been used to determine the brain's role in humor. The first used individuals who had suffered damage to the cerebral cortex as a result of either a stroke or accident. The idea here was to determine the nature of any deficits that resulted from damage to specific areas of the brain. If several studies confirmed that damage to a given area was associated with a humor deficit (while those with that brain area intact showed normal humor comprehension), it was concluded that the damaged area must play an important role in understanding humor. A major problem with this kind of research, however, is that other areas of brain damage that the researcher is unaware of may also have resulted from the stroke or accident, and these other areas may actually be responsible for the humor deficits found. Nonetheless, the early studies of humor and the brain based on this approach provided a major step forward in understanding the brain's role in humor.

The second approach used recently developed neuroimaging techniques to determine areas of the brain (in individuals with no brain damage) that are actively engaged when we experience humor. A variety of such techniques is now available. The most exciting one is called functional magnetic resonance imaging or fMRI. This technique is based on measuring differences in blood flow to the brain. When a particular area of the brain is being used, it consumes more oxygen. Blood flow to that area is increased in order to supply the oxygen required. An fMRI procedure measures the extent of this increased blood flow to the active brain area.

Before talking about this new research (done in the past decade), it should be noted that brain areas activated during humor might be assumed to also be activated by other forms of intellectual activity. Basic mental processes, such as reading or listening to language—which engage both short- and long-term memory—are involved in other (serious) mental activities, as well as in humor. We have long known that humor involves an active comparison of memories or knowledge of prior events with some new (and incongruous, bizarre, inappropriate, etc.) idea or event. So areas of the brain that do this for non-humorous experiences would be expected to also do so for humor. As we shall see below, this is, indeed, the case.

A widely accepted view of the intellectual processes involved in humor is that the brain must first identify information that is incongruous—inconsistent in some way with prior experience—and then find other information/knowledge that allows for the resolution (or making sense) of the incongruity.[3] Of course, some humor is funny precisely because it is sheer nonsense; there is nothing to (at least fully) resolve the incongruity we see. Many people love such nonsense humor, while others do not—precisely because there is no way of ultimately making sense out of it. This resolution—i.e., the insight that occurs when you "get" the unexpected other meaning of a word or identify other information that makes the incongruity coherent again—generates the experience of humor. As discussed below, a similar process occurs when we struggle to make sense of other forms of (nonhumorous) figurative or ambiguous language.

BUILD YOUR HUMOR SKILLS

[Work on all three jokes before checking the answers.]

[Note: Understanding the skill-building jokes in this chapter requires some background knowledge of the brain. So don't worry if some make no sense.]

1. What kind of neurological tests to veterinarians do? ____ _____.

1st *clue*: What's the general name you use to refer to the cat or dog that lives in your house?
2nd *clue*: It's a kind of scan.

2. What do you get if you attach a light bulb to your cerebral cortex? A _____ _____.
1st *clue*: It's a certain kind of thought.
2nd *clue*: What is the effect of putting a higher wattage light bulb in your lamp?

3. What happens if you drop a brain scanner? It's a _____.

1st *clue*: Find a word for an extreme disaster.
2nd *clue*: A feline pet.

In most jokes or cartoons, then, we are initially puzzled by key information in the punch line. We first make a judgment about which parts of our past experience and knowledge are pertinent and then scan those memories for key information that enables us to make sense in a new way of the unexpected or incongruous features of the joke. Seeing this new connection enables us to appreciate the joke. Reflect for a moment about how this process works in your own mind as you read the following joke.

A thoughtful wife has pork chops ready when her husband comes home from _____.

In this case, if you think of a traditional family with a stay-at-home wife, your mind automatically fills in "work" to complete the sentence. There is no humor here, of course, since there is nothing unexpected or incongruous. Think (before you read on) about how you might complete the sentence to make a joke out of it. Ah ah! Don't peak at the next paragraph! Give yourself a full minute or so to work on this. You have to think of a word or phrase that—at first glance—is unexpected and incongruous, but which—at the same time—enables you to find a funny reinterpretation of something that comes before the punch line.

Many words other than "work" can be added here and still make perfectly good sense (e.g., bowling, jogging or cutting the grass). Now end the sentence with "fishing." Suddenly, a whole new set of ideas rush forth. As you will soon see, it is this network of relevant information related to past efforts at fishing, including a pessimistic outlook about her husband's fishing skills or luck (different people hearing this joke may also bring some unique associations to it, in addition to the notion of expecting him to catch no fish), that the RB is especially good at accessing and bringing to bear on the joke.

Apply the incongruity-resolution theory of humor to this joke.

A 90-year-old man is driving down the freeway when his cell phone rings. It's his wife. She frantically tells her husband, "John, be careful! I just heard on the radio that there's some madman driving the wrong way down the freeway you're on."

John answers, "I know! I know! But it's not just one madman. It looks like hundreds of them!"

The key question for most of this chapter centers around how the brain goes about finding the information required to see the humor in this and other funny situations in which we finally make some sense out of what is initially unexpected, bizarre, incongruous, etc.

Humor Deficits in Brain-Damaged Individuals

A large body of research on individuals who have suffered brain damage supports the generally-held conclusion that the LB is generally sufficient for basic or simpler aspects of language while the RB plays a more important role in specialized and more sophisticated uses of language—especially uses that require putting verbal information in a specific context. Thus, when the LB is damaged (but not the right), basic and severe forms of speech production, object naming and language comprehension show deficits.[4] When the damage is to the RB, these deficits do not show up. Instead, more subtle deficits appear (as discussed in the next section); these include, but are not restricted to, deficits in one's sense of humor. One early clue to what 20+ years of subsequent research has subsequently confirmed was the finding in the 1980s that RB damage causes deficits in understanding nonliteral uses of language while LB damage results in difficulty in understanding literal language.[5]

ANSWERS TO JOKES

1. PET scan   2. bright idea, brilliant thought, etc.
3. CATastrophy (think CAT scan)

An easy way to determine one's ability to understand humor is to provide a choice of funny captions or punch lines. For example, researchers provided a series of cartoons with four possible captions to individuals with either normal brains or RB damage; the task was to simply choose the funniest caption.[6] The choices included the real joking caption, a straightforward sad or straightforward neutral caption, and a *non sequitur* (a statement that does not follow logically from anything previously said or depicted in the cartoon). In comparison with the normal control group, the RB damage patients chose fewer joking captions and more *non sequiturs* as the funniest caption. They also showed a reduced ability to provide a verbal explanation of what made the cartoon funny. Other studies produced similar findings with *non sequiturs.*[7]

The following joke is typical of the kind of humor an individual with RB damage would have difficulty understanding.

"I let my accountant do my taxes because it saves time. Last spring it saved me ten years."

The authors of this study concluded that the tendency to choose *non sequiturs* as the funniest "suggests that patients with RB damage recognize the importance of the form of a joke, but they have difficulty fully interpreting a joke's content."[8] That is, both the correct and *non sequitur* caption satisfied the normal prerequisite for humor in the cartoons, in that they did not directly follow from information provided in the cartoon. However, *the non sequitur lacked the meaningful coherence that a punch line provides. So these individuals with RB damage could not distinguish between a coherent and non-coherent incongruous caption.* Further evidence of their lack of comprehension of the cartoons could be seen in their greater tendency (relative to subjects without brain damage) to give comparable funniness ratings to all four types of captions.

With respect to the two-stage (incongruity + resolution) model of humor discussed above, Howard Gardner (who conducted much of the early research in this area) and his associates noted that RB patients were able to achieve the first step, but not the second. In a study using jokes, RB patients were similarly able to detect surprise in the punch line, but were unable to pick which surprising ending was also funny as a result of that ending's essential coherence with the body of the joke.[9] The following is one of the jokes used.

The neighborhood borrower approached Mr. Smith one Sunday afternoon and inquired, "Say Smith, are you using your lawnmower this afternoon?"

"Yes, I am," Smith replied warily.
Then the neighborhood borrower replied:

Joking ending: **"Fine, then you won't be wanting your golf clubs. I'll just borrow them."**

Non sequitur ending: **"You know, the grass is always greener on the other side."**

Straightforward ending: **"Do you think I could use it (the lawnmower) when you're done?"**

Again, *non-sequitur* endings were considered just as funny as the joking endings. So even though they were surprised, individuals with RB damage were unable to integrate the punch line information with the information from the rest of the joke or cartoon in order to provide a coherent overall package of meanings.

These researchers suggested that for jokes, "Integration in this context requires a listener to review the elements of the joke and to identify a new, internally consistent, line of reasoning from which the punch line could well follow as part of a coherent narrative . . . This pattern of deficits also clarifies an earlier claim that right hemisphere patients' narrative deficit is due to an inability to integrate content across parts of a narrative unit." Given the similar impact of RB damage on other forms of complex linguistic material (discussed below), it may be that *disruption of one's sense of humor as a result of RB damage is simply one additional byproduct of a general deficit in the ability to integrate divergent information.*

So these two early studies of RB damage patients showed the same deficit for both cartoons and jokes. Another study specifically compared nonverbal cartoons to jokes. Both humorous and non-humorous versions of each were presented, and subjects chose the funniest ending. Here is an example of the jokes used.

A woman is taking a shower. All of a sudden, her doorbell rings. She yells, "Who's there?" and a man answers, "Blind man." Well, she's a charitable lady so she runs out the door of the shower naked and opens the door.

Straightforward ending: **"Can you spare a little change for a blind man?"**

Humorous ending: **"Where should I put these blinds, lady?"**

Non sequitur ending: **"I really enjoy going to the symphony."**

For the cartoons, four-panel drawings from the old *"Ferd'nand"* comic strip were modified to similarly provide a humorous, straightforward or non sequitur final panel. The ability to select the humorous ending was disrupted among RB damage patients for both cartoons and jokes.[10] So this early brain damage research suggested that *it is the basic kind of thinking involved in humor that is affected by RB damage*, not the way (visual vs. auditory) in which the information is presented. Consistent with earlier research, these patients did retain the awareness that an element of surprise is important for humor, but they lost the ability to integrate information from different parts of the joke so as to make it coherent.

A doctor was giving a talk on nutrition to the general community. He said, "Most of us have no idea that the things we're putting into our stomach are slowly killing us. We all know about the problems with red meat. And soft drinks corrode you stomach lining and leach calcium from your system. Sugary foods are creating a diabetic country, and junk foods are making us obese. But there is one food that is more dangerous than any other we eat. It can cause you grief and suffering long after you eat it. Does anyone have an idea what that food might be?"
After several seconds, a 75-year-old man raised his hand and said, "Wedding cake."

Most studies of humor and brain damage are consistent with this general pattern of findings. Other evidence suggests that when

RB patients do make attempts at humor, their efforts tend to be inappropriate or make no sense at all.[11]

Deficits in Other Complex Mental Functions. People with RB damage also show deficits in the following mental activities.

1) Deception and Distinction between Lies and Jokes

Normal functioning of the RB is required for individuals to understand deception and to distinguish between a lie and a joke.[12] When confronted with a non-literal statement, individuals with RB damage have difficulty determining whether the communicative intent was to lie, joke or be sarcastic.[13]

2) Comprehension of Irony

A reduced comprehension of irony occurs among individuals with RB damage. This would be expected, since irony is a complex, indirect form of communication. In irony, you intend to say just the opposite of what you literally say. If you rent a beach condo on your only free weekend of the summer and find that it's cold and rainy, you might say to your spouse, "Ah, we chose the perfect weekend to get a tan." You obviously mean you'll get no tan at all.[14]

3) Ability to Detect Sarcasm

Sarcasm is a stronger form of irony which is generally meant to communicate criticism or some other negative feeling. If you say to someone, "Sam, you work too hard," you might really saying that Sam is goofing off again. RB patients are generally unable to detect and interpret sarcasm.[15] LB patients do not show this deficit.

4) Interpretation of Intonation

Sometimes an important part of vocally communicated humor stems from the intonation with which it is delivered. (The rhythmic and intonational aspects of speech are generally referred to as "prosody.") Subtle nuances of emotional tone can switch the communication from a straightforward one to one which is clearly tongue-in-cheek, a put-down, etc. Among patients who have suffered strokes or some other form of brain damage, it is those with RB (and not LB) damage who have difficulty judging the emotional tone of speech produced by others; they also tend to speak with flattened intonation themselves.[16]

5) Comprehension of Indirect Requests

RB patients have difficulty understanding any kind of indirect request, where some inference has to be made about what the person is really asking.[17] My wife is very fond of such requests. "Do you think we should get those toys from the back yard in case it rains?" This means "Please go out and bring the toys in." RB patients tend to respond to indirect commands in a literal fashion; they are also unable to use contextual cues to determine the appropriate response to a command or suggestion.[18]

6) Comprehension of Metaphors

RB damage patients have difficulty understanding metaphoric statements like the following:[19]

"Life is a journey."
"She has a heavy heart."
"A loved one's voice is a symphony."

These individuals generally interpret metaphors literally. They are, however, often able to understand familiar metaphors—those they have heard in different contexts in the past.

7) Comprehension of Idiomatic Phrases

The RB plays an important role in understanding unfamiliar or complex idioms.[20]

8) Ability to Make Inferences

As noted above, RB patients show a general deficit in making inferences.[21] Inference-making abilities are crucial to making sense of conversations—and of the world in general—when we have incomplete information about something. These patients similarly have difficulty grasping the main point of a narrative passage.[22]

9) Interpretation of Ongoing Conversations

RB patients have difficulty extracting key ideas from an ongoing conversation.[23] This limits their ability to assess the coherence of the steady pace of new information as the conversation continues.

While most of the research on humor and other more sophisticated forms of thought and language points to the special importance of the RB for these mental activities, it should be noted that there are also a smaller number of findings with brain-damaged patients that suggest a balanced involvement of the two hemispheres in humor, indirect requests, pictorial and verbal metaphors, inferences, sarcasm, alternative word meanings and comprehension of narratives.[24] This is more consistent with the findings discussed below (using neuroimaging techniques) and suggests that humor studies using patients with brain damage may not fully reflect the ways in which healthy brains are processing humor.

Humor in the Healthy Brain

As informative as the data for brain-injured individuals are, the strongest case for the idea that the RB plays a specialized role in humor and other sophisticated uses of language requires evidence of the relative contributions of the two hemispheres in individuals with healthy brains.

As noted earlier, recently-developed brain imaging technologies have finally allowed researchers to obtain this information. The number of humor studies using these procedures, however, is still small (although growing). Since a considerably larger number of studies along these lines has been completed on other forms of non-literal language that have clear implications for humor—comparable to those just discussed for "other complex, mental functions" in connection with brain damage—that research is reviewed here first. The results of this work will then provide a strong basis for prediction of expected outcomes for humor.

Lateralization for Complex Mental Functions Other than Humor. Several areas of research (not focusing on humor) have a direct bearing on our discussion of hemispheric differences in the brain's functioning during humor.

1) Frequency of Use and Context of Word Meaning

Both the frequency of occurrence of a word or phrase and the context in which it occurs influence the degree of activation of the two hemispheres. These factors play a key role in resolving any form of linguistic ambiguity—whether humorous or not. (Context, of course, is always crucial in humor.) The LB responds more to "local" contextual cues provided within a sentence—cues which make sense out of the sentence using the most commonly occurring meanings for the key ideas represented.[25] As one group of researchers put it, *the LB allocates its attention to the "dominant" or most common meaning of a word and generally comes up with that meaning,* all the while inhibiting the RB's tendency to look for alternative meanings.[26] There is no reason to search further most of the time, since the usual meaning renders the sentence coherent. This difference in operation of the two hemispheres "might have the purpose of freeing the left hemisphere to concentrate on the most likely word meaning, while preserving a capacity in the brain to access alternative meanings if they should be later required."[27]

These findings from linguistic ambiguity studies are especially important for our understanding of humor, so I'll provide a lengthy quote from the researchers to be sure the distinctions are clear.

"Meaning frequency is evidently an important factor in hemispheric processing of word meaning . . . [our] results suggest that the right hemisphere automatically retrieves all meanings of a word, irrespective of their relative importance in language, while the left hemisphere focuses upon the most frequent or dominant meaning of a word . . . The results support the view that the right hemisphere activates a larger semantic field than the left hemisphere . . . the right hemisphere has a critical role in ensuring a proper utilization of *context* in the comprehension of discourse. . . . it is possible that this pattern of effects reflects a mechanism designed to allow the left hemisphere to process language rapidly on the assumption that the dominant meaning of a word is, by definition, usually the appropriate one. The *function of the right hemisphere may be to make all of the alternative meanings available, in order to provide for rapid access to those meanings on those occasions [as in jokes] where a less frequent meaning turns out to be appropriate to the context.*"[28] (Italics are McGhee's.)

If the RB does, in fact, specialize in activating a larger semantic field and finding less common alternative meanings, it should be activated to some extent in most forms of humor. So these findings lead to the prediction that both LB and RB activation should be the norm. It is not clear from these findings whether a pattern of simultaneous engagement of the two hemispheres should occur or one of initial primary LB engagement followed by RB engagement when the expected meaning does not work.

One group of researchers has suggested that while each hemisphere (in a healthy brain) is engaged in providing possible meanings of a word or phrase, ". . . constructing the message of the sentence takes place only within the LH [left hemisphere]. In the LH contextually inappropriate meanings are suppressed and only meanings consistent with the message remain active."[29] This suggests that the RB may not be heavily engaged until difficulty in finding meaning is experienced. The same may also apply to humor.

2) Weak or Unusual Associations

Some early neuroimaging studies suggested that only the LB is involved in processing the meaning of words,[30] while others pointed to the activation of both hemispheres during semantic tasks.[31] One of the earliest studies to help clarify the linguistic contributions of the right cerebral cortex suggested that the RB may specialize in finding weaker or more challenging meanings (a finding that is consistent with the view proposed below that the RB becomes more important for more challenging forms of humor). Words which have either very strong or weak associations to a target word were presented in a way that caused them to go to either the RB or LB first. For example, the word *pound* has a strong meaningful connection to *hammer,* while *drop* has a weak one. After first being presented with a strong- or weak–association word, the target word was then presented so that it arrived first at either the LB or RB. Recognition of the target word by the LB was aided only by prior presentation of strong, frequent association words, while the right was aided by prior exposure to even weak association words.[32]

Similarly, when individuals were asked to provide associations to a list of words, the RB was more likely to be engaged when they thought of less common associations than when they came up with common ones.[33] In many forms of verbal humor (like puns), of course, this same processes occurs in searching for an association which is uncommon within the specific context set up in the joke, but is required to understand the joke. These and other findings again suggest that the LB has as its strong suit the processing of straightforward uses of language, while the right is more adept at metaphorical, creative *and humorous* aspects of language.

3) Resolving Ambiguity

The RB plays a key role in interpreting or resolving ambiguous sentences.[34] Ambiguity is one of the cornerstones of humor.

4) Fixing Grammatically Incorrect Sentences

The RB becomes more actively engaged when you are asked to mentally repair or correct sentences that are obviously incorrect grammatically.[35] An example of such a sentence is, "The spy is in the caught." There are many ways of correcting this grammatically, of course, but the act of doing so engages the RB more than thinking about a sentence that is grammatically correct. The LB mainly takes over in the latter case. While grammatically incorrect sentences are generally not funny, the mental process of identifying the feature that is "out of kilter" and fixing it has a clear parallel to identifying features that are distorted or incorrectly presented in humor.

5) Understanding Metaphors

RB areas roughly equivalent to LB areas that are known to process basic language functions have been shown to be activated as one tries to understand metaphors. This did not occur when looking for literal meanings of sentences.[36] It is worth noting, however, that when simpler and familiar metaphors were presented, LB areas were mainly activated, with minimal RB involvement.[37] Examples of the metaphors used in these studies are:

"The alarm clock is a torturer."
"My job is a jail."
"The camel is a desert taxi."
"Their cross mother was an elastic band."

The degree of simplicity/complexity, then, seems to be the key in determining the extent of RB involvement needed to understand metaphors. The relative novelty or familiarity of the metaphor also contributes to ease of interpretation, so that the LB can make sense out of familiar or conventional metaphors, while the RB is called upon to understand novel ones.[38] Even more complex metaphors may be understandable by the LB if they are familiar.

All metaphors involve placing ideas in a new context; and while the LB does have the ability to consider the context in which particular ideas or meanings occur, the RB is better at activating contextually inappropriate meanings.[39] The most common view among researchers studying this topic is that *it is the complexity of mental processing required to get meaning from metaphor that determines the extent of the RB's engagement*—not the demands imposed by the figurative nature of the language per se.[40]

The fact that increased RB activation occurs in a broad range of tasks as the task becomes more difficult[41] is consistent with this view. The LB also typically remains engaged to varying extents as the mental task becomes more difficult. Humor is simply one additional kind of complex mental task, one that has a clear parallel to metaphor. These findings suggest that degree of RB activation in response to humor should similarly be a direct function of difficulty level of the humor.

6) Integrating Information in Complex Narratives

As the context in which verbal information is presented becomes more complex, the RB becomes increasingly active. Thus, the RB is highly engaged in an ongoing narrative in which the listener must keep track of the story information presented and tie it into new information. "While both left and right hemispheres were active at the beginning of a story, right hemisphere activity increased dramatically at the end, when narrative details must be synthesized into a coherent whole."[42] Since a lot of humor occurs in the context of a story, the RB should similarly be engaged in this kind of humor.

7) Detection of Surprising Events

Consistent with the special role of the RB in processing unusual or less frequent meanings, it is also activated more by surprising events[43] and events that are inconsistent within a story.[44] Again, surprise and inconsistency are key aspects of most forms of humor.

8) Novelty and Violation of Expectation

The specific brain areas involved in non-humorous violations of expectation have also been studied.[45] Expectations were set up experimentally by providing a sequence of numbers to subjects in an identifiable pattern. An area of the RB was found to be involved in "the active maintenance of context information for prediction." A different RB area was activated when an unexpected or incongruous sequence of numbers then violated the learned sequence. There is a clear parallel here between encountering an unexpected number in an established sequence or pattern of numbers and encountering an unexpected ending in the punch line of a joke.

"You cannot hold back a good laugh any more than you can the tide. Both are forces of nature."   William Rotsler

One pair of neuropsychologists, Elkhonon Goldberg and Louis Costa, have argued that the relative amount of novelty of a task is crucial in determining the relative degree of participation of the two hemispheres—regardless of the specific nature of the task.[46] The LB is especially efficient in processing information that relates to highly routinized or familiar verbal or motor tasks; the RB gets more engaged when the task is highly novel, and there is no backlog of experience to call on to make sense of the situation or execute the task. They argue that the LB again gets more engaged when ideas and actions associated with the task become more familiar; i.e., when the processing of the information becomes more routine. *This means that for many activities, we can expect a gradual shift from RB to LB engagement as the novel aspects of the activity become more familiar. This may also occur with repetitions of humor.*

9) Detection of Discrepancy between Visual and Tactile Perception

Cross-modal perception refers to what happens when an object is first presented in one sensory modality (e.g., visually) and then presented along with other objects in a second modality (e.g., touch alone). The goal is to find the original object. The RB is engaged when the information from the two systems is conflicting—i.e., when there is no match.[47] Again, this points to a specialization in the RB for finding meaning where no meaning is initially present.

10) Perception of Objects with Unnatural Colors

The RB similarly is activated in connection with objects which do not have their natural or usual colors.[48] We recognize that something is out of kilter here and the RB tries to determine just what it is. While color distortion is rarely a basis for humor, this is consistent with the familiar theme of the RB specializing in making sense out of things that are disjointed or that initially make no sense.

11) Detection of Emotional Tone

The same word can carry quite different meaning, depending on the intonation with which it is uttered. The RB plays the key role in processing the emotional intonation of language.[49] Again, intonation is often used to carry subtleties of meaning in humor.

12) Making Inferences

When an event is inferred in an ongoing text, the key information related to the inference is more accessible in the RB than the LB.[50] When listening to a story that requires an inference to be made, neural activity in the RB occurs earlier than neural activity in the same region of the LB. This suggests that the RB may not always require a LB assessment before jumping into action. Certain areas of the LB are sure to be activated as the story is read, however, so we may again have a picture of some LB areas (or LB and RB areas) being engaged as the story unfolds, while key RB areas are activated only when an inference must be made.

There is presently (in 2010) an explosion of interest in brain mechanisms involved in the comprehension of figurative language. There is no agreement yet on just how to make sense out of all the data, but two recent reviewers of this research have emphasized that the complexity of the mental processing required appears to be one key in determining the extent of engagement of the RB.

"Taken together, the evidence yielded in imaging studies suggests that the processing of figurative language consistently activates fronto–temporal networks known to be involved in language processing per se. As to the question of lateralization, both hemispheres contribute to the processing of figurative language, albeit in different ways. The *RH appears to be relatively more involved in processing complex syntactic and semantic structures* and in accessing the meaning of novel or generally salient metaphors, while the *LH seems to contribute more to the decoding of word meaning* in a metaphoric context."[51] (Italics are McGhee's.)

The same researchers reached the following conclusion following a review of research in which key verbal information is first made available to one hemisphere (by presenting it to either the left or right visual field alone; words presented to the right visual field arrive directly at the LB first—and vice versa) before it is accessible to the other hemisphere via the corpus callosum.

". . . the evidence . . . suggests that the RH seems to be more engaged in activating distant semantic associations. Thus, the RH also activates more alternative interpretations, particularly in the case of unfamiliar figurative expressions and maintains their activation for longer time periods."[52]

It would be a most startling finding if the basic processing of information in humor were found to be different from the way in which information is processed in this wide-ranging set of non-humor studies. *If semantic complexity or other indicators of mental challenge are key determinants of extent of RB engagement in the absence of humor, they should be pivotal in influencing relative hemisphere engagement for humor, as well.*

fMRI Studies of Humor. Neuroimaging studies outside the realm of humor suggest that bilateral engagement of the hemispheres can be expected, with progressively greater involvement of the RB with increased mental challenge or complexity, ambiguity, novelty of key elements of the joke, and increased demand for integrating information or making inferences. As this section shows, humor researchers have generally not focused on these dimensions; their work has focused on areas of brain activation in response to other dimensions of the cartoons or jokes presented. Also, researchers have been primarily interested in identifying the specific brain areas engaged by humor within each hemisphere, not in the relative engagement of the two hemispheres.

Since the main focus of this chapter is the relative importance of the two hemispheres for humor, the findings from these studies relative to specific areas activated within each hemisphere in response to humor are generally not discussed. We are a long way from having any real consensus regarding the role of specific brain areas in humor. This is to be expected, since a wide range of features of any given cartoon, joke or funny circumstance can be expected to influence the specific brain area activated.

The first functional MRI study of humor (published in 2000) required individuals to listen to a tape recording of three different types of verbal texts: jokes, a (non-humorous) newspaper article and a complicated philosophical text. Since these all involved the use of language, the area of the LB long known to mediate basic language functions (the temporal lobe, including Wernicke's area) would be expected to be activated. This was found to be the case for all three listening tasks—with activation occurring in both the LB and RB.[53] So this initial finding for humor was consistent with the non-humor studies just discussed, although complexity levels of the materials presented was not assessed. And although the philosophical text might be assumed to be more complex, the relative engagement of the two hemispheres for the different materials was not discussed.

The second fMRI study, published the next year, took into consideration the fact that important distinctions can be made within the general category of "verbal" humor. Subjects listened to either puns or "semantic" jokes. The former is a simple form of humor, while the latter is more complex, relying for its humor on factors other than mere word play.

Semantic jokes: **What do engineers use for birth control? Their personalities.**

Puns (phonological jokes): **Why did the golfer wear two pairs of pants? He got a hole in one.**

Consistent with the non-humor studies, only the LB was activated by puns, while both hemispheres were activated by semantic jokes. Thus, the RB was engaged only for more complex jokes.[54] These researchers emphasized that the two types of humor engaged the brain differently. Simple puns used a "left hemisphere network centered around speech production regions (especially Broca's area)," while semantic incongruities engaged a network of neurons in both hemispheres.

In the case of simple puns, where the ambiguity is generally carried by a single word, the LB alone was sufficient to understand the ambiguity carried by the joke. This presumably reflects the fact that *the left temporal area of the cortex holds the memories of the extra meanings required to understand basic puns. In the case of more complex forms of humor, however, where previously unrelated domains of our experience are brought together for the first time, pertinent information might be stored in any number of other areas of the brain—areas which may even have little or no connection with language. In this case, the right hemisphere comes into play.*

Similarly, other researchers used a measure of electrical activity in the brain and concluded that the LB has an initial advantage when it comes to understanding puns, although "pun-related information is eventually available to both hemispheres."[55] The following are examples of the puns used in this study.

An archaeologist's career ended in ruins.
A psychiatrist on a hike fell into a depression.
A reporter was at the ice cream store getting the scoop.
Selling coffee has its perks.
Drilling for oil is boring.

Using the same measure of electrical activity in the brain, they found that this advantage switches to the RB when the complexity of the humor moves beyond simple puns.[56] Other fMRI studies have similarly demonstrated more active engagement of the right temporal lobe for more complex forms of humor[57] or bilateral activity in response to humor, with greater activity in the RB.[58]

One Italian team of researchers suspected that the engagement of the LB in humor may simply reflect the fact that the humor generally involved the use of language in prior studies. To check this out, they used captionless nonverbal cartoons in an fMRI study in which understanding the humor required making complex inferences about the intentions of a key character in the cartoon.[59] However, even in the absence of words, both the LB and RB were engaged.

This finding is supported by other evidence that (nonverbal) "sight gags" (*Far Side* cartoons, in which the humor was based on visual information in the cartoon—not on the caption) engage both halves of the brain.[60] *This suggests that the LB plays a general role in humor that is independent of the use of language in carrying the humor. As discussed below, it may be that an analytical process is occurring in which the LB makes the primary initial effort to understand humor, while the RB becomes relatively more engaged when the LB encounters difficulty in understanding what is depicted.*

BUILD YOUR HUMOR SKILLS

[Work on all three before checking the answers.]

1. Why do employers love to hire neurons? Because they keep on working no matter how many times they're _____.
1st *clue*: What can happen if an employee's work is not satisfactory?
2nd *clue*: What happens almost every year in the southwest if there's a lack of rain?

2. Why do neurons grown in a laboratory dish love the arts so much? Because they've grown up very _____.
1st *clue*: What kind of differences do anthropologists study?
2nd *clue*: It rhymes with "vulture."

3. What does a friendly brain do when it sees a neighbor across the way while shopping? It gives a _____ _____.
1st *clue*: Electrical activity in the brain.
2nd *clue*: EEG.

A German research group, however, also used nonverbal *Far Side* cartoons, but found only LB activation of certain brain areas and bilateral activation of other areas.[61] Yet another study found the largest cortical activation in response to funny cartoons with captions to occur in the LB.[62] And the degree of activation shown within a subject was greater for cartoons rated by that subject to be funnier. While their cartoons were rated in advance on their degree of simplicity-complexity, differences in activation of different brain areas as a function of complexity were not reported.

A European research team obtained fMRI data while presenting three different types of nonverbal cartoons (containing no caption or other kind of verbal information) to healthy individuals.[63] Areas of brain activation in response to these cartoons were compared to areas engaged by a fourth category of cartoons that clearly were incongruous, but provided no incongruity-resolution information. They called these "irresolvable cartoons." These cartoons were used as a control condition, not as a humor category. (They were clearly different from "nonsense" cartoons reported in a separate study—discussed next.) The example provided in the article showed a person sitting in a doctor's office with large dark spots (like those on a leopard) covering his body. The image is a bit funny (a preschooler would find it funny to see a person with leopard spots), but there is no punch line—no way of getting the "point" of the joke. This type of cartoon was consistently rated as "not funny at all."

They found a predominantly "left-sided network" of activation for all three main categories of cartoons (all of which contained resolution information), although both hemispheres were engaged to some extent. Their most crucial finding, in terms of hemisphere differences, was that *for cartoons with irresolvable incongruities, RB activation was dominant* (in sharp contrast to the strong LB engagement by the three humor categories). "It is striking that the left frontal cortex is involved in successful humor processing, whereas *the INC condition [irresolvable incongruities] evoked activation only in the right frontal cortex.*"[64] (Italics are McGhee's.)

In this case, the researchers did rate their three categories of cartoons for complexity, but did not relate complexity data to their findings. So it is difficult to comment on whether their findings do or do not support the notion that the RB becomes increasingly important for humor as complexity increases. They do note that their three humor categories were of comparable levels of complexity, but do not report what level of complexity that was.

> *"The kind of humor I like is the thing that makes me laugh for five seconds and then think for five minutes."*   William Davis

While the researchers doing this study showed little interest in the irresolvable incongruity cartoon category (it was used as a basis of comparison with the other cartoon categories), it is actually quite important. These cartoons present individuals with precisely the kind of cognitive task for which the *RB would be expected to be maximally engaged by the effort to understand what is going on.* The initial efforts to make sense of it do not work, so you must continue to look at it and think about it, trying to find the point of the cartoon (the punch line) . . . until you finally give up because you just don't get it. Consistent with this notion, they report that subjects ". . . need[ed] more time to process the INC condition: It might reflect cognitive effort required to decide definitively that there is no joke in the picture. . . Subjects have to continuously generate new hypotheses as to how the picture could be interpreted as a funny stimulus."[65] Consistent with this need for greater time to process the INC cartoons, subjects rated these cartoons as having higher levels of "residual incongruity."

ANSWERS TO JOKES

| 1. fired | 2. cultured | 3. brain wave |

Finally, the same research team, led by Andrea Samson, reanalyzed this same set of data by selecting only those cartoons which could be classified as examples of either incongruity-resolution humor or nonsense humor. In incongruity-resolution cartoons, as already noted, information is available in one part of the cartoon which allows for the complete resolution of an incongruity elsewhere in the cartoon. Once this resolution information is identified, the cartoon is understood—what initially makes no sense does then make sense in an unexpected way.

In nonsense cartoons, no information is available which enables one to make sense of the incongruous situation presented; or a partial resolution is possible, but you are still left with some type of unexplained incongruity.[66] Consistent with the general pattern of findings discussed above, several brain areas were activated bilaterally in response to incongruity-resolution humor; surprisingly, however, no specific area of activation was found for nonsense humor—in either hemisphere. Again, while the two types of cartoons were said to be of comparable levels of complexity, no information is provided on how complex these cartoons were perceived to be.

Taken together, then, the research on healthy brains confirms the findings from studies of people with brain injuries that the RB is especially important for many forms of humor. However, it clearly does not work alone in the mental processing of humor. Consistent with the findings for non-humorous forms of more sophisticated kinds of thought, the two hemispheres work together in most (if not all) humor. In many cases, the initial emphasis is on left hemisphere processing; but bilateral processing also appears to occur from the outset in other cases.

The extent of RB engagement exists along a continuum, ranging from minimal involvement to primary engagement. There is some evidence to support the view that complexity of the materials presented influences the relative engagement of the hemispheres, but this issue has not yet been satisfactorily tested. While a range of complexity has been present in the cartoons and jokes used, researchers have not specifically related complexity ratings to extent of engagement of the two hemispheres. Clearly, simple puns can be understood and enjoyed by engagement of the LB alone, but it is not yet clear just how much complexity the LB can handle on its own.

Other fMRI studies of complex—but non-humorous—materials, however, (discussed above), clearly point to networks of neural activation that are very different for different kinds of complexity.[67] That evidence shows that *more complex material activates more neural tissue and more complex networks than simpler material. Since this holds for thinking and problem solving in a general sense, the engagement of wider neural networks for complex than for simple humor is to be expected.*

Engagement of Recently-Evolved Neurons by Humor. Certain kinds of cells within the cortex have been hypothesized to have evolved more recently than others. These cells are called von Economo cells[68] (previously known as "spindle neurons") and have been found only in two regions of the cortex. They are estimated to have evolved in the last 15 million years,[69] and are found only in humans and the great apes.

Both regions of the brain containing these neurons have been shown to be activated in response to verbal and nonverbal cartoons.

And the extent of activation (in both regions) was positively related to the funniness of the cartoons presented.[70] The investigators who did this study suggested that these cells may play an important role in the very rapid and intuitive assessments that occur when we appreciate the humor of a joke or cartoon (or any other funny situation).

It has long been observed that the optimal conditions for humor are when the "point" or "punch line" is quickly gotten. At the same time, it can't be so simple and obvious that there is no mental challenge at all to getting the joke. Also, if it's so difficult that it takes a lot of reflective thought to get the punch line, this reduces its funniness.[71] *It is often only after this intuitive and spontaneous understanding of the joke occurs that we become consciously aware of what we're laughing at.* The researchers believe it is these newly-evolved von Economo cells that mediate this first level of intuitive insight into the joke.

The Importance of Communication between the Two Hemispheres

The view that the LB plays the key role in basic language functions (at least among right-handed individuals) while the RB is essential for more sophisticated language functions is, of course, an over-simplified view of what actually happens in the brain during humor or any other experience. Many different areas of the brain are active at the same time, and communication between neurons both within and between the two hemispheres is constantly occurring. *Thus, both hemispheres can be expected to be engaged to some extent in responding to most forms of humor—even in cases where the LB alone may be sufficient for comprehension.* In the case of a joke, the LB probably initially plays the most important role as the joke is read or listened to. But this hemisphere is more limited in finding the unexpected meaning associated with many incongruities (especially those that are more complex or challenging) or unexpected events at the heart of the joke, so the special skills of the RB come into play and help us get the joke. But there is every reason to think that the two hemispheres are constantly "talking" back and forth with each other throughout this process. (See the next section for a discussion of this issue.)

One way to document the importance (for humor) of this ongoing dialog between the two hemispheres is to look at the impact of neurological conditions which interfere with inter-hemispheric communication. The primary channel through which the right and left hemispheres talk to each other is the corpus callosum. This is the so-called "white matter" separating the two hemispheres. It is white because of the fatty substance (the myelin sheath, which speeds up neural transmission at greater distances) covering the axons connecting distant neurons in the two hemispheres.

Individuals who show normal intelligence, but lack a corpus callosum (this condition results from a birth defect called "agenesis of the corpus callosum") find it difficult to understand a broad range of "second order" meanings, including jokes, proverbs and nonliteral language.[72] This is the very same conclusion reached above from studies of damaged and healthy brains regarding the importance of the RB.

It is also worth noting that individuals lacking a corpus callosum show no difficulty in understanding puns—even though they do show deficits in understanding more complex forms of verbal humor.[73] Again, this is consistent with the fMRI data just discussed and suggests that the LB alone may be sufficient to understand this simple form of verbal humor. Alternate meanings of words (the basis for puns), then, must be stored in the same (left) hemisphere; *only in the case of more complex forms of language-mediated humor does the LB have to communicate with the right to make coherent what initially makes no sense.* It is worth noting that these deficits in understanding complex forms of verbal humor among individuals lacking the main neural path for sharing information between the two hemispheres cannot be the result of a lower IQ generally, since the patients used in the study were matched with individuals with intact brains and comparable IQs—(including verbal IQ) and the latter group showed no humor deficits.

Bill Gates and the president of General Motors are talking over lunch and Bill is going on and on about computer technology. "If you guys had kept pace with computer technology, we'd all be driving a V-16 instead of a V-8 or V-6, and it would have a top speed

of 500 miles per hour," says Gates. "Or you could
have an economy car that weighs 500 pounds and gets
700 miles to a gallon gas. In either case, the sticker
price of a new car would be less than a few hundred
dollars. Why haven't you guys kept up?"

The president of GM smiles and says, "Because the
government won't let us build cars that crash every
day."

The same study that showed LB comprehension of puns in
people lacking a corpus callosum found that the LB was sufficient for
understanding simple (captionless) cartoons. These cartoons were not
complex enough to require RB engagement.

So this is a third kind of data showing that *both hemispheres
are required to fully understand and enjoy humor that goes beyond simple
reinterpretation of key words.* While the LB controls the basic processing
of the joke or other language-based humor in these individuals
with no corpus callosum, it alone cannot directly access information
present elsewhere in the brain which lends coherence to the initial
incongruities or unexpected events represented in the joke. As
one research team put it, ". . . information necessary for adequate
humor processing would be trapped in the right hemisphere by the
absence of the very large band of interhemispheric fibers of the corpus
callosum. . . . This [is] . . . consistent with the implications of deficits
in individuals with RHD [RB damage] in the comprehension of
both nonliteral language . . . and humor . . ."[74]

*In the case of individuals with RB damage, the corpus callosum presumably
tries to communicate with regions of the (right) brain where key information
required to get the joke is stored, but the injury has either removed the
knowledge/memories necessary for comprehension or made it inaccessible. The
net result is the same.*

It is tempting to conclude that a sequential engagement of the
two hemispheres occurs. The LB starts by processing the basic
information in a joke, but then must switch over to the RB (via
the corpus callosum) to seek out a context which resolves the
incongruity or generates a sense of coherence. It would, however, be
oversimplified to think that the hemispheres operate in an "either or"

fashion—i.e., either the left or the right is doing the work. Rather—as suggested above—they appear to work together in a coordinated fashion. For example, there is evidence that both hemispheres are actively engaged while reading (or listening to) a narrative[75] and understanding "natural language."[76]

The extent of RB activation in this scenario would depend on the success of the left in finding coherent meaning in what is being read. Right-hemisphere engagement would increase sharply when confronted by (more complex) jokes, cartoons, metaphors, sarcasm, etc., since the left hemisphere would be unable on its own to generate any sense of coherence in the information presented. When a story or series of paragraphs is being read (or listened to), we automatically engage in an ongoing process of sustaining a thread of meaningful coherence as new information is presented. This occurs even for normal, straightforward communication which contains no incongruity or figurative language. The RB appears to handle this task in all communications; it is suggested here that it is simply more actively engaged when the challenge to creating coherence is escalated (as in humor, metaphor, etc.).

> "Our results . . . clearly show that right hemisphere engagement during sentence comprehension is not specific to the processing of figurative language. Rather, right hemisphere engagement appears to be a more general phenomenon that occurs routinely as readers attempt to construct a unitary coherent model of a discourse and discover the producer's intent."[77]

Rapid Alternation between Left and Right Brain Processing. It is clear that the areas of the brain engaged fluctuate rapidly, depending on the demands imposed by a mental task—especially in terms of lateralization of brain activity.[78] "When the brain processes words, for example, it is likely that neural systems involving both left and right hemispheres will be differentially engaged when the words are processed in isolation, in a syntactic structure, or in a coherent narrative, since each of these contexts supports a different, increasingly complex level of semantic representation."[79]

BUILD YOUR HUMOR SKILLS

[Work on all three before checking the answers.]

1. What are the only fish allowed to do neurosurgery? _____.

1st *clue*: Caviar.
2nd *clue*: What kind of fish produces the eggs for caviar?

2. Why was the young neuron always getting in trouble at school? Because it couldn't control its _____.
1st *clue*: This is a common problem with kids—especially hyperactive kids.
2nd *clue*: Part of this word is a way of referring to your heartbeat.

3. What did the right hemisphere say to the left hemisphere when they just couldn't get along any more? "Let's _____."
1st *clue*: "Let's get out of here"
2nd *clue*: A dessert with bananas, ice cream and whipped cream.

With humor, as with ordinary non-humorous forms of discourse, we must make inferences as more and more information is presented in order to integrate the information in a coherent fashion. Key points may be ambiguous, and we must come up with our own interpretation of what is meant. The RB becomes increasingly engaged as this process of integration or interpretation occurs. For example, while listening to brief narratives from Aesop's fables, the LB is initially more prominently engaged; but by the end of the story, when information allowing an integration of previously-presented information is presented (making possible a coherent understanding), the RB is more prominently engaged.[80]

In fact, many different areas beyond basic LB language areas are activated. A large network of neurons is engaged in varying areas of the brain, depending on the specific information presented in the narrative. *The RB becomes specifically prominent when some kind of interpretative or synthesizing process is required—especially when the information becomes increasingly complex.*

Other studies of non-humorous language ambiguity similarly point to this sequencing of relative involvement of the hemispheres. For example, one research team created a bias toward one (more likely) interpretation of a key word and then provided information toward the end of the sentence that made it clear that the first interpretation was incorrect.[81] Examples of the items used are:

"Unfortunately, the table was too large for him to copy it into his notebook."

"Actually, the port was popular even though it had a strange flavor."

"Unfortunately, the bank was rather dirty even though the town took care to keep the river itself clean."

In the first example, most people initially interpret "table" to mean a piece of furniture. The last phrase, however, makes it clear that this meaning is wrong. The key question, then, is which hemisphere plays the greatest role in both generating the first (incorrect) meaning and seeking out other meanings once it becomes clear that that first meaning is wrong.

The LB was first activated. When the biased meaning proved incorrect, the RB became engaged as other meanings were sought out. The RB was not engaged in this fashion for unambiguous sentences (such as "The total was too large for him to copy into his notebook." Or "Actually, the soup was popular even though it had a strange flavor."). A bilateral involvement of both the LB and RB then followed in order to—in the view of the researchers—assess the coherence of the second meaning that had been found.

So these findings are consistent with the notion that the LB is most commonly engaged in seeking out common or "expected" meanings, while the RB quickly comes in to help out if the LB is either unsuccessful or concludes that it has been led down the wrong semantic path. Both hemispheres remain engaged as the brain verifies that it has "got it right" this time.

Creating Humor: A Better Test of the Role of Complexity in RB Specialization

As noted above, researchers have not yet tested the notion that the special capacities of the RB become increasingly relied upon for comprehension of more complex forms of humor. In most of the studies completed, no effort was made to assess difficulty level of the jokes, cartoons, metaphors, etc. used before obtaining brain imaging or brain-damage data. If complexity is a key factor in determining the relative engagement of the two hemispheres, inconsistent findings across studies is exactly what one would expect, since a wide range of difficulty levels appears to be present in the specific items used.

ANSWERS TO JOKES

1. Neurosturgeons   2. impulses   3. split (Some readers will be familiar with the notion of a "split brain." If you're not, this makes no sense.)

Because of this oversight in fMRI studies of humor, I suggested recently in an article written for researchers that it is essential to measure complexity in advance and use a wide range of difficulty levels of cartoons, jokes, etc. in future studies along these lines.[82]

I also suggested that researchers should conduct neuroimaging experiments which go beyond simply observing brain activity while subjects seek to understand a punch line presented to them. If the goal is to offer a true mental challenge in the context of humor, the best approach would be to do the very thing you are required to do when reading the humor skill-building examples presented in the boxes throughout this book. In those examples, instead of simply trying to understand the information presented in the punch line, you have to generate the key information that carries the humor.

And even when asking subjects to create their own humor, the difficulty level of the jokes or cartoons presented must still be considered. While creating humor by filling in a missing key part of the punch line is more difficult than merely understanding the same punch line when it is provided, completing a missing part of the punch line for simple puns is less mentally demanding than doing so for more complicated forms of humor. My books *Stumble Bees and Pelephones* and *Small Medium at Large* provide both children (in the former case) and adults (in the latter case) several hundred opportunities to exercise and challenge both sides of the brain in generating their own humor using one or more clues.[83] (See www. LaughterRemedy.com to order either book.) One example from each book is shown below.

What happens to little canoes when they're bad? They get _____."
1ˢᵗ clue: **It's a kind of spanking.**
2ⁿᵈ clue: **Find another word for "oar."**
3ʳᵈ clue: **Only one word works for both clues 1 and 2.**

A man goes ice fishing. He cuts a hole in the ice, but then hears a loud booming voice say, "There are no fish there!"
Although startled at this, he moves over to another location and begins cutting a new hole. Again, a voice booms, "There are no fish there!"
He tries a new spot, and the voice repeats, "I said there are no fish there!"
"Who is that?" he cries out. "Who's talking to me?"
"The _____," says the voice.
1ˢᵗ clue: **It's not God. In this joke, you're trying to make the ice cutter appear pretty simple-minded.**

2ⁿᵈ *clue*: Think of a situation where there's ice, but where there couldn't possibly be fish below.

Adults clearly can be expected to show a greater level of RB engagement in coming up with answers to jokes like the second example than to jokes like the children's riddle.

Which Hemisphere Explains Why it's Funny?

We've all had the experience at some point of being the only one not laughing at something. Chances are you've also had the opposite experience of having a fall-down belly laugh at something in the presence of someone who failed to see any humor in it at all. When they ask, "I don't get it, what's so funny?" you have a hard time explaining it in a way that enables them to get the same hearty yucks that you got. You may not even know why it strikes you as funny. This is a common experience that many people report. They quickly get the point and laugh, but have a difficult time explaining *why* they laughed. This quick processing of humor seems to be crucial to its enjoyment (although it won't be very funny if it's too easy and we get it too quickly), but it doesn't necessarily give us any insight into just *why* we think it's funny.

ANSWERS TO ADULT JOKES ON PREVIOUS PAGE

paddled   rink manager

Some individuals consistently have a hard time explaining why anything is funny. These may be people who are simply less inclined to be analytical in their reasoning about most things. But explaining humor is not as easy as you might think. Try telling the following two jokes (or any others you might choose) to a small group of people and ask them to write down just what makes the joke funny. You will be amazed at how differently people respond.

A man suspected of having SARS is lying in bed with a mask over his mouth. A young nurse comes by to sponge his face and hands. He mumbles from behind his mask, "Nurse, are my testicles black?"

Embarrassed, the nurse says, "I don't know, Mr. Thompson, I'm only here to wash your face and hands."

He again struggles to ask, "Are my testicles black?" Again, the nurse says, "I can't tell. I'm just here to wash your face and hands."

The Head Nurse was passing by at that moment and notices the man getting distraught; so she walks over and asks what's wrong. Again, the man mumbles, "Are my testicles black?"

Given her years of experience, the Head Nurse just whips the sheet back, pulls down his pajamas and underwear, pulls his penis out of the way, has a good look, then pulls the clothes and sheet back up and announces, "Nope! Nothing wrong with your testicles."

At this, the man pulls off his mask and again asks, "I said . . . are my test results back?"

Three tough bikers walk into a truck stop diner and go up to an older man at the counter eating his breakfast. The first biker takes his cigarette and drops it into the man's coffee. But the man doesn't say a word and just keeps eating his breakfast. The second biker tips over the man's orange juice. Still no reaction. The third biker dumps the guy's plate of eggs and bacon on the floor. But the older man just gets up without saying a word, pays his bill and leaves the diner.

The leader of the bikers says, "Well, he wasn't much of a man, was he?"

"No," says the waitress, "and not much of a truck driver either. He just ran over three Harleys in the parking lot.

I argued 25 years ago that different processes are involved in understanding a joke or other humor and explaining why it's funny. Although there were virtually no pertinent data available, I suggested that if one is asked to reflect about why a joke is funny, the more analytical LB takes the prominent role in coming up with an explanation. *The RB, while better at spontaneously getting the joke, is less adept at explaining what it just got.*[84] One study has showed that patients with RB damage have difficulty explaining why material presented to them was funny.[85] But is this because the RB normally has the role of explaining humor or because of the lack of access of the LB to the key information it needed to explain why it was funny? Studies using neuroimaging techniques have not yet focused on which areas of the brain are active during attempts to explain funniness.

The difficulty we have in putting into words why something is funny helps explain why researchers have often found only low to moderate positive correlations between measures of the appreciation and comprehension of humor. The RB plays the key role of detecting and appreciating (more complicated forms of) humor, but is not very good at explaining its own amusement.

My own view is that it is the LB which takes the RB's insight into the point of the joke (at least for more complicated jokes) and comes up with an explanation for its perceived funniness. The LB has to search around for rule violations or unexpected, incongruous or "taboo" content which might have triggered the rapid insight that occurred in the RB. *When a rationale for the laughter is found that makes sense, it is offered by the LB as an explanation for funniness of the joke or situation whose enjoyment was made possible by the RB.* This is consistent with the conclusion among researchers that the LB is better at analytic functions, while the RB is better at obtaining a more holistic understanding of things.[86]

The notion that the LB becomes more actively engaged when asked to explain humor is consistent with a finding regarding how the brain processes music. While music has long been assumed to be processed mainly by the RB, trained musicians (who are more analytical when listening to music) showed better recognition of melodies played though the right ear (received first by the LB) than through the left ear (received first by the RB). Musically naïve listeners, however, showed better recognition through the left ear.[87] If the LB plays a more active role in analyzing music, it may well also do so with humor.

Many researchers over the past few decades (myself included) have assumed that it is possible to measure the comprehension of humor by simply determining an individual's ability to come up with the same reasons for funniness that have been agreed upon by a panel of adult judges prior to undertaking the research project. The limits of this approach are clear. If the RB is calling upon other neural connections and associations with which the LB is not immediately aware, is it valid to say that the person who can give reasons that match the experimenter's explanations for funniness experiences greater appreciation of humor than the person whose left hemisphere is unable to access the basis for a great guffaw?

It may be, then, that *the brain experiences two different kinds of appreciation of humor.* The first stems from a more holistic and intuitive level of understanding that directly and quickly triggers laughter and the awareness, "that's funny." The second results from a more reasoned, reflective or analytical level of comprehension. I am not suggesting that the latter reflects a deeper or truer level of humor comprehension (although this may sometimes be the case). They are simply different; or at least they are often different. In any particular case, there is no way of knowing just how these two aspects of comprehension differ, since we have no way of accessing the first without asking the person—which will generate a LB logical or analytical answer.

Conclusion: Humor Engages a Neural Network—There is No Humor Center

Most people have long assumed that humans are the only species capable of humor (I do not think that is the case), and some researchers have wondered whether there might be some special area in the brain devoted exclusively to humor—an area that could be labeled as the "humor center." We can finally say that there is no such center. William Fry was among the first to emphasize this point in 2002, noting that researchers who had long assumed that such a center would eventually be identified were clearly on the wrong track.[88] He suggested that complex networks of neurons are probably always involved in humor. Different networks may even prove to be activated by different features of the same joke, cartoon or funny real-life event. The specific network activated may depend on just where information represented in the joke or cartoon is stored, the extent of visual or auditory imagery generated, the extent to which sexual or hostile content is represented, and a host of other factors that vary from joke to joke. The LB (in right-handed individuals), of course, would be expected to always be activated to the extent that language is involved.

At this point, as we have seen, it appears that the LB alone can appreciate simpler forms of humor, such as puns. More complex forms of humorous and non-humorous uses of language require the unique skills of the RB. We don't yet know if repeated or otherwise long-familiar forms of humor come to be mediated by the LB as they become more familiar. Since other routinized tasks tend to shift to the LB (as noted below), highly familiar humor may do so, as well.

In retrospect, of course, this makes perfect sense. It is much more efficient for the brain to function in a manner that allows it to use particular brain areas (in this case, regions within the RB) for a broad range of functions that have certain things in common. This is precisely what happens as the brain uses a wide-ranging network of neurons in the cortex to understand and enjoy humor, metaphor, and other non-literal uses of language.

The Functional and Structural Basis for the Right Brain's Special Role in Complex Humor

Is it a coincidence that the RB plays a key role in our most sophisticated mental abilities (one of which is humor)? Or does the RB have specific features which make it ideally suited to support our capacity for humor and other forms of sophisticated thought?

Right Brain Functions

The two frontal lobes (right *and* left) of the brain have long been linked to a variety of cognitive functions or processes—especially the capacity for abstract thought—that are crucial to appreciation of humor. [89] For example, in the case of humor beyond simple puns or slapstick, a skill generally referred to as "working memory" is required. This is the ability to hold key information in mind while engaging in some mental task, and it is dependent on the frontal lobes of the cortex.[90]

Many occurrences of humor have a special emotional salience for the recipient of the humor; that is, they tie significantly into our unique personal experience in some way. (Put-down humor and humor involving some personal embarrassment are also examples of this.) The frontal region of the RB has been shown to be especially active during the retrieval of such past personal events.[91] And self-awareness in general has been linked to the frontal lobes—especially the right frontal lobe.[92]

In addition to this specialization for emotionally salient humor, two more general specialized functions of the RB are especially important for our understanding of hemisphere differences in humor.

Specialization for Novelty and Discrepancy. A great deal of attention has been given by researchers to the fact that the right hemisphere is especially effective in processing novel information. Elkhonon Goldberg, a neuropsychologist at the New York University School of Medicine, has argued (as noted earlier) for the past 25 years that the RB is specialized for processing novelty, while the left is geared more to processing "routine" information.[93] The early stages of learning, he points out, always involve some degree of newness or novelty. As learning proceeds, objects, tasks and actions become increasingly familiar and routinized. Our entire life is spent going through this sequence. The transfer of routinized information to the LB, in his view, makes for more efficient learning since it leaves the RB to specialize in novel information. Humor, of course, can be viewed as one form of novelty (unless you've heard the joke or experienced the funny situation before).

In support of his view of the increased efficiency of this division of hemispheric labor into novel and routine, he notes that highly sophisticated computer systems have been developed to simulate the operation of the human brain. They are called "formal neural nets," and are composed of an enormous number of simple units. They are true learning machines, in that they can store and accumulate information about their environment—as long as their actions generate feedback which is available to the system. One pioneer of neural net modeling, Stephen Grossberg, supported Goldberg's view in his finding that *a computer system is more efficient if it is split into two parts, one handling routine inputs and the other novel inputs.*[94] If such splitting provides a computational advantage to a computer, it may also do so for a living brain.

This view of the brain, of course, means that a constant shifting must occur in the specific information which is handled by the two hemispheres. What was novel, surprising or incongruous yesterday is old news and easily processed today. So the RB would need to be constantly shifting information to the left; and this is precisely what happens, according to Goldberg. As one acquires more and more experience with anything, processing of future related information should increasingly be handled by the LB.

In support of this view, Goldberg notes that such a shift can be demonstrated in the case of the brain's processing of music. As noted earlier, music has long been assumed to be processed in the RB. This is, indeed, the case among right-handed people with no musical training. Among trained musicians, however, music is processed mainly in the left hemisphere.[95] Similarly, the processing of images of faces has long been assumed to be a specialty of the RB. Familiar faces, however, are processed mainly in the LB, while unfamiliar faces are processed in the right.[96]

My own guess is that a similar shift occurs with humor. That is, when first presented with any joke, cartoon or other funny event with some moderate or high level of complexity, the RB should initially play the major role in processing the information presented (even though the LB can also be expected to be engaged to some extent). If the same humor is then presented days or weeks later, the level of RB engagement should drop at the same time that LB engagement increases. This shift would obviously be much weaker—if it occurs at all—for simpler forms of humor.

Unique Way of Processing Information. It was assumed for many years that nonverbal functions are mainly handled by the RB. Research in the 1970s and 1980s, however, refined this view, showing that the two hemispheres actually differ in the way they process information. The LB was shown to be specialized for analytical processing and the right for holistic processing.[97] Springer and Deutsch, the authors of several editions of *Left Brain/Right Brain* (for many years, the best known text on right and left brain differences), also argued that the hemispheres differ not in the kind of stimuli they process, but in the kind of mental operations performed. The greater the extent to which an analytical function is required, the greater the likely involvement of the LB. The greater the extent to which holistic processing of information from diverse sources is required, the more likely the RB is to be engaged.

> *"Keep me away from the wisdom which does not cry, the philosophy which does not laugh. . ."*   Kahlil Gibran

Even within language, we're generally in the position of not merely making sense out of strings of written or spoken words, but of integrating or synthesizing the basic ideas represented in all those words (something we have already noted to be a specialty of the RB). We need to simultaneously have access to many pieces of information to grasp systems of relationships. The RB is ideally suited to considering information in a more holistic sense. As noted above, we probably shift back and forth continually between the two hemispheres and between these two types of processing in dealing with the normal problems of everyday life.

"The right-holistic mode is particularly good at grasping patterns of relations between the component parts of a stimulus array, integrating many inputs simultaneously to eventually arrive at a complete configuration . . ."[98] It is this ability to grasp patterns and integrate diverse elements (that may initially appear to be unrelated) that makes the RB an ideal candidate for mediating humor that is not easily understood. In most humor, information is sequentially presented until an unexpected and incongruous punch line comes at the end. To get the joke, you must integrate the various pieces that make up the incongruity and find some meaningful link. The RB excels at precisely this kind of meaningful integration.

Right-Brain Anatomy/Structure

Given the clear pattern of findings showing greater engagement of the RB for more complex forms of thought, the obvious question to be raised is whether there are LB/RB structural differences which account for the functional differences found for the two hemispheres. Research along these lines has focused on the relative amount of gray and white matter,[99] dentritic branching,[100] size of neurons,[101] patterns of interconnectivity between neurons,[102] width of (and distance between) "microcolumns" of neurons,[103] number of interconnected "macrocolumn" systems of neurons,[104] and amount of cortex devoted to "association areas"—that is, brain areas involved with higher level integrative functions,[105] among other structural features.

Although considerable research attention has now been given to this issue, one pair of researchers noted in 2003 that ". . . we can only speculate about the functional consequences of structural asymmetries in language cortex."[106] While their comments were restricted to areas of the cortex related to language, the same conclusion applies to other areas of the brain. As late as 2009, another group of researchers concluded that while ". . . important progress has been made with regards to understanding how the brain consists of interconnected networks that underlie cognitive processing, there is very little clear evidence linking brain asymmetries with functional lateralization."[107]   Given the lack of any clear conclusions regarding structural hemisphere asymmetry at this point, this research will not be discussed here.

Enjoying Humor: Why it Feels so Good

Once we understand or "get" the joke, we immediately experience amusement—an emotional rush that is best characterized as joy or exhilaration—and we feel both pleasure and the urge to laugh. This urge to laugh seems to be both a built-in means of releasing tension and an important communication tool that developed during our early evolution; but why do we get such pleasure from humor? Why does it feel so good? And does this good feeling only occur when we laugh, or can the feel-good side of humor also occur in response to the mere experience of humor—whether we laugh or not?

The research on this issue is still limited, but by 2009, a half dozen studies had shown that the rewarding or pleasurable feeling that goes along with the appreciation of humor is a result of the activation of known (sub cortical) reward or pleasure centers in the brain—actually a network of brain regions, not a localized center.[108] This network is located in (phyologenetically) older regions of the brain and involves several distinct, but interconnected, dopamine-enriched (dopamine is a neurotransmitter) structures, including the nucleus accumbens and amygdala (the amygdala plays a key role in emotion in general). This network has been referred to as the "mesolimbic dopaminergic reward system" because it utilizes known dopamine-based reward or pleasure pathways.

One particular area within this reward system—the nucleus accumbens—appears to be especially important for the pleasure experienced in humor. This is the same area of the brain that lights up (is activated) in response to cocaine and methamphetamine, as well as other sources of "psychological reward."[109] This area mediates the euphoria or "high" induced by these drugs; and it may well be the activation of this reward/pleasure center that is responsible for the natural high we experience as a result of humor and a good belly laugh. When the nucleus acumbens is directly stimulated electrically, smiling occurs and people report feelings of euphoria.[110]

BUILD YOUR HUMOR SKILLS

[Work on all three before checking the answers.]

1. What's the one time you can expect a lot of thunder and lightening in your head? During a _____ _____.
1st clue: When do thunder and lightening normally occur?
2nd clue: A rush of really good ideas.

2. Which of a neuron's mathematical skills get worse as it gets older? _____ and _____.
1st clue: Our neurons do an amazing amount of this during infant development.
2nd clue: Times tables in school.

3. What nerve in your head is named after a famous gambling city? The _____ nerve.
1st clue: Viva . . .
2nd clue: It's in Nevada.

The first study documenting the connection between humor and this reward system further found that the degree of activation of the nucleus accumbens was directly related to the funniness of the cartoons presented. The funnier the cartoons, the greater the level of pleasure experienced.[111] Similarly, degree of activation of the (left) amygdala was positively related to the rated funniness of nonverbal cartoons.[112]

So now we know why humor makes us feel so good. This also helps explain humor's amazing power to pull us out of a negative emotional state and substitute a more positive emotion in its place (see Chapter 1 for a discussion of this research). And it goes a long way in explaining how humor helps us cope. Activation of this reward system creates a positive shift of mood and attitude which enables us to take active steps to deal with the problem causing stress at the moment. It helps produce the optimistic attitude that leads us to believe that we can overcome and survive the problem.

As with the research discussed in Chapter 2 regarding humor and health, we don't know how much of the feel-good side of humor (resulting from activation of pleasure centers in the brain) is due to the mental and emotional experience of humor and how much is due to the act of laughing itself. You cannot obtain good neuroimaging data if your subjects are allowed to have a real let-go belly laugh as you monitor their brain activity, since the "laughing head" would be moving around too much. But we know from our own experience that it just somehow feels good to have a real belly laugh.

In my keynotes to both corporate and healthcare groups, I always do a "laughter exercise" which is built into a fun routine and culminates in 20-30 seconds of non-stop belly laughter. When I ask people right afterwards what they notice about changes in body states or feelings relative to before the laughter, someone almost always says that they just feel "good" or "better." And people who participate in the hundreds of laughter clubs around the world that get together to laugh "for no reason" similarly say that it just feels good to laugh with friends (and strangers too, although most people feel more comfortable doing this kind of laughter among friends).

It was noted 30 years ago that simply getting your body to engage in the behaviors associated with a given emotion is enough to cause you to experience that emotion, and that this includes the experience of positive feelings in response to forced laughter.[113] In fact, even simply imagining oneself laughing—without actually doing so—increases feelings of happiness.[114]

Jaak Panksepp has argued that there is a very good reason for why this should occur: "My reading of the evidence is that the mechanisms of raw emotional feelings are very closely linked to the emotional-instinctual action systems of the brain. If so, the feeling of mirth might be closely linked to brain systems that generate the full and sincere pattern of laughter within the brain." In his view, the joy and good feeling that comes from shared play and laughter occur in other species (including rats), as well. He has shown that this same mesolimbic dopaminergic pleasure system is activated in response to the tickling of rats,[115] suggesting that the pleasure we

PAUL MCGHEE, PhD

get from humor and laughter is mediated by neurological reward or pleasure systems that evolved long ago.

Additional Sources of Pleasure via the Dopamine Reward System

As one would expect, humor is just one among many sources of pleasure mediated by this dopamine-based reward system. Pleasure experienced in response to activation of this system has also been shown to result from food,[116] sex,[117] drugs,[118] winning money,[119] maternal behavior (in rats),[120] music[121] and even animal play.[122] While this system may initially have served to sustain basic survival needs (e.g., via the experience of pleasure associated with sex and eating), the same centers came to be extended to psychological forms of reward.

ANSWERS TO JOKES

1. brain storm   2. Multiplication and division   3. vagus

It is especially interesting that the play behavior of lower species (e.g., rats) activates these reward centers. This suggests that the pleasurable nature of play behavior was established early on in evolution. My own view of humor is that it is merely a sophisticated form of play behavior—intellectual play, or play with ideas. Humor is the evolutionary end result of a general tendency among higher-order species to play with existing capacities (when no strong biological urges or perceived threats are present). *The neurophysiological foundation for enjoyment of humor, then, is the same as that found for social or object play among lower animals.* This also means that just as there is no humor "center" uniquely devoted to understanding humor, so there is no center uniquely devoted to the pleasure experienced in connection with humor.

Influences on Degree of Reward Center Activation

At this point, no effort has been made to refine the finding that humor activates known reward/pleasure centers and look at which kinds of humor are most/least effective in activating these centers. We have long known, however, that certain qualities of the humorous event—ranging from features of the joke/cartoon/funny situation itself to the nature of the social context in which it occurs—increase laughter or the perceived funniness of the event while others reduce it. Since we do have some initial evidence indicating (as we would expect) that the rated funniness of a humorous event is positively related to the level of activation of the reward centers, we might expect that already-demonstrated factors which boost funniness should also boost the level of activation of these reward centers. The same should hold for laughter. Although we often laugh for reasons that have nothing to do with humor, my own guess is that well-established sources of increased laughter will be associated with increased activation of the mesolimbic-dopaminergic reward center. Research in the coming years will determine whether this guess is a good one.

Most researchers studying humor have long assumed that the laughter that occurs when we find something funny is a reflection of—i.e., a result of—the pleasure associated with the experience of humor. Even after decades of research on many different aspects of humor, however, we still have not sorted out the relative importance of the mental-emotional experience of humor and the actual act of laughing when it comes to the pleasure and enjoyment of humor. If two people give similar funniness ratings to a cartoon or joke, but one lets out a real belly laugh while the other just shows a wide grin, which one experiences more pleasure? Most people would probably choose the person who laughed more. Part of the problem in studying this issue lies in the fact that anyone participating in this kind of study has to remain still while the brain scan is occurring. Since our bodies (and brains) move around a lot when we laugh, subjects have to restrain their laughter in order to get good measures.

It is also important to remember that a strong social component appears to have been present in the evolutionary origins of laughter.

All things being equal, we generally laugh more when humor is experienced in a social context. Again, it is not clear just how this might influence the degree of activation of pleasure-mediating reward centers of the brain.

Preliminary data suggest that women may derive more pleasure from humor than men. In the first study to examine sex differences, even though men and women used the same areas of the brain to understand cartoons, and rated them similarly for funniness, women showed greater activation of the nucleus acumbens. This suggests that women derived more pleasure than men from the cartoons, even though they did not rate them as funnier than men did.[123]

Also, this reward center showed greater activation among women as they gave increasingly higher funniness ratings to the cartoons. Surprisingly, this pattern did not occur for men. This suggests that among women, the mental experience of increased funniness is associated with progressively greater pleasure. While the same humor is experienced as pleasurable among men, a progressively greater mental experience of funniness does not generate a greater and greater euphoric experience. In other words, the emotional enjoyment component of humor may be elevated in women, in comparison to men. Obviously, more research is needed to confirm this finding.

REFERENCES

The following abbreviations are used below: Abstr. = Abstracts, Amer. = American, Assn. = Association, Beh. = Behavior or Behavioral, Bull. = Bulletin, Cog. = Cognition or Cognitive, Clin. = Clinical, Dev. = Development, Diff. = Difference or Differences, Dissert. = Dissertation, Exp. = Experimental, Int. = International, J. = Journal, Lang. = Language, Med. = Medicine or Medical, Neurol. = Neurology or Neurological, Pers. = Personality, Psych. = Psychology or Psychological, Psychol. = Psychologist, Psychosom. = Psychosomatic, Rehab. = Rehabilitation, Rep. = Reports, Res. = Research, Rev. = Review, Sci. = Science or Sciences, Soc. = Social.

Introduction

1. Ryff, C.D. & Singer, B. (1998). The contours of positive human health. *Psych. Inquiry*, 9, 1-28.
Seligman, M.E.P. & Csikszentmihalyi, M. (2000). Positive psychology: An introduction. *Amer. Psychol.*, 55, 5-14.
2. Maslow, A.H. (1970). *Motivation and Personality* (2nd ed.). New York: Harper & Row.
3. Biswas-Diener, R. (2009). Personal coaching as positive intervention. *J. of Clin. Psych.*, 65(5), 544-553.
Stober, D. & Grant, A.M. (2006). *Evidence-Based Coaching Handbook*. Hoboken, NJ: Wiley.
4. Fredrickson, B.L. (2003). Positive emotions and upward spirals in organizations. In K.S. Cameron, et al. (Eds.), *Positive Organizational Scholarships: Foundations of a New Discipline*. San Francisco: Berrett-Koehler, pp. 163-175.
Peterson, C. & Park, N. (2006). Character strengths in organizations. *J. of Organiz. Beh.*, 27, 1149-1154.
5. Fredrickson (2003).
6. Seligman, M.E.P., et al. (2005). Positive psychology progress: Empirical validation of intervenetions. *Amer. Psychol.*, 60, 410-421.
7. Peterson, C. & Seligman, M.E.P. (2004). *Character Strengths and Virtues: A Handbook and Classification*. New York: Oxford Univ. Press.
8. Shimai, S., et al. (2006). Convergence of character strengths in American and Japanese young adults. *J. of Happiness Studies*, 7, 311-322.
9. Devereux, P.G. & Heffner, K.L. (2007). Psychophysiological approaches to the study of laughter. In A.D. Ong & M.H.M. van Dulmen (Eds.), *Oxford Handbook of Methods in Positive Psychology*. New York: Oxford Univ. Press.
10. Diener, E. & Biswas-Diener, R. (2008). *Happiness: Unlocking the Mysteries of Psychological Wealth*. New York: Blackwell.

11. Fredrickson, B.L., et al. (2003). What good are positive emotions in crisis? A prospective study of resilience and emotions following the terrorist attacks on the United States on September 11, 2001. *J. Pers. & Soc. Psych.*, 84(2), 365-376. Stein, N., et al., (1997). Appraisal and goal processes as predictors of psychological well-being in bereaved caregivers. *J. Pers. & Soc. Psych.*, 72(4), 872-884.

12. Dunn, J.R. & Schweitzer, M.E. (2005). Feeling and believing: The influence of emotion on trust. *J. Pers. & Soc. Psych.*, 88(5), 736-748.

13. Waugh, C.E. & Fredrickson, B.L. (2006). Nice to know you: Positive emotions, self-other overlap, and complex understanding in the formation of new relationships. *J. Pos. Psych.*, 1, 93-106.

14. Diener, E., et al. (2002). Dispositional affect and positive outcomes. *Soc. Indicators Res.* 59, 229-259.

15. Danner, D.D., et al. (2001). Positive emotions in early life and longevity: Findings from the nun study. *J. Pers. & Soc. Psych.*, 80(5), 804-813.

16. Fredrickson, B.L., et al. (2008). Open hearts build lives: positive emotions, induced through loving kindness meditation, build consequential personal resources. *J. Pers. & Soc. Psych.*, 95(5), 1045-1062.

17. Fredrickson, B.L. & Joiner, T. (2002). Positive emotions trigger upward spirals toward emotional well-being. *Psych. Sci.*, 13, 172-175.

18. Fredrickson, et al. (2003).

19. Fredrickson, et al., (2003).

20. Steptoe, A., et al. (2005). Positive affect and health-related neuroendocrine, cardiovascular and inflammatory responses. *Proceedings of the Nat. Acad. of Sci., USA*, 102, 6508-6512.

21. Gil, K.M., et al. (2004). Daily mood and stress predict pain, health care use, and work activity in African American adults with sickle-cell disease. *Health Psych.*, 23, 267-274.

22. Cohen, S., et al. (2003). Emotional style and susceptibility to the common cold. *Psychosom. Med.*, 65, 652-657.

23. Ostir, G.V., et al. (2001). The associations between emotional well-being and the incidence of stroke in older adults. *Psychosom. Med.*, 63, 210-215.

24. Danner, et al. (2001). Moskowitz, J.T. (2003). Positive affect predicts lower risk of AIDS mortality. *Psychosom. Med.*, 65, 620-626. Ostir, G.V., et al. (2000). Emotional well-being predicts subsequent functional independence and survival. *J. of the Amer. Geriatrics Soc.*, 48, 473-478.

25. Chida, Y. & Steptoe, A. (2008). Positive psychological well-being and mortality: A quantitative review of prospective observational studies. *Psychosom. Med.*, 70, 741-756. (Quote on p. 741.)

26. Fredrickson, B.L. (2001). The role of positive emotions in positive psychology: The broaden-and-build theory of positive emotions. *Amer. Psychol.*, 56, 218-226.

27. Cohn, M.A. & Fredrickson, B.L. (2009). Positive emotions. In S.J. Lopez & C.R. Snyder (Eds.), *Oxford Handbook of Positive Psychology*, New York: Oxford Univ. Press.

28. Wadlinger, H.A. & Isaacowitz, D.M. (2006). Positive affect broadens visual attention to positive stimuli. *Mot. & Emot.*, 30, 89-101.

29. Isen, A.M. & Daubman, K.A. (1984). The influence of affect on categorization. *J. of Pers. & Soc. Psych.*, 47, 1206-1217.

30. Isen, A.M., et al., (1987). Positive affect facilitates creative problem solving. *J. of Pers. & Soc. Psych.*, 52, 1122-1131.

31. Estrada, C.A., et al. (1997). Positive affect facilitates integration of information and decreases anchoring in reasoning among physicians. *Organiz. Beh. & Human Decision Processes*, 72, 117-135.

32. Aspinwall, L. (1998). Rethinking the role of positive affect in self-regulation. *Mot. & Emot.*, 22(1), 1-32.

33. Dunn, J. & Schweitzer, M. (2005). Feeling and believing: The influence of emotion on trust. *J. of Pers. & Soc. Psych.*, 88(6), 736-748.

34. Gable, S.L., et al. (2004). What do you do when things go right? The intrapersonal and interpersonal benefits of sharing positive events. *J. of Pers. & Soc. Psych.*, 87, 228-245.

35. Aldis, O. (1975). *Play Fighting.* New York: Academic Press.
Gervais, M. & Wilson, D.S. (2005). The evolution and functions of laughter and humor: A synthetic approach. *Quart. Rev. of Biol.*, 80, 395-451.

36. McGhee, P.E. (1979). *Humor: Its Origin and Development.* San Francisco, W.H. Freeman.

37. Ashby, F.G., et al. (1999). A neuropsychological theory of positive affect and its influence on cognition. *Psych. Rev.*, 106(3), 529-550.

38. Burns, A.B., et al. (2007). Upward spirals of positive emotion and coping: Replication, extension, and initial exploration of neurochemical substrates. *Pers. & Indiv. Diffs.*, 44, 360-370.
Fredrickson, B.L. & Joiner, T.E., Jr. (2002). Positive emotions trigger upward spirals toward emotional well-being. *Psych. Sci.*, 13(2), 172-175.

39. Block, J. & Kremen, A.M. (1996). IQ and egoresiliency: Conceptual and empirical connections and separateness. *J. Pers. & Soc. Psych.*, 70(2), 349-361.
Lazarus, R.S. (1993). From psychological stress to the emotions: A history of changing outlooks. *Annual Rev. of Psych.*, 44, 1-21.

40 Frankl, V. (1966). *Man's Search for Meaning.* New York: Washington Square Press.

41. Tedeschi, R.G. & Calhoun, L.G. (2004). Posttraumatic growth: Conceptual foundations and empirical evidence. *Pych. Inquiry*, 15(1), 1-18.
Werner, E.E. & Smith, R.S. (2001). *Journies from Childhood to Midlife: Risk, Resilience and Recovery.* Ithica, NY: Cornell Univ. Press.

42. Florian, V., et al. (1995). Does hardiness contribute to mental health during a stressful real-life situation? The roles of appraisal and coping. *J. Pers. & Soc. Psych.*, 68(4), 687-695.
Fredrickson, et al. (2003).
Moskowitz, J.T., et al. (1996). Coping and mood during AIDS-related caregiving and bereavement. *Annals of Beh. Med.*, 18, 49-57.

Taylor, S.E., et al. (2000). Psychological resources, positive illusions and health. *Amer. Psychol.*, 55(1), 99-109.

43. Waugh, C.E., et al. (2006). Adapting to life's slings and arrows: Individual differences in resilience when recovering from an anticipated threat. *J. Res. in Pers.*, 42, 1031-1046.

44. Tugade, M.M. & Fredrickson, B.F. (2002). Positive emotions and emotional intelligence. In L.F. Barrett & P. Salovey (Eds.), *The Wisdom of Feelings*. New York: Guilford, pp. 319-340.

Tugade, M.M. & Fredrickson, B.F. (2004). Emotions: Positive emotions and health. In N. Anderson (Ed.), *Encyclopedia of Health and Behavior*. Thousand Oaks, CA: Sage., pp. 306-310.

Tugade, M.M. & Fredrickson, B.F. (2007). Regulation of positive emotions: Emotion regulation strategies that promote resilience. *J. of Happiness Studies*, 8, 311-333.

45. Fredrickson, et al. (2003).

Ong, A.D., et al. (2006). Psychological resilience, positive emotions and successful adaptation to stress in later life. *J. Pers. & Soc. Psychol.*, 91, 730-749.

Tugade, M. M. & Fredrickson, B.L. (2004). Resilient individuals use positive emotions to bounce back from negative emotional experiences. *J. Pers. & Soc. Psych.*, 86, 320-333.

46. Fredrickson, B.L. & Losada, F. (2005). Positive affect and the complex dynamics of human flourishing. *Amer. Psychol.*, 60, 678-686.

47. Folkman, S. (2008). The case for positive emotions in the stress process. *Anxiety, Stress & Coping: An Internat. J.*, 21(1), 3-14.

48. Fredrickson, B.L. (2009). Positivity: The path to flourishing. Paper presented at the First World Congress on Positive Psychology, Philadelphia, July 20.
Fredrickson, & Joiner (2002).

49. Folkman, S. & Moskowitz, J.T. (2000). Positive affect and the other side of coping. *Amer. Psychol.*, 55, 647-654.

50. Folkman, S. (1997). Positive psychological states and coping with severe stress. *Soc. Sci. Med.*, 45, 1207-1221.

51. Wortman, C. & Silver, R. (1987). *Coping with Irrevocable Loss*. Washington, DC: Amer. Psychol. Assn.

52. Viney, L.L. (1986). Expression of positive emotion by people who are physically ill: Is it evidence of defending or coping? *J. Psychosom. Res.*, 30, 27-34.

53. Werner, & Smith (1992).
Wolin, S.J. & Wolin, S. (1993). *Bound and Determined: Growing Up Resilient in a Troubled Family*. New York: Villard.

54. Masten, A.S., et al. (1990). Resilience and development: Contributions from the study of children who overcome adversity. *Dev. & Psychopathol.*, 2, pp. 425-444.

55. Culver, J.L., et al. (2002). Coping and distress among women under treatment for early stage breast cancer: Comparing African Americans, Hispanics and non-Hispanic whites. *Psychooncol.*, 11, 295-301.

56. Carver, C.S., et al. (1993). How coping mediates the effect of optimism on stress: A study of women with early stage breast cancer. *J. Pers. & Soc. Psych.*, 65, 375-390.

57. Hendin, H. & Haas, H. (1984). *Wounds of War.* New York: Basic Books.

58. Keyes, C.L.M. & Lopez, S. (2002). *Toward a Science of Mental Health: Positive Direction in Diagnosis and Intervention.* New York: Oxford Univ. Press.

59. Keyes and Lopez (2002).

60. Keyes, C.L.M. (2002). The mental health continuum: From languishing to flourishing in life. *J. of Health & Soc. Beh.*, 43(2), 207-222.

61. Diener, E. & Emmons, R.A. (1985). The independence of positive and negative affect. *J. of Pers. & Soc. Psych.*, 47, 1105-1117.

62. Diener, E. (2000). Subjective well-being: The science of happiness and a proposal for a national index. *Amer. Psychol.*, 55, 34-43.

63. Larson, R.J., et al., (1985). An evaluation of subjective well-being measures. *Soc. Indicators Res.*, 17, 1-18.

64. Diener, E. (2000). Subjective well-being: The science of happiness and a proposal for a national index. *Amer. Psychol.*, 55, 34-43.

65. Schwartz, R.M., et al. (2002). Optimal and normal affect balance in psychotherapy of major depression: Evaluation of the balanced states of mind model. *Beh. & Cog. Psychotherapy*, 30(4), 439-450.

66. Gottman, J.M. (1994). *What Predicts Divorce? The Relationship between Marital Processes and Marital Outcomes.* Mahwah, NJ: Erlbaum.

67. Fredrickson, B.L. & Losada, M.F. (2005). Positive affect and the complex dynamics of human flourishing. *Amer. Psychol.*, 60, 678-686.

68. Emmons, R.A. & McCullough, M.E. (2003). Counting blessings vs. burdens: An experimental investigation of gratitude and subjective well-being in daily life. *J. of Pers. & Soc. Psych.*, 84, 377-389.

Folkman & Moskowitz (2000).

69. Szabo, A. (2003). The acute effects of humor and exercise on mood and anxiety. *J. of Leisure Res.*, 35(2), 152-162.

70. Foley, E., et al. (2002). Effect of forced laughter on mood. *Psych. Rep.*, 90(1), 184. Neuhoff, C.C. & Schaefer, C. (2002). Effects of laughing, smiling and howling on mood. *Psych. Rep.*, 91(3, Pt. 2), 1079-1080.

71. Ito, T.A. & Cacioppo, J.T. (2005). Variations on a human universal: Individual differences in positivity offset and negative bias. *Cog. & Emot.*, 19, 1-26.

Larson, R.J. (2002). Differential contributions of positive and negative affect to subjective well-being. In J.A. DaSilva, et al. (Eds.), *Meeting of the Int. Soc. For Psychophysics*, vol. 18, Rio de Janeiro, Brazil: Editora Legis Summa Ltd., pp. 186-190.

Rozin, P. & Royzman, E.B. (2001). Negativity bias, negativity dominance, and contagion. *Pers. & Soc. Psych. Rev.*, 5, 296-320.

72. Larsen (2002).

73. Emmons, R.A. & McCullough, M.E. (2003). Counting blessings vs. burdens: An experimental investigation of gratitude and subjective well-being in daily life. *J. of Pers. & Soc. Psych.*, 84, 377-389.

74. Wegener, D.T. & Petty, R.E. (1994). Mood management across affective states: The hedonic contingency hypothesis. *J. of Pers. & Soc. Psych.*, 66, 1034-1048.

75. Lyubomirsky, S., et al. (2005). Pursuing happiness: The architecture of sustainable change. *Rev. of Gen. Psych.*, 9, 111-131.

76. Myers, D.G. (2008). Religion and human flourishing. In M. Eid & R.J. Larsen (Eds.), *The Science of Subjective Well-Being.* New York: Guilford Press, pp. 323-343.

77. Suldo, S.M. & Huebner, E.S. (2004). Does life satisfaction moderate the effects of stressful life events on psychopathological behavior during adolescence? *School Psych. Quart.*, 19, 93-105.

78. Rusting, C.L. & Larsen, R.J. (1997). Extraversion, neuroticism, and susceptibility to positive and negative affect: A test of two theoretical models. *Pers. & Indiv. Diffs.*, 22, 607-612.

79. DeNeve, K.M. & Cooper, H. (1998). The happy personality: A meta-analysis of 137 personality traits and subjective well-being.

Lucas, R.E., et al., 1996). Discriminant validity of well-being measures. *J. Pers. & Soc. Psychol.*, 71, 616-628.

80. Lykken, D. & Tellegen, A. (1996). Happiness is a stochastic phenomenon. *Psych. Sci.*, 7, 186-189.

81. Kuppens, P., et al. (2008). The role of positive and negative emotions in life satisfaction judgment across nations. *J. of Pers. & Soc. Psych.*, 95(1), 66-75.

82. Cohn, M.A. (2009). Happiness unpacked: Positive emotions increase life satisfaction by building resilience. *Emot.*, 9, 361-368. (Quote on p. 361.)

83. Crawford, S. Humor skills enhancement: A positive approach to emotional well-being. Unpublished Doctoral Dissert., James Cook Univ., North Queensland, Australia.

Rusch, S. & Stolz, H. (2009). Can a sense of humor be trained: Evidence from the 8-Step Program. Unpublished Masters Thesis, Univ. of Zurich, Switzerland.

84. McGhee, P.E. (2010). *Humor as Survival Training for a Stressed-Out World.* Bloomington, IN: Author House, in press.

Chapter 1

1. Nathan, R.G., et al. (1987). *The Doctors' Guide to Instant Stress Relief.* New York: G. P. Putnam Sons, p, 39.

2. Salovey, P., et al. (2000). Emotional states and physical health. *Amer. Psychol.*, 55(1), 110-121.

3. Everson, S.A., et al. (1997). Hostility and increased risk of mortality and acute myocardial infarction: the mediating role of behavioral risk factors. *Amer. J. of Epidemiol.*, 146, 142-152.

4. Nathan, et al. (1987).

5. Salovey, et al. (2000).

6. Pratt, L.A., et al. (1996). Depression, psychotropic medication, and risk of myocardial infarction. *Circulation*, 94, 3123-3129.

7. Herrmann, C., et al. (1998). Diagnostic groups and depressed moods as predictors of 22-month mortality in medical inpatients. *Psychosom. Med.*, 60, 570-577.

8. Segerstrom, S.V. & Miller, G.E. (2004). Psychological stress and the human immune system: A meta-analytic study of 30 years of inquiry. *Psych. Bull.*, 130(4), 601-630.

9. Kiecolt-Glaser, J.K., et al. (2002). Emotions, morbidity, and mortality: New perspectives from psychoneuroimmunology. *Annual Rev. of Psych.*, 53, 83-107.

10. Kiecolt-Glaser, et al. (2002).

11. Dhabhar, F.S. & McEwan, B.S. (1997). Acute stress enhances while chronic stress suppresses cell-mediated immunity *in vivo*: a potential role for leukocyte trafficking. *Brain, Beh., & Immunity*, 11, 286-306.

12. Fredrickson, B. L. (1998). What good are positive emotions? *Rev. of Gen. Psych.: Special Issue: New Directions in Res. on Emot.*, 2, 300-319.

13. Kiecolt-Glaser, et al. (2002). p. 97.

14. Kobasa, S.C. (1979). Stressful life events, personality and health: An inquiry into hardiness. *J. of Pers. & Soc. Psych.*, 37, 1-11.

Schaffer, M. (1982). *Life after Stress*. New York: Plenum.

15. Kuiper, N.A., et al. (1993). Coping humor, stress, and cognitive appraisals. *Canadian J. of Beh. Sci.*, 25, 81-96.

16. Kuiper, N.A., et al. (1995). Cognitive appraisals and individual differences in sense of humor: Motivational and affective implications. *Pers. & Indiv. Diff.*, 19(3), 359-372.

17. Block, J. & Kremen, A.M. (1996). IQ and ego-resiliency: Conceptual and empirical connections and separateness. *J. of Pers. & Soc. Psych.*, 70, 349-361.

Carver, C.S. (1998). Resilience and thriving: Issues, models and linkages. *J. of Soc. Issues*, 54, 245-266.

Lazarus, R.S. (1993). From psychological stress to the emotions: A history of changing outlooks. *Annual Rev. of Psych.*, 44, 1-21.

18. Tugade, M.M. & Fredrickson, B.L. (2004). Resilient individuals use positive emotions to bounce back from negative emotional experiences. *J. of Pers. & Soc. Psych.*, 86, 320-333.

19. Fredrickson, B.L., et al. (2003). What good are positive emotions in crisis? A prospective study of resilience and emotions following the terrorist attacks on the United States on September 11, 2001. *J. of Pers. & Soc. Psych.*, 84, 365-376.

20. Smith, A.S. & Baum, A. (2003). The influence of psychological factors on restorative function in health and illness. In J. Suls & K.A. Wallston (Eds.), *Social Psychological Foundations of Health and Illness*. Malden, MA: Blackwell, pp. 431-457.

21. Rozanski, A, et al. (1999). Impact of psychological factors on the pathogenesis of cardiovascular disease and implications for therapy. *Circulation*, 99, 2192-2217.

22. Baum, A. & Anderson, B.L. (Eds.). (2001). *Psychological Interventions for Cancer.* Washington, DC: American Psychological Association.

23. Affleck, G., et al. (1997). A dual pathway model of daily stressor effects on rheumatoid arthritis. *Annals of Behav. Med.,* 19, 161-170.

24. Ionescu-Tirgonstei, C., et al. (1987). The signification of stress in aetiopathogenesis of Type-sub-2 diabetes mellitus. *Stress Med.,* 3, 277-284.

25. Biondi, M. & Zannino, L. (1997). Psychological stress, neuroimmodulation, and susceptibility to infectious diseases in animals and man. *Psychotherapy & Psychosomatics,* 66, 3-26.

26. Damasio, A.R. (1995). *Decartes' Error: Emotion, Reason, and the Human Brain.* New York: Avon.

LeDoux, J. (1998). *The Emotional Brain.* New York: Simon & Schuster.

27. Mayer, J.D. & Salovey, P. (1997). What is emotional intelligence? In P. Salovey & D.J. Sluyter (Eds.), *Emotional Development and Emotional Intelligence: Educational Implications.* New York: Basic Books, pp. 3-31.

Mayer, J.D., et al. (2000). Models of emotional intelligence. In R.J. Sternberg(Ed.), *Handbook of Intelligence.* Cambridge: Cambridge Univ. Press, pp. 396-420.

28. Goleman, D. (1995). *Emotional Intelligence.* New York: Bantam.

29. Salovey, P., et al. (1999). Coping intelligently: Emotional intelligence and the coping process. In C.R. Snyder (Ed.), *Coping: The Psychology of What Works.* New York: Oxford, pp. 141-164.

30. Feldman B.L., et al. (2001). Knowing what you're feeling and knowing what to do about it: Mapping the relation between emotion differentiation and emotion regulation. *Cog. & Emot.,* 15, 713-724.

31. Giuliani, N.R., et al. (2008). The up- and down-regulation of amusement: Experiential, behavioral and autonomic consequences. *Emotion,* 8, 714-719.

32. Thayer, R.E., et al. (1994). Self-regulation of mood: Strategies for changing a bad mood, raising energy, and reducing tension. *J. of Pers. & Soc. Psych.,* 67, 910-925.

33. Baron, R.A. & Ball, R.L. (1974). The aggression-inhibiting influence of nonhostile humor. *J. of Exp. Soc. Psych.,* 10, 23-33.

Dworkin, E. & Efran, J. (1967). The angered: Their susceptibility to varieties of humor. *J. of Pers. & Soc. Psych.,* 6(2), 233-236.

Leak, G. (1974). Effects of hostility arousal and aggressive humor on catharsis and humor preference. *J. of Pers. & Soc. Psych.,* 30(6), 736-740.

Prerost, F. (1976). Reduction of aggression as a function of related content of humor. *Psych. Rep.,* 38, 771-777.

34. Cann, A., et al. (1999). The roles of humor and sense of humor in responses to stressors. *Humor: Int. J. of Humor Res.,* 12(2), 177-193.

Yovetich, N.J., et al. (1990). Benefits of humor in reduction of threat-induced anxiety. *Psych. Rep.,* 66, 51-58.

35. Danzer, A.J., et al. (1990). Effect of exposure to humorous stimuli on induced depression. *Psych. Rep.,* 66, 1027-1036.

Mussman, S., et al. (1992). Depression: Is laughter a good medicine? Paper presented at meeting of the Southeastern Psychological Assn., Atlanta, GA.

36. White, S. & Winzelberg, A. (1992). Laughter and stress. *Humor: Int. J. of Humor Res.*, 5(4), 343-355.

37. Cann, A., et al. (1999).

38. Newman, M.G. & Stone, A.A. (1996). Does humor moderate the effects of experimentally-induced stress? *Annals of Beh. Med.*, 18(2), 101-109.

39. Lehman, K.M., et al. (2001). A reformulation of the moderating effects of productive humor. *Humor: Int. J. of Humor Res.*, 14(2) 131-161.

40. Smyth, J. et al. (1998). Stressors and mood measured on a momentary basis are associated with salivary cortisol secretion. *Psychoneuroendocrinol.*, 23(4), 353-370.

41. Smyth, et al. (1998). p. 365.

42. Lehman, et al. (2001).

Martin, R.A. & Lefcourt, H.M. (1983). Sense of humor as a moderator of the relation between stressors and moods. *J. of Pers. & Soc. Psych.*, 45, 1313-1324.

43. Yovetich, et al. (1990).

44. Martin & Lefcourt (1983).

45. Deaner, S.L. & McConatha, J.T. (1993). The relation of humor to depression and personality. *Psych. Rep.*, 72, 755-763.

Nezu, A.M., et al. (1988). Sense of humor as a moderator of the relation between stressful events and psychological distress: A prospective analysis. *J. of Pers. & Soc. Psych.*, 54, 520-525.

Skevington, S.M. & White, A. (1998). Is laughter the best medicine? *Psych. & Health*, 13(1), 157-169.

46. Lefcourt, H.M & Martin, R.A. (1986). *Humor and Life Stress: Antidote to Adversity*. New York: Springer-Verlag.

47. Kuiper, et al. (1993).

48. Kuiper, N.A. & Martin, R.A. (1998a). Laughter and stress in daily life: relation to positive and negative affect. *Mot. & Emot.*, 22, 133-153.

Moran, C.C. & Massam, M.M. (1999). Differential influences of coping humor and humor bias on mood. *Beh. Med.*, 25(1), 36-42.

49. Lebowitz, K.R. (2002). The effects of humor on cardiopulmonary functioning, psychological well-being, and health status among older adults with chronic obstructive pulmonary disease. *Dissert. Abstr. Int. Section B: Sciences & Engineering*, 63(4-B), 2063.

50. Carver, C.S., et al. (1993). How coping mediates the effect of optimism on distress: A study of women with early stage breast cancer. *J. of Pers. & Soc. Psych.*, 65(2), 375-390.

51. Skevington & White (1998).

52. Ong, A.D. (2004). The role of daily positive emotions during conjugal bereavement. *J. of Gerontology. Series B: Psych. Sci. & Soc. Sci.*, 59B(4), 168-176.

53. Meiselman, J.L. (2003). Relocation to a residential care facility for the elderly: Examining the impact of coping processes on adaptation. *Dissert. Abstr. Int. Section A: Humanities & Soc. Sci.*, 64(1-A), 247.

54. Trice, A.D. & Price-Greathouse, J. (1986). Joking under the drill: A validity study of the coping humor scale. *J. of Soc. Beh. & Pers.*, 2, 163-166.

55. Davidson, J.R.T., et al. (2005). *Int. Clinical Psychopharmacol.*, 20(1), 43-48.

56. Deaner, S. & McConatha, J. (1993). The relation of humor to depression and personality. *Psych. Rep.*, 72, 755-763.

Kuiper, N.A. & Martin, R. (1998b). Is sense of humor a positive personality characteristic? In W. Ruch (Ed.), *The sense of humor: Explorations of a Personality Characteristic.* New York: Mouton de Gruyter, 159-178.

Overholser, J. (1992). Sense of humor when coping with life stress. *Pers. & Indiv. Diff.*, 13(7), 799-804.

57. Freknall, P. (1994). Good humour: A qualitative study of the uses of humour in everyday life. *Psych.: A J. of Human Beh.*, 31, 12-21.

Kuiper & Martin (1998b).

58. Kelly, W.E. (2002). An investigation of worry and sense of humor. *J. of Psych.: Interdisciplinary & Applied*, 136(6), 657-666.

59. Killian, J.G. (2005). Career and technical education teacher burnout: Impact of humor-coping style and job-related stress. *Dissert. Abstr., Int.: Section A: Humanities & Soc. Sci.*, 65 (9-A).

60. Kuiper, N. & Martin, R. (1993). Humor and self-concept. *Humor: Int. J. of Humor Res.*, 6(3), 251-270.

61. Kuiper, N.A., et al. (1992). Sense of humor and enhanced quality of life. *Pers. & Indiv. Diff.*, 13, 1273-1283.

Kuiper & Martin (1998a).

62. Abel, M.H. & Maxwell, D. (2002). Humor and affective consequences of a stressful task. *J. of Soc. & Clin. Psych.*, 21(2), 165-190.

Cann, et al. (1999).

63. Moran, C.C. & Massam, M.M. (1999). Differential influences of coping humor and humor bias on mood. *Beh. Med.*, 25(1), 36-42.

64. Kuiper & Martin (1998a)

65. Kuiper & Martin (1998a).

66. Maas. C.L. (2003). Sense of humor and spirituality as correlates of psychological well-being in men with and without Human Immunodeficiency Virus (HIV). *Dissert. Abstr. Int. Section B:Sci. & Engineering*, 64(6-B), 2899.

67. Panish, J.R. (2002). Life satisfaction in the elderly: The role of sexuality, sense of humor and health. *Dissert. Abstr. Int. Section B: Sci. & Engineering*, 63(5-B), 2598.

68. Lebowitz, K.R. (2002). The effects of humor on cardiopulmonary functioning, psychological well-being, and health status among older adults with chronic obstructive pulmonary disease. *Dissert. Abstr. Int. Section B: Sci. & Engineering*, 63(4-B), 2063.

69. Maas (2003).

70. Anson, K. & Ponsford, J. (2006). Coping and emotional adjustment following traumatic brain injury. *J. of Head Trauma Rehab.*, 21(3), 248-259.

Freknall (1994).

Kuiper, et al. (1992).

Kuiper, et al. (1993).

Martin, R.A., et al. (1993). Humor, coping with stress, self-concept, and psychological well-being. *Humor: Int. J. of Humor Res.*, 6(1), 89-94.

71. Kuiper & Martin (1993).

72. Skevington & White (1998).

73. Campbell, M.E. & Chow, P. (2000). Preliminary development of the Body Image Affect Scale. *Psych. Rep.*, 86(2), 539-540.

Gurnakova, J. (2000). Negative self-esteem and preferred coping strategies in Slovak university students. *Studia Psychologica*, 42(1-2), 75-86.

74. Fickova, E. & Korcova, N. (2000). Psychometric relations between self-esteem and measures of coping with stress. *Studia Psychologica*, 42(3), 237-242.

75. Daniel, H.J. et al. (1990). Values in mate selection: A 1984 campus survey. *College Student J.*, 1985, 19, 44-50.

Goodwin, R. (1990). Sex differences among partner preferences: Are the sexes really very similar? *Sex Roles*, 23, 501-513.

McGee, E. & Shevlin, M. (2009). Effect of humor on interpersonal attraction and mate selection. *J. of Psych.*, 143(1), 67-77.

76. Buss, D.M. (1988). The evolution of human intrasexual competition: Tactics of mate attraction. *J. of Pers. & Soc. Psych.*, 54, 616-628.

77. Murstein, B.I. & Brust, R.G. (1985). Humor and interpersonal attraction. *J. of Pers. Assessment*, 49, 637-640.

78. Cann, et al. (1999).

79. Fraley, B. & Aron, A. (2004). The effect of shared experience on closeness of initial encounters. *Personal Relationships*, 11, 61-78.

80. Glenn, N.D., & Weaver, C.N. (1981). The contribution of marital happiness to global happiness. *J. of Marriage & the Family*, 43, 161-168.

81. Sarason, I.G. & Sarason, B. (Eds.) (1985). *Social Support: Theory, Research, and Application.* The Hague: Nijhoff.

82. Bazinni, D., et al. (2007). The effect of reminiscing about laughter on relationship satisfaction. *Mot. & Emot.*, 31, 25-34.

83. Lauer, R., et al. (1990). The long-term marriage: Perceptions of stability and satisfaction. *Int. J. of Aging & Human Dev.*, 31(3), 189-195.

84. Ziv, A. & Gadish, O. (1989). Humor and marital satisfaction. *J. of Soc. Psych.*, 129, 759-768.

85. Johansen, A.B. & Cano, A. (2007). A preliminary investigation of affective interaction in chronic pain couples. *Pain*, 132, S86–S95.

86. Rust, J. & Goldstein, J. (1989). Humor in marital counseling. *Humor: Int. J. of Humor Res.*, 2, 217-224.

Ziv, A. (1988). Humor's role in married life. *Humor: Int. J. of Humor Res.*, 1, 223-229.

Ziv & Gadish (1989).

87. Rust & Goldstein (1989).

88. Jacobs, E. (1985). The functions of humor in marital adjustment. *Dissert. Abstr.*, 46 (5-B), 1688.

89. Lefcourt, H.M., & Martin, R.A. (1986). *Humor and Life Stress: Antidote to Adversity.* New York: Springer-Verlag.

90. Kelly, H.H. (1983). Love and commitment. In H.H. Kelly, et al. (Eds.), *Close Relationships*. New York: W. H. Freeman, pp. 265-314.

91. Gottman, J. (1998). What makes marriage work? In E.J. Coats & R.S. Feldman (Eds.), *Classic and Contemporary Readings in Social Psychology*. New Jersey: Prentice-Hall, pp. 140-147.

92. Cann, A. & Etzel, K.C. (2008). Remembering and anticipating stressors: Positive personality mediates the relationship with sense of humor. *Humor: Int. J. of Humor Res.*, 21(2), 157-178.

93. Kirsh, G. & Kuiper, N.A. (2003). Positive and negative aspects of sense of humor: associations with the constructs of individualism and relatedness. *Humor: Int. J. of Humor Res.*, 16(1), 33-62.

Kuiper, N.A., et al. (2004). Humor is not always the best medicine: Specific components of sense of humor and psychological well-being. *Humor: Int. J. of Humor Res.*, 17(1/2), 135-168.

Martin, R.A., et al. (2003). Individual differences in uses of humor and their relation to psychological well-being: Development of the humor styles questionnaire. *J. of Res. in Pers.*, 37(1), 48-75.

94. Kuiper, et al. (2004).

Martin, et al. (2003).

95. Kuiper, et al. (2004). p. 140.

96. Martin & Lefcourt (1983).

97. Huber, T., et al. (2007). Sulky and Angry laughter: The search for distinct facial displays. In D. Peham & E. Banninger-Huber (Eds.)., *Proceedings of the FACS-Workshop*, Innsbruck, Austria: Innsbruck University Press.

Ruch, W. & Ekman, P. (2001). The expressive pattern of laughter. In A.W. Kaszniak (Ed.), *Emotions, Qualia, and Consciousness*. Tokyo: Word Scientific Publisher, pp. 426-443.

Zweyer, K., et al. (2004). Do cheerfulness, exhilaration, and humor production moderate pain tolerance? *Humor: Int. J. of Humor Res.*, 17(1/2), 85-119.

98. Keltner, D. & Bonanno, G.A. (1997). A study of laughter and dissociation: distinct correlates of laughter and smiling during bereavement. *J. of Pers. & Soc. Psych.*, 73, 687-702.

99. Bachorowski, J.A. & Owren, M.J. (2001.) Not all laughs are alike: voiced but not unvoiced laughter readily elicits positive affect. *Psychol. Sci.*, 12, 252-257.

Smolski, M.J. & Bachorowski, J.A. (2003). Antiphonal laughter in developing friendships. *Annals of the New York Acad. of Sci.*, 1000, 300-303.

100. Hays, T. (2006). Riders rescued from N. Y. cable car after 11 hours. Associated Press article, April 20.

101. Alexander, P. (2008). 9-foot hole forces plane to land. Associated Press article, July 26.

102. Dowling, J.S., et al. (2003). Sense of humor, childhood cancer stressors and outcomes of psychological adjustment, immune function, and infection. *J. of Pediatric Oncol. Nursing*, 20(6), 271-292.

Keene, N., et al. (2000). *Childhood Cancer Survivors: A Practical Guide to Your Future*. Sebastopol, GA: O'Reilly.

103. Broeckel, J.A. (2000). Emotional functioning, coping, and optimism among long-term breast cancer survivors. *Dissert. Abstr. Int. Section B: Sci. & Engineering*, 60(8-B), 4204.

104. Fulbright, B.A. (1996). The use of humor and its mediation of depression in cancer patients and primary caregivers. *Dissert. Abstr. Int. Section A: Humanities & Soc. Sci.*, 57(5-A), Nov., 1969.

105. Aarstad, A.K.H., et al. (2008). Personality and choice of coping predict quality of life in head and neck cancer patients during follow-up. *Acta Oncologica*, 47(5), 879-890.

Kershaw, T., et al. (2004). Coping strategies and quality of life in women with advanced breast cancer and their family caregivers. *Psych. & Health*, 19(2), 139-155.

106. Roussi, P., et al. (2007). Patterns of coping, flexibility in coping and psychological distress in women diagnosed with breast caner. *Cog. Therapy Res.*, 31, 97-109.

107. Christie, W. & Moore, C. (2005). The impact of humor on patients with cancer. *Clin. J. of Oncol. Nursing*, 9(2), 211-218.

108. Wong, C.F. (2005). Regulation of negative emotions in response to an acute stressor among breast cancer survivors. *Dissert. Abstr. Int.: Section B: Sci. & Engineering*, 66, (4-B), p. 2342.

109. Johnson, P. (2002). The use of humor and its influences on spirituality and coping in breast cancer survivors. *Oncol. Nursing Forum*, 29(4), 691-695. Quote on p. 694.

110. Kershaw, T., et al. (2004). Coping strategies and quality of life in women with advanced breast cancer and their family caregivers. *Psych. & Health*, 19(2), 139-155.

111. Lengacher, C., et al. (2002). Frequency of use of complementary/alternative medicine (CAM) in women with breast cancer. *Oncol. Nursing Forum*, 29, 1445-1452.

112. Bennett, M.P. & Lengacher, C. (1999). Use of complementary therapies in a rural cancer population. *Oncol. Nursing Forum*, 26, 1287-1294.

113. Manne, S., et al. (2003). Coping and the course of mother's depressive symptoms during and after pediatric bone marrow transplantation. *J. of the Amer. Acad. of Child & Adol. Psychiatry*, 42(9), 1055-1068.

114. Dowling, J.S. (2001). Sense of humor, childhood cancer stressors and outcomes of psychosocial adjustment, Immune function and infection. *Dissert. Abstr. Int. Section B: Sci. & Engineering*, Vol. 61 (70B), 3505.

115. Le Vieux, J.S. (2003). Use of humor in pediatric oncology patients as a coping mechanism. *Dissert. Abstr. Int. Section B: Sci. & Engineering*, 63(7-B), 3496.

116. Riegner, E.J. (1997). The relationship of role strain, perceived social support, and humor to quality of life among couples experiencing the life-limiting illness of chronic obstructive pulmonary disease. *Dissert. Abstr. Int. Section B: Sci. & Engineering*, 57(10-B), 6173.

117. Makoae, L.N. (2008). Coping with HIV-related stigma in five African countries. *J. of the Assn. of Nurses in AIDS Care*, 19(2), 137-146.

118. Penson, R.T., et al. (2005). Laughter: The best medicine? *The Oncologist*, 10, 651-660. (Quote on p. 654.)

119. Francis, L., et al. (1999). A laughing matter? The uses of humor in medical interactions. *Mot. & Emot.*, 23(2), 155-174

Lipson, J.G. & Koehler, S.L. (1986). The psychiatric emergency room: Staff subculture. *Issues in Mental Health Nursing*, 8, 237-246.

Zussman, R. (1992). *Intensive Care*. Chicago: University of Chicago Press.

120. Francis, et al. (1999).

121. Robinson, V. (1991). *Humor and the Health Professions*. Thorofare, NJ: Slack.

122. Schulman-Green, D. (2003). Coping mechanisms of physicians who routinely work with dying patients. *Omega: J. of Death & Dying*, 47(3), 253-264.

123. Johnson, W. (1985). To the ones left behind. *Amer. J. of Nursing*, (August), p. 936.

124. Alvarado, I.A. (2001). Psychological well-being in pediatric professionals. *Dissert. Abstr. Int. Section B: Sci. & Engineering*, 61(8-B), 4386.

125. Keller, K. (1989). Management of stress and prevention of burnout in emergency nurses. *J. of Emergency Nurses*, 16, 90-95.

Wanzer, M., et al. (2005). "If we didn't use humor, we'd cry: Humorous coping communication in health care settings. *J. of Health Communic.*, 10, 105-125.

126. Francis, et al. (1999).

127. Francis, et al. (1999). p. 166.

128. Sim, K., et al. (2004). Severe acute respiratory syndrome-related psychiatric and posttraumatic morbidities and coping responses in medical staff within a primary health care setting in Singapore. *J. of Clin. Psychiatry*, 65(8), 1120-1127

129. Mesmer, P.J. (2001). Use of humor as a stress coping strategy by paraprofessional youth care workers employed in residential group care facilities. *Dissert. Abstr. Int.*, 62(1-B), 587.

130. Jacobs, D.C. (2003). The coping skills of child protection workers exposed to primary and secondary trauma in the workplace. *Dissert. Abst. Int. Section A: Humanities & Soc. Sci.*, 64(6-A), 2003.

131. Peterson, A.K. (2005). Gallows humor usage by crisis mental health clinicians: A funny way to cope with stress. *Dissert. Abstr. Int.: Section B: Sci. & Engineering*, 65, (12-B), p. 6669.

132. Scott, T. (2007). Expression of humour by emergency personnel involved in sudden deathwork. *Mortality*. 12(4), 350-364.

133. Herrman, J.D. (1989). Sudden death and the police officer. *Issues in Comprehensive Ped. Nursing*, 12, 327-332.

Scott (2007).

134. Scott (2007).

135. Durham, T.W., et al. (1985). The psychological impact of disaster on rescue personnel. *Annals of Emergency Med.*, 14, 664-668.

Rosenberg, L. (1991). A qualitative investigation of the use of humor by emergency personnel as a strategy for coping with stress. *J. of Emergency Nursing*, 17, 197-203.

136. Coughlin, J.J. (2002). Gallows humor and its use among police officers. *Dissert. Abstr. Int. Section B: Sci. & Engineering*, 63(2-B), 1018.

137. Burkle, F.M. (1983). Coping with stress under conditions of disaster refugee care. *Military Med.*, (Oct.), 148, 800-803.

138. Shuler, S. (2001). Talking community at 911: The centrality of communication in coping with emotional labor. In G.J. Shepherd & E.W. Rothenbuhler (Eds.), *Communication and Community*. Mahwah, NJ: Lawrence Erlbaum Associates, pp. 53-77.

139. McCarroll, J.E., et al. (1993). Handling bodies after violent death: Strategies for coping. *Amer. J. of Orthopsychiatry*, 63(2), 209-214.

140. Ritz, S.E. (2001). Surviving humor: The role of humor in coping with disasters. In W.A. Salameh & W.F. Fry, Jr., (Eds.), Humor and Wellness in Clinical Intervention. Westport, CT: Praeger, pp. 165-203.

141. Weinrich, S., et al. (1990). Nurses respond to Hurricane Hugo victims' disaster stress. *Archives of Psychiatric Nursing*, 4, 195-205.

142. Obrdlik, A.J. (1942). "Gallows humor"—A sociological phenomenon. *Amer. J. of Sociol.*, 47, 709-716.

143. Hendin, H. & Hass, H. (1984). *Wounds of War*. New York: Basic Books.

144. Nevo, O., & Levine, J. (1993). Jewish humor strikes again: The outburst of humor in Israel during the Gulf war. *Humor: Int. J. of Humor Res.*

Nevo, O. (1994). The psychological contribution of humor during the Gulf War. *Psychologia: Israeli J. of Psych.*, 4(1-2), 41-50.

145. Palmer, L. (1993). The nurses of Vietnam, still wounded. *New York Times Magazine*, Nov. 7, pp. 36-43, 68, & 72-73.

146. Bizi, S., et al. (1988). Humor and coping with stress: A test under real-life conditions. *Pers. & Indiv. Diff.*, 9, 951-956.

147. Coffee, G. (1990). *Beyond Survival*. New York: Putnam, pp. 131-132.

148. Anderson, T. (1993). *Den of Lyons*. New York: Crown.

149. Nice, S., et al. (1996). Long-term health outcomes and medical effects of torture among U.S. Navy prisoners of war in Vietnam. *J. of the Amer. Med. Assn.*, 276, 375-381.

150. Henman, L.D. (2001). Humor as a coping lesson: Lessons from POWs. *Humor: Int. J. of Humor Res.*, 14 (1), 83-94.

151. Henman (2001). p. 92

152. Gaither, R. (1973). *With God in a P.O.W. Camp*. Nashville: Broddman Press.

153. Frankel, V. (1984). *Man's Search for Meaning*. New York: Washington Square Press.

Nardini, J. (1952). Survival factors of American prisoners of war of the Japanese. *Amer. J. of Psychiatry*, 109, 241-248.

154. Ford, C. & Spaulding, R. (1973). The Pueblo incident. *Archives of Gen. Psych.*, 29, 340-343.

155. Victoroff, D. (1969). New approaches to the psychology of humor. *Impact of Society on Sci.*, 19, 291-298.

156. Martin & Lefcourt (1983).

157. Abel, M.H. & Maxwell, D. (2002). Humor and affective consequences of a stressful task. *J. of Soc. & Clin. Psych.*, 21(2), 165-190.

158. Lefcourt, H.M., et al. (1997). Humor as a stress moderator in the prediction of blood pressure obtained during five stressful tasks. *J. of Res. in Pers.*, 31, 523-542.

159. Folkman, S. & Moskowitz, J.T. (2000). Positive affect and the other side of coping. *Amer. Psychol.*, 55, 647-654.

160. Tugade & Fredrickson (2004).
Tugade, M.M., et al., (2004). Psychological Resilience and positive emotional granularity: Examining the benefits of positive emotions on coping and health. *J. of Pers.*, 72(6), 1161-1190.

161. Middleton, R.A. & Byrd, E.K. (1996). Psychological factors and hospital readmission status of older persons with cardiovascular disease. *J. of Applied Rehab. Counseling*, 27, 3-10.

162. Danner, D.D., et al. (2001). Positive emotions in early life and longevity: Findings from the nun study. *J. of Pers. & Soc. Psych.*, 80, 804-813.

163. Ostir, G.V., et al. (2001). The association between emotional well-being and the incidence of stroke in older adults. *Psychosom. Med.*, 63, 210-215.

164. Folkman, S. & Moskowitz, J.T. (2000). Positive affect and the other side of coping. *Amer. Psychol.*, 55, 647-654.

165. Folkman & Moskowitz (2000).

166. Bachorowski, J. & Owren, M.J. (2001). Not all laughs are alike: Voiced but not unvoiced laughter readily elicits positive affect. *Psychol. Sci.*, 12, 252-257.

167. Ruch, W. (1993). Exhilaration and humor. In M. Lewis & J.M. Haviland (Eds.), *The Handbook of Emotions*. New York: Guilford Press.

168. Fredrickson (1998).
Fredrickson, B.L. (2001). The role of positive emotions in positive psychology: The broaden-and-build theory of positive emotions. *Amer. Psychol.: Special Issue*, 56, 218-226.

169. Isen, A.M. (1999). Positive affect. *Handbook of Cognition and Emotion*. New York: Wiley, pp. 521-539.

170. Isen, A.M., et al. (1987). Positive affect facilitates creative problem solving. *J. of Pers. & Soc. Psychol.*, 52, 1122-1131.

171. Fredrickson, B.L. & Levinson, R.W. (1998). Positive emotions speed recovery from the cardiovascular sequelae of negative emotions. *Cog. & Emot.*, 12, 191-220.
Fredrickson, B.L., et al. (2000). The undoing effect of positive emotions. *Mot. & Emot.*, 24, 237-258.

172. Fredrickson, et al. (2000).

173. Tugade & Fredrickson (2004).

174. Blascovich, J.J. & Katkin, E.S. (1993). *Cardiovascular Reactivity to Psychological Stress and Disease*. Washington, D. C.: American Psychological Association.

175. Dienstbier, R. (1989). Arousal and physiological toughness: Implications for mental and physical health. *Psych. Rev.*, 96, 84-100.

176. Folkman, S. & Lazarus, R. (1985). If it changes it must be a process: Study of emotion and coping during three stages of a college examination. *J. of Pers. & Soc. Psych.*, 48, 150-170.

Pearlin, L.I. & Schooler, C. (1978). The structure of coping. *J. of Health & Soc. Beh.*, 19, 2-21.

177. Lefcourt, H.M., et al. (1995). Perspective taking humor: Accounting for stress moderation. *J. of Soc. & Clin. Psych.*, 14(4), 373-391.

178. Thayer, R.E., et al. (1994). Self-regulation of mood: Strategies for changing a bad mood, raising energy, and reducing tension. *J. of Pers. & Soc. Psych.*, 67, 910-925.

179. Baron, R.A. (1976). The reduction of aggression: A field study of the influence of incompatible reactions. *J. of Applied Soc. Psych.*, 6, 260-274.

180. Schelde, J.T.M. (1998). Major depression: Behavioral markers of depression and recovery. *J. of Nervous & Mental Disease*, 186(3), 133-140.

181. Thayer, et al. (1994).

182. Cousins, N. (1989). *Head First: The Biology of Hope*. New York: Dutton, p. 138.

183. Martin & Lefcourt (1983).

184. Lefcourt & Martin (1986).

185. Caesar, S. (1988). Comments made at the Power of Humor and Play Conference, Anaheim.

186. Danzer, A.J., et al. (1990). Effect of exposure to humorous stimuli on induced depression. *Psych. Rep.*, 66, 1027-1036.

Nezu, A.M., et al. (1988). Sense of humor as a moderator of the relation between stressful events and psychological distress: A prospective analysis. *J. of Pers. & Soc. Psych.*, 54, 520-525.

187. Nezu, et al. (1988).

188. Meadowcraft, J.M. & Zillmann, D. (1987). Women's comedy preferences during the menstrual cycle. *Communication Res.*, 14, 204-218.

189. Schmitt, N. (1990). Patients' perception of laughter in a rehabilitation hospital. *Rehab. Nursing*, 15 (No. 3), 143-146.

190. Cousins (1989). p. 126.

191. Korotkov, D. & Hanna, T.E. (1994). Extraversion and emotionality as proposed superordinate stress moderators: A prospective analysis. *Pers. & Indiv. Diff.*, 16, 787-792.

192. Snyder, C. R. (1994). *The Psychology of Hope: You Can Get There from Here.* New York: Free Press.

193. Carver, et al. (1993).

194. Herth, K. (1993). Hope in older adults in community and institutional settings. *Issues in Mental Health Nursing*, 14, 139-156.

195. Vilaythong, A.P., et al. (2003). Humor and hope: Can humor increase hope? *Humor: Int. J. of Humor Res.*, 16(1), 79-89.

196. Westburg, N.G. (1999). Humor and hope: Using the hope scale in outcome studies. *Psych. Rep.*, 84, 1014-1020.

197. Vilaythong, A.P., et al. (2003). Humor and hope: Can humor increase hope? *Humor: Int. J. of Humor Res.*, 16(1), 79-89.

198. Kuiper & Martin (1998b).

199. Fredrickson & Levinson (1998).

Fredrickson, et al. (2000).

Tugade & Fredrickson (2004).

200. Tyson, P.D. (1998). Physiological arousal, reactive aggression, and the induction of an incompatible relaxation response. *Aggr. & Violent Beh.*, 3(2), 143-158.

201. Fry, P.S. (1995). Perfectionism, humor and optimism as moderators of health outcomes and determinants of coping styles of women executives. *Gen. Psych. Monogr.*, 121, 213-245.

202. Kuiper & Martin (1998b). p, 162.

203. Abel, M.H. (2002). Humor, stress, and coping strategies. *Humor: Int. J. of Humor Res.*, 15(4), 365-381 (quote on p. 377).

204. Goleman, D. (1995). *Emotional Intelligence.* New York: Bantam.

205. Gervais, M. & Wilson, D.S. (2005). The evolution and functions of laughter and humor: A synthetic approach. *Quart. Rev. of Biol.*, 80(4), 395-430.

206. Dixon, N.F. (1980). Humor: A cognitive alternative to stress. In C.D. Spielberger & I.G. Sarason (Eds.), *Anxiety and Stress*, pp. 281-289. Vol. 7. Washington, D.C.: Hemisphere.

207. Lefcourt, H.M., et al. (1995). Perspective-taking humor: Accounting for stress moderation. *J. of Soc. & Clin. Psych.*, 14, 373-391.

208. Bizi, et al. (1988).

209. Wooten, P. (1991). Effect of humor training for health professionals. Paper presented at 8th International Conference on Humor.

210. Abel (2002).

211. Justice, B. (1987). *Who Gets Sick: How Beliefs, Moods, and Thoughts Affect Your Health.* Los Angeles: Tarcher, p. 307.

212. Dienstbier, R.A. (1995). The impact of humor on energy, tension, task choices, and attributions: Exploring hypotheses from toughness theory. *Mot. & Emot.*, 19(4), 255-267.

213. Martin, R.A. (2001). Humor, laughter, and physical health: Methodological issues and research findings. *Psych. Bull.*, 127(4), 504-519.

214. Hampes, W.P. (1992). Relation between humor and intimacy. *Psych. Rep.*, 71, 127-130.

Kuiper & Martin (1993).

215. Korotkov, D. & Hanna, T.E. (1994). Extraversion and emotionality as proposed superordinate stress moderators: A prospective analysis. *Pers. & Indiv. Diff.*, 16, 787-792.

Ruch, W. (1994). Temperament, Eysenck's PEN system, and humor-related traits. *Humor: Int. J. of Humor Res.*, 7, 209-244.

216. Ruch, W. & Carrell, A. (1998). Trait cheerfulness and the sense of humour. *Pers. & Indiv. Diffs.*, 24, 551-558.

217. Kuiper & Martin (1998b).

218. Ruch, W. (1997). State and trait cheerfulness and the induction of exhilaration. *European Psych.*, 2(4), 328-341.

219. Foley, E., et al. (2002). Effect of forced laughter on mood. *Psych. Rep.*, 90(1), 184.

Neuhoff, C.C. & Schaefer, C. (2002). Effects of lauaghing, smiling and howling on mood. *Psych. Rep.*, 91(3, Pt. 2), 1079-1080.

220. Block, J. & Kremen, A.M. (1996). IQ and ego-resiliency: Conceptual and empirical connections and separateness. *J. of Pers. & Soc. Psychol.*, 70(2), 349-361.

221. Bonanno, G.A. (2004). The importance of being flexible: The ability to both enhance and suppress emotional expression predicts long-term adjustment. *Psychol. Sci.*, 15(7), 482-487.

222. Phelps, E.A. & LeDous, J.E. (2005). Contributions of the amygdala to emotional processing: From animal models to human behavior. *Neuron*, 48(2), 175-187.

223. Siegle, G.J., et al. (2002). Can't shake that feeling: event-related fMRI assessment of sustained amygdala activity in response to emotional information in depressed individuals. *Biol. Psychiatry*, 51(9), 693-707.

224. Waugh, C.E., et al. (2008). The neural correlates of trait resilience when anticipating and recovering from threat. *Soc., Cog. & Affective Neurosci.*, 3(4), 322-332.

225. Werner, E.E. & Smith, R.S. (2001). *Journies from Childhood to Midlife: Risk, Resilience and Recovery*. Ithica, NY: Cornell Univ. Press.

Wolin, S.J. & Wolin, S. (1993). *Bound and Determined: Growing Up Resilient in a Troubled Family*. New York: Villard.

226. Masten, A.S., et al. (1990). Resilience and development: Contributions from the study of children who overcome adversity. *Dev. & Psychopathol.*, 2, pp. 425-444.

227. Culver, J.L., et al. (2002). Coping and distress among women under treatment for early stage breast cancer: Comparing African Americans, Hispanics and non-Hispanic whites. *Psychooncol.*, 11, 295-301.

228. Carver, C.S., et al. (1993). How coping mediates the effect of optimism on stress: A study of women with early stage breast cancer. *J. Pers. & Soc. Psych.*, 65, 375-390.

229. Hendin, H. & Haas, H. (1984). *Wounds of War*. New York: Basic Books.

230. Fredrickson (1998).

Fredrickson, B.L. (2001). The role of positive emotions in positive psychology: The broaden-and-build theory of positive emotions. *Amer. Psychol.*, 56, 218-226.

231. Levy, B.R., et al. (2002). Longevity increased by positive self-perceptions of aging. *J. of Pers. & Soc. Psychol.*, 83, 261-270.

Ostir, G.V., et al. (2000). Emotional well-being predicts subsequent functional independence and survival. *J. of the Amer. Geriatrics Soc.*, 48, 473-478.

232. Fredrickson, B.L. & Joiner, T.E., Jr. (2002). Positive emotion triggers upward spirals toward emotional well-being. *Psychol. Sci.*, 13(2), 172-175.

Burns, A.B., et al. (2008). Upward spirals of positive emotion and coping: Replication, extension, and initial exploration of neurochemical substrates. *Pers. & Indiv. Diffs.*, 44, 360-370.

233. Fredrickson, B.L. (2009). Positive emotions. Video on www.Youtube.com. Produced by the Carolina News Studio, uncnews.unc.edu/broadcast-studios.html.

234. Kok, B.E., et al. (2008). The broadening, building, buffering effects of positive emotions. In S.J. Lopez (Ed.), *Positive Psychology: Exploring the Best People*: Vol. 3. *Capitalizing on Emotional Experiences*. Westport, CT: Greenwood Publishing Co., pp. 1-19. Quote on p. 4.

235. McGhee, P.E. (1979). *Humor: Its Origin and Development*. San Francisco: W. H. Freeman.

McGhee, P.E. (2004). *Understanding and Promoting the Development of Children's Humor*. Dubuque, IA: Kendall/Hunt.

236. Ruch, W. & Kohler, G. (1998). A temperament approach to humor. In W. Ruch (Ed.), *The Sense of Humor: Explorations of a Personality Characteristic*. New York: Mouton de Gruyter. pp. 203-228.

237. Cohn, M.A. & Fredrickson, B.L. (2009). Positive emotions. In S.J. Lopez & C.R. Snyder (Eds.), *Oxford Handbook of Positive Psychology*, New York: Oxford Univ. Press.

238. Emmons, R.A. & McCullough, M.E. (2003). Counting blessings vs. burdens: An experimental investigation of gratitude and subjective well-being in daily life. *J. of Pers. & Soc. Psych.*, 84, 377-389.

Seligman, M.E.P., et al., (2005). Positive psychology progress: Empirical validation of interventions. *Amer. Psychol.*, 60, 410-421.

239. Seligman, M.E.P., et al., (2005). Positive psychology progress: Empirical validation of interventions. *Amer. Psychol.*, 60, 410-421.

240. Fredrickson, B.L. & Losada, F. (2005). Positive affect and the complex dynamics of human flourishing. *Amer. Psychol.*, 60, 678-686.

241. Sheldon, K.M. & Lyubomirsky, S. (2004). Achieving sustainable new happiness: Projects, practices, and prescriptions. In P.A. Linley & S. Joseph (Eds.), *Positive Psychology in Practice*. Hoboken, NJ, Wiley.

242. Gunderson, A.L. (1998). A comparison of the effect of two humor programs on self-reported coping capabilities and pain among the elderly. Unpublished Master's Thesis, Montclair State Univ.

243. Crawford, S. (2009). Humor skills enhancement: A positive approach to emotional well-being. Unpublished Doctoral Dissert., James Cook Univ., North Queensland, Australia.

Rusch, S. & Stolz, H. (2009). Ist sinn fur humor lernbar? Eine anwendung und evaluation des 8 Stupfen Programs (McGhee, 1999). Can a sense of humor be learned? An application and evaluation of the 8-Step Program (McGhee, 1999). Unpublished Masters Thesis, Univ. of Zurich, Switzerland.

Sassenrath, S. (2001). Humor und lichen als stressbewaltigungsstrategie. Unpublished Masters Thesis, Univ. of Vienna, Austria.

244. Rusch & Stolz, (2009).

245. Crawford (2009).

246. McGhee, P.E. (2010). *Humor as Survival Training for a Stressed-Out World.* Bloomington, IN: Author House. (Available about March, 2010.)

247. Nevo, O., et al. (1998). The development and evaluation of a systematic program for improving your sense of humor. In W. Ruch (Ed.), *The Sense of Humor: Explorations of a Personality Characteristic.* New York: Mouton de Gruyter.

Lowis, M.J. & Niewoudt, J.M. (1994). Humor as a coping aid for stress. *Soc. Work*, 30, 124-131.

248. Franzini, L.R. (2001). Humor in therapy: The case for training therapists in its uses and risks. *J. of Gen. Psych.*, 128(2), 170-193.

Fry, W.F. & Salameh, W. (Eds.) (1993). *Advances in Humor and Psychotherapy.* Sarasota, FL: Professional Resource Press.

Strean, H.S. (Ed.) (1994). *The Use of Humor in Psychotherapy*, Northvale, NJ: Jason Aronson.

249. Rosenheim, E. & Golan, G. (1986). Patients' reactions to humorous interventions in psychotherapy. *Amer. J. of Psychotherapy*, 40(1), 110-124.

250. Sultanof, S. (2002). Integrating humor into psychotherapy. In C. Schaefer (Ed.), *Play Therapy with Adults.* New York: Wiley, quote on p. 120.

251. Crawford (2009).

252. Wilbers, J. (2009). Humour appreciation and emotion regulation: Training humour abilities in depressive patients. Unpublished Masters Thesis, Maastricht Univ., Netherlands.

253. Sultanoff (2002).

254. Johnson, P. (2007). The use of humor and its influence on spirituality in breast cancer survivors. *Oncol. Nursing Forum*, 29(4), 691-695.

255. Rew, L., et al. (2004). The relationship between prayer, health behaviors, and protective resources in school-age children. *Issues in Comprehensive Pediatric Nursing*, 27, 245-255.

256. Belt, J.L. (2006). The relationship between humor, stress, coping strategies, and spirituality. *Dissert. Abst. Int.: Section B: Sci. & Engineering*, 67, (6-B), p. 3439.

257. Ostling, R.H. (1994). Laughing for the Lord. *Time*, August 15, p. 38.

258. Peterson, C. (2006). *A Primer in Positive Psychology.* New York: Oxford University Press.

Seligman, M.E.P. (2002). *Authentic Happiness.* New York: Free Press.

259. Seligman (2002).

260. Peterson, C. & Seligman, M.E.P. (2004). *Character Strengths and Virtues: A classification and Handbook.* New York: Oxford University Press.

Peterson (2007).

261. Hooda, D., et al., (2009). Social intelligence as a predictor of positive psychological health. *J. of the Indian Acad. of Applied Psych.*, 35(1), 143-150.

Shefet, O.M. (2007). Subjectivewell-being and psychodynamic psychology. *Dissert. Abstr. Int., Section B: Sci. & Engineering*, 68(6-B), 4167.

262. Gordon, N.S. (2003). The neural basis for joy and sadness: A functional magnetic resonance imaging study of the neuroaffective effects of music, laughter and crying. *Dissert. Abstr. Int.: Section B: Sci. & Engineering*, 64(2-B), 997.

263. Nettle, D. (2005). *Happiness: The Science Behind Your Smile*. Oxford Univ. Press. Oxford, UK.

264. Lyubomirsky, S., et al. (2005). Pursuing happiness: The architecture of sustainable change. *Rev. of Gen. Psych.*, 9(2), 111-131.

265. Diener, E., et al. (1999). Subjective well-being: Three decades of progress. *Psych. Bull.*, 125, 276-302.

Lykken, D. & Tellegen, A. (1996). Happiness is a stochastic phenomenon. *Psych. Sci.*, 7, 186-189.

266. McCrae, R.R. & Costa, P.T. (1990). *Personality in Adulthood*. New York: Guilford Press.

267. Diener, E., et al. (2006). Beyond the hedonic treadmill: Revising the adaptation theory of well-being. *Amer. Psychol.*, 61, 305-314.

268. Diener, et al. (2006).

Sheldon, K.M. & Lyubomirsky, S. (2006). Achieving sustainable gains in happiness: Change your actions, not your circumstances. *J. of Happiness Studies*, 7, 55-86.

269. Crawford (2009).

Sassenrath (2001).

270. Rusch & Stolz (2009).

271. Crawford (2009).

272. Sassenrath (2001).

273. Crawford (2009).

274. Rush & Stolz (2009).

275. Bisconti, T.L., et al. (2004). Emotional well-being in recently bereaved widows: A dynamical systems approach. *J. of Gerontol.: Psych. Sci.*, 59B, 158-167.

Bonanno, G.A. & Kaltman, S. (1999). Toward an integrative perspective on bereavement. *Psych. Bull.*, 125, 769-776.

276. Hill, R.D. (2005). *Positive Aging*. New York: W.W. Norton.

Ong, A.D., et al. (2006). Psychological resilience, positive emotions and successful adaptation to stress later in life. *J. Pers. & Soc. Psych.*, 91(4), 730-749.

277. Ong, A.D., et al. (2004). The role of daily positive emotions during conjugal bereavement. *J. of Gerontol.: Psych. Sci. & Soc. Sci.*, 59B, 168-176.

278. Lund, D.A., et al. (2008). Humor, laughter and happiness in the daily lives of recently bereaved spouses. *Omega (Westport)*, 58(2), 87-105.

279. Southwick, S.M., et al. (2005). The psychobiology of depression and resilience to stress: Implications for prevention and treatment. *Ann. Rev. of Clin. Psych.*, 1, 255-291.

280. Chemali, Z.N., et al. (2008). On happiness: A minimalist perspective on a complex neural circuitry and its psychosocial constructs. *J. Happiness Stud.*, 9, 489-501.

281. Park, N., et al. (2004). Strengths of character and well-being. *J. of Soc. & Clin. Psychol.*, 23(5), 603-619.

Peterson, C., et al. (2007). Strengths of character, orientations to happiness, and life satisfaction. *J. of Positive Psych.*, 2.

282. Meiselman, J.L. (2003). Relocation to a residential care facility for the elderly: Examining the impact of coping processes on adaptation. *Dissert. Abstr. Int., Section A*, 64(1-A), 247.

Panish, J.R. (2002). Life satisfaction in the elderly: The role of sexuality, sense of humor and health. *Dissert. Abstr. Int., Section B.* 63(5-B), 2598.

283. Wanzer, M.B., et al. (2009). Humorous communication within the lives of older adults: The relationships among humor, coping efficacy, age and life satisfaction. *Health Communic.*, 24, 128-136.

284. Mathieu, S. (2008). Happiness and humor group promotes life satisfaction for senior center participants. *Activities, Adaptation & Aging*, 32(2), 134-148.

285. Peterson, C., et al. (2006). Greater strengths of character and recovery from illness. *J. of Pos. Psych.*, 1(1), 17-26.

Chapter 2

1. Goldstein, J.H. (1987). Therapeutic effects of laughter. In W.F. Fry & W.A. Salameh (Eds.), *Handbook of Humor and Psychotherapy*. Sarasota, FL: Professional Resource Exchange.

2. Klopfer, B. (1957). Psychological variables in human cancer. *J. of Projective Techniques*, 21, 331-340.

3. Bellinger, D.L., et al. (1992). A longitudinal study of age-related loss of noradrenergic nerves and lymphoid cells in the rat spleen. *Exp. Neurol.*, 116, 295.

4. Pert, C. (1993). The chemical communications. In B. Moyers, *Healing and the Mind* (quote on p. 176).

5. Pert (1993). p. 190.

6. Helsing, K.J., et al. (1981). Factors associated with mortality after widowhood. *Amer. J. of Pub. Health*, 71, 802-809.

Rees, W.D. & Lutkins, S.G. (1967). Mortality of bereavement. *Brit. Med. J.*, 4, 13-16.

7. Shekelle, R.B. (1981). Psychological depression and 17-year risk of death from cancer. *Psychosom. Med.*, 43, 117-125.

8. Temoshok, L. (1986). Clinical psychoneuroimmunology in AIDS. Paper presented at annual meeting of the Society of Beh. Med., San Francisco.

9. Associated Press. (1994). Pessimism can be deadly for heart patients. *The New York Times*, April 16, p. 8.

10. Associated Press. (1994). Pessimism can be deadly for heart patients. *The New York Times,* April 16, p. 8.

11. Luborsky, L., et al. (1976). Herpes simplex virus and moods: A longitudinal study. *J. of Psychosom. Res.,* 20, 543-548.

12. Scheier, M.F. & Carver, C.S. (1985). Optimism, coping and health: Assessment and implications of generalized outcome expectancies. *Health Psych.,* 4, 219-247.

13. Cohen, R., et al. (1991). Psychological stress and susceptibility to the common cold. *New England J. of Med.,* 325, 606-612.

14. Cluff, L.E., et al. (1966). Asian influenza: Infection, disease and psychological factors. *Archives of Int. Med.,* 117, 159-164.

15. Verthein, U. & Kohler, T. (1997). The correlation between everyday stress and angina pectoris: A longitudinal study. *J. of Psych. Res.,* 43, 241-245.

16. Pressman, S.D. & Cohen, S. (2005). Does positive affect influence health? *Psych. Bull.,* 131, 925-971.

17. Moskowitz, J.T. (2003). Positive affect predicts lower risk of AIDS mortality. *Psychosom. Med.,* 65, 620-626.

Ostir, G.V., et al. (2000). Emotional well-being predicts subsequent functional independence and survival. *J. of the Amer. Geriatrics Soc.,* 48, 473-478.266.

Danner, D.D., et al. (2001). Positive emotions in early life and longevity: Findings from the nun study. *J. of Pers. & Soc. Psych.,* 80, 804-813.

18. Pressman & Cohen (2005).

19. Levy, S.M., et al. (1988). Survival hazards analysis in first recurrent breast cancer patients: Seven-year follow-up. *Psychosom. Med.,* 50, 520-528.

Moskowitz, J.T. (2003). Positive affect predicts lower risk of AIDS mortality. *Psychosom. Med.,* 65, 620-626.

20. Moskowitz (2003).

21. Gottshalk, L.A. (1985). Hope and other deterrents of illness. *Amer. J. of Psychother.,* 39, 515-524.

22. Green, E. & Green, A. (1975). *Beyond Biofeedback.* New York: Delta.

23. Mossey, J. A. & Shapiro, E. (1982). Self-rated health: A predictor of mortality among the elderly. *Amer. J. of Public Health,* 72, 800-808.

24. Cohen, S., et al. (2003). Emotional style and susceptibility to the common cold. *Psychosom. Med.,* 65, 652-657.

25. Pressman & Cohen (2005). p. 933.

26. Mason, T., et al. (1969). Acceptance and healing. *J. of Religion & Health,* 8, 123-142.

27. Melnechuk, T. (1988). Emotions, brain, immunity and health: A review. In M. Clynes & J. Panksepp (Eds.), *Emotions & Psychopathology.* New York: Plenum, pp. 181-247.

28. Peterson, C., et al. (1988). Pessimistic explanatory style is a risk factor for physical illness: A thirty-five year longitudinal study. *J. of Pers. & Soc. Psych.,* 55, 23-27.

29. Weiss, J.M. (1971). Effects of coping behavior in different warning-signal conditions on stress pathology in rats. *J. of Compar. & Physiol. Psych.,* 77, 1-13.

30. Seligman, M.E.P., et al. (1971). Unpredictable and uncontrollable aversive events. In F. R. Brush (Ed.), *Aversive Conditioning and Learning.* New York: Academic Press, pp. 347-400.

31. Haldeman, S. (1991). Failure of the pathology model to predict back pain. *Spine*, 15, 718-724.

Svebak, S., et al. (2006). One-year prevalence of chronic musculoskeletal pain in a large Norwegian county population: Relations with age and gender—The HUNT study. *J. of Musculoskeletal Pain*, 14(1), 21-28.

32. Bongers, P.M., et al. (1993). Psychosocial factors and musculoskeletal disease. *Scandinavial J. of Work Env. & Health*, 19, 73-84.

Westgaard, R.H. & Jansen, T. (1992). Individual and work-related factors associated with symptoms of musculoskeletal complaints. II: Different risk factors among sewing machine operators. *British J. of Industrial Med.*, 49, 154-162.

33. Bru, E., et al. (1997). Back pain, dysphoric versus euphoric moods and the experience of stress and effort in female hospital staff. *Pers. & Indiv. Diffs.*, 22(4), 565-573.

34. Carter, L., et al. (2002). *Pain Res. & Management*, 7(1), 21-30.

Riley, J.L., III. (1999). The role of emotion in pain. In R.J. Gatchel & D.C. Turk (Eds.), *Psychosocial Factors in Pain: Critical Perspectives.* New York: Guilford Press, pp. 74-88.

35. Mahoney, D.L., et al. (2001). The effects of laughter on discomfort thresholds: Does expectation become reality? *J. of Gen. Psych.*, 128(2), 2170226.

Nevo, O., et al. (1993). Humor and pain tolerance. *Humor: Int. J. of Humor Res.*, 1993, 6, 71-78.

Weisenberg, M., et al. (1995). Humor as a cognitive technique for increasing pain tolerance. *Pain*, 1995, 63, 207-212.

36. Cogan, R., et al. (1987). Effects of laughter and relaxation on discomfort thresholds. *J. of Beh. Med.*, 10, 139-144.

Zillmann, D., et al. (1993). Does humor facilitate coping with physical discomfort? *Mot. & Emot.*, 17, 1-21.

37. Stuber, M., et al. (2007). Laughter, humor and pain perception in children: A pilot study. *Evidence-Based Comp. & Alt. Med.*, Published electronically, Oct. 5, 2007, 1-6.

38. Zweyer, K., et al. (2004). Do cheerfulness, exhilaration, and humor production moderate pain tolerance? *Humor: Int. J. of Humor Res.*, 17(1/2), 85-119.

39. Zweyer et al. (2004).

40. Weisenberg et al. (1995).

Zillmann, D., et al. (1993). Does humor facilitate coping with physical discomfort? *Mot. & Emot.*, 17, 1-21.

41. Hodes, R.L., et al. (1990). The effects of distraction on responses to cold pressor pain. *Pain*, 41, 109-114.

42. Hudak, D.A., et al. (1991). Effects of humorous stimuli and sense of humor on discomfort. *Psych. Rep.*, 69, 779-786.

43. Mahoney, et al. (2001).

339

44. Guadagnoli, E. & Mor, V. (1989). Measuring cancer patients' positive affect: Revision and psychometric properties of the profile of mood states (POMS). *Psych. Assessment*, 1, 150-154.

45. Potter, P.T., et al. (2000). Stressful events and information processing dispositions moderate the relationship between positive and negative affect: Implications for pain patients. *Annals of Beh. Med.*, 22, 191-198.

46. Potter, et al. (2000).

47. Kvaal, S.A. & Patodia, S. (2000). Relations among positive affect, negative affect and somatic symptoms in a medically ill patient sample. *Psych. Rep.*, 87, 227-233.

48. Yoshino, S., et al. (1996). Effects of mirthful laughter on neuroendocrine and immune systems in patients with rheumatoid arthritis. *J. of Rheumatol.*, 23, 793-794.

49. Leise, C.M. (1993). The correlation between humor and the chronic pain of arthritis. *J. of Holistic Nursing*, 11, 82-95.

50. Schmitt, N. (1990). Patients' perception of laughter in a rehabilitation hospital. *Rehab. Nursing*, 15 (No. 3), 143-146.

51. Adams, E.R. & McGuire, F.A. (1986). Is laughter the best medicine? A study of the effects of humor on perceived pain and affect. *Activities, Adaptation, & Aging*, 8, 157-175.

52. Rotton, J. & Shaats, M. (1996). Effects of state humor, expectancies and choice on post-surgical mood and self-medication: a field experiment. *J. of Applied Soc. Psych.*, 26(20), 1775-1794.

53. Kelly, M.L., et al. (1984). Decreasing burned children's pain behavior: Impacting the trauma of hydrotherapy. *J. of Applied Beh. Analysis*, 17, 147-158.

Trice, A.D. & Price-Greathouse, J. (1986). Joking under the drill: A validity study of the humor coping scale. *J. of Soc. Beh. & Pers.*, 1, 265-266.

54. McCaffery, M. (1990). Nursing approaches to non-pharmacological pain control. *Int. J. of Nursing Studies*, 27, 1-5.

55. Ljungdahl, L. (1989). Laugh if this is a joke. *J. of the Amer. Med. Assn.*, 261, 558.

56. Jerrett, M.D. (1985). Children and their pain experience. *Children's Health Care*, 14, 83-89.

57. D'Antonio, I.J. (1988). The use of humor with children in hospital settings. *J. of Children in Contemp. Society*, 23(4), 79-90.

Matz, A. & Brown, S.T. (1998). Humor and pain management: A review of current literature. *J. of Holistic Nursing*, 16(1), 68-75.

Smith, D.P. (1986). Using humor to help children with pain. *Children's Health Care*, 14, 187-188.

58. WebMDLive Events Transcript (2007). Humor and laughter for health, with S. Hilber, M. Stuber and L. Zeltzer. Taken from MedicineNet.com November 11, 2007.

59. Goodenough, B., et al. (2001). Children's self-reported use of humor as a coping strategy for acute pain. Paper presented at 22nd meeting of the Australian Pain Society, Cairns, Australia.

Goodenough, B. & Ford, J. (2005). Self-reported use of humor by hospitalized pre-adolescent children to cope with pain-related distress from a medical intervention. *Humor: Int. J. of Humor Res.*, 18(3), 279-298.

60. Goodenough & Ford (2005).

61. Stuber, et al. (2007).

62. WebMDLive Events Transcript (2007).

63. McCaul, K.D. & Malott, J.M. (1984). Distraction and coping with pain. *Psych. Bull.*, 95, 516-533.

Villemure, C. & Bushnell, M.C. (2002). Cognitive modulation of pain: how do attention and emotion influence pain processing? *Pain*, 95, 195-199.

64. Mitchell, L.A., et al. (2006). A comparison of the effects of preferred music, arithmetic, and humour on cold pressor pain. *European J. of Pain*, 10(4), 343-351.

65. Berk, L.S., et al. (1989). Neuroendocrine and stress hormone changes during mirthful laughter. *Amer. J. of Med. Sci.*, 298(6), 390-396.

Yoshino, et al. (1996).

66. Berk, L.S. & Tan, S.A. (2006). [beta]-Endorphin and HGH increase are associated with both the anticipation and experience of mirthful laughter. *The FASEB J.*, 2006, 20, A382.

67. Kogan, R. & Kluthe, K.B. (1981). The role of learning in pain reduction associated with relaxation and patterned breathing. *J. of Psychosom. Res.*, 25, 535-539.

68. Overeem, S., et al. (2004). Is motor inhibition during laughter due to emotional or respiratory influences? *Psychophysiol.*, 41, 254-258.

69. Becessa, L., et al. (2001). Reward circuitry activation by noxious thermal stimuli. *Neuron*, 32, 927-946.

70. Cohen, S., et al. (1993). Negative life events, perceived stress, negative affect, and susceptibility to the common cold. *J. of Pers. & Soc. Psych.*, 64, 131-140.

Segerstrom, S.Z. & Miller, G.E. (2004). Psychological stress and the human immune system: A meta-analytic study of 30 years of inquiry. *Psych. Bull.*, 130(4), 601-630.

Vollhardt, L.T. (1991). Psychoneuroimmunology: A literature review. *Amer. J. of Orthopsychiatry*, 61, 35-47.

71. Ader, R. & Cohen, N. (1993). Psychoneuroimmunology: Conditioning and stress. *Annual Rev. of Psych.*, 44, 53-85.

72. Dillon, K.M., et al. (1985). Positive emotional states and enhancement of the immune system. *Int. J. of Psychiatry in Med.*, 5, 13-18.

Lefcourt, H., et al. (1990). Humor and immune system functioning. *Humor: Int. J. of Humor Res.*, 3, 305-321.

McClelland, D. & Cheriff, A.D. (1997). The immunoenhancing effects of humor on secretory IgA and resistance to respiratory infections. *Psych. & Health*, 12, 329-344.

Perera, S., et al. (1998). Increases in salivary lysozyme and IgA concentrations and secretory rates independent of salivary flow rates following viewing of a humorous videotape. *Int. J. of Beh. Med.*, 5, 118-128.

73. Berk, L.S., et al. (1991). Immune system changes during humor associated with laughter. *Clin. Res.,* 39, 124A.

Berk, L.S., et al. (2001). Modulation of neuroimmune parameters during the eustress of humor-associated mirthful laughter. *Alt. Therapies in Health & Med.,* 7, 62-76.

74. Lambert, R.B. & Lambert, N.K. (1995). The effects of humor on secretory immunoglobulin A levels in school-aged children. *Ped. Nursing,* 21(1), 16-19.

75. Harrison, L.K., et al., (2000). Cardiovascular and secretory immunoglobulin A reactions to humorous, exciting and didactic film presentations. *Biol. Psych.,* 52(2), 113-126.

76. Pressman & Cohen (2005).

77. Mouton, C., et al. (1989). Salivary IgA is a weak stress marker. *Ann. Behav. Med.,* 15, 179-185.

Stone, A., et al. (1987). Secretory IgA as a measure of immunocompetence. *J. Human Stress,* 13, 136-140.

78. Schulz, R., et al. (1990). Psychiatric and physical morbidity effects of care giving. *J. Gerontol.,* 45, 181-191.

79. Berk, et al. (1989).

Berk, et al. (2001).

Takahashi, K., et al. (2001). The elevation of natural killer cell activity induced by laughter in a crossover designed study. *Int. J. of Molecular Med.,* 8, 645-650.

80. Bennett, M.P., et al. (2003). The effect of mirthful laughter on stress and natural killer cell activity. *Alt. Therapies in Health & Med.,* 9(2), 38-45.

81. Ishihara, S., et al. (1999). Immune function and psychological factors in patients with coronary heart disease. *Japanese Circulation J.,* 63, 704-709.

82. Wise, B. (1989). Comparison of immune response to mirth and to distress in women at risk for recurrent breast cancer. *Dissert. Abstr. Int.,* 49, 2918.

83. Itami, J., et al. (1994). Laughter and immunity. *Japanese J. of Psychosom. Med.,* 34, 565-571.

Kamei, T., et al. (1997). Changes of immunoregulatory cells associated with psychological stress and humor. *Percep. & Motor Skills,* 84, 1296-1298.

84. Takahashi, et al. (2001).

85. Hayashi, T., et al. (2007a). Laughter up-regulates the genes related to NK cell activity in diabetes. *Biomed. Res.,* 28(6), 281-285.

86. Levy, S.M., et al. (1985). Prognostic risk assessments in primary breast cancer by behavior and immunological parameters. *Health Psych.,* 4, 99-113.

87. Bellert, J.L. (1989). Humor: A therapeutic approach in oncology nursing. *Cancer Nursing,* 12, 65-70.

88. Kemeny, M. (1993). Emotions and the immune system. In B. Moyers (Ed), *Healing and the Mind.* New York.

89. Immunotherapy Shows Promise in Cancer Treatment. (2006). Article posted at www.roswellpark.org, May 9, 2006.

90. Berk, L.S., et al. (1993). Eustress of humor associated with laughter modulates specific immune system components. *Annals of Beh. Med.,* 15 (supplement), p. S111.

Berk, et al. (2001).

91. Berk, et al. (1993).

92. Berk, et al. (1993).

93. Berk, et al. (1989).

Berk, et al., (1993).

94. Kiecolt-Glaser, J., et al. (1986). Modulation of cellular immunity in medical students. *J. of Beh. Med.*, 9, 5-21.

95. Gruber, B.L., et al. (1988). Immune system and psychologic changes in metastatic cancer patients while using ritualized relaxation and guided imagery: A pilot study. *Scand. J. of Beh. Therapy*, 17, 25-46.

96. Callen, M. (1990). *Surviving AIDS*. New York: Harper Collins.

97. Berk, L.S. & Tan, S.A. (1996). A positive emotion, the eustress of mirthful laughter, modulates the immune system lymphokine interferon-Gamma. Research Perspectives in Psychoneuroimmunology. *PNI Res. Society Prog. Abstr.*, June.

98. Atsumi, T., et al. (2004). Pleasant feeling from watching a comical video enhances free radical-scavenging capacity in human whole saliva. *J. of Psychosom. Res.*, 56, 377-379.

Atsumi, T., et al. (2008). Salivary free radical scavenging capacity is affected by physical and mental activities. *Oral Dis.*, 14(6), 490-496.

99. Dillon, K.M., et al. (1985). Positive emotional states and enhancement of the immune system. *Int. J. of Psychiatry in Med.*, 5, 13-18.

100. Ishihara, et al. (1999).

Wise (1989).

101. Lefcourt, et al. (1990).

McClelland & Cheriff (1997).

102. Martin, R.A. & Dobbin, J.P. (1988). Sense of humor, hassles, and immunoglobulin A: Evidence for a stress-moderating effect of humor. *Int. J. of Psychiatry in Med.*, 18, 93-105.

103. Stone, A.A., et al. (1987). Evidence that secretory IgA is associated with daily mood. *J. of Pers. & Soc. Psych.*, 52, 988-993.

104. Irwin, M., et al. (1987). Life events, depressive symptoms and immune function. *Amer. J. of Psychiatry*, 144, 437-441.

105. Linn, B.S., et al. (1981). Anxiety and immune responsiveness. *Psych. Rep.*, 49, 969-970.

106. Jabaaij, L., et al. (1993). Influences of perceived psychological stress and distress on antibody response to lose dose rDNA hepatitis B vaccine. *J. of Psychosom. Res.*, 37, 361-369.

107. Stone, et al. (1987).

108. Martin, R.A. & Lefcourt, H. (1983). Sense of humor as a moderator of the relation between stressors and moods. *J. of Pers. & Soc. Psych.*, 45, 1313-1324.

109. Siegel, B.S. (1989). *Peace, Love and Healing*. New York: Harper & Row.

110. Labbott, S.M., et al. (1990). The physical and psychological effects of the expression and inhibition of emotion. *Beh. Med.*, 16, 182-189.

111. Zweyer, et al. (2004).

112. McClelland & Cheriff (1997).

113. Cousins, N. (1979). *Anatomy of an Illness*. New York: Norton.

114. Cousins, N. (1989). *Head First: The Biology of Hope*. New York: Dutton.

115. Berk, L.S., et al. (2008). Mirthful laughter, as an adjunct therapy in diabetic care, attenuates catecholamines, inflammatory cytokines, C-RP, and myocardial infarction occurrence. *The FASEB J.*, 22:1226.2.

Berk, L.S. & Tan, S. (2009). Mirthful laughter as an adjunct therapy in diabetic care, increases HDL cholesterol and attenuates inflammatory cytokines and hs-CRP and possible CVD risk. Paper presented at Meeting of the Amer. Physiological Society, New Orleans, April 18-22.

116. Matsuzaki, T., et al. (2006). Mirthful laughter differentially affects serum pro-and anti-inflammatory cytokine levels depending on the level of disease activity in patients with rheumatoid arthritis. *Rheumatol.*, 45(2), 182-186.

117. Duman, R.S. (2004). Depression: a case of neuronal life and death? *Biol. Psychiatry*, 56(3), 140-145.

Warner-Schmidt, J.L. & Duman, R.S. (2006). Hippocampal neurogenesis: opposing effects of stress and anti-depressant treatment. *Hippocampus*, 16(3), 239-249.

118. Epel, E.S., et al. (2004). Accelerated telomere shortening in response to life stress. *Proceedings of the Nat. Acad. of Sci.*, 101(49), 17312-17315.

119. Overeem, S., et al. (1999). Weak with laughter. *Lancet*, 354, 838.

Overeem, S., et al. (2004). Is motor inhibition during laughter due to emotional or respiratory influences? *Psychophysiol.*, 41, 254-258.

Prerost, F.J. & Ruma, C. (1987). Exposure to humorous stimuli as an adjunct to muscle relaxation training. *Psych: A Quart. J. of Human Beh.*, 24, 70-74.

Zweyer, et al. (2004).

120. Overeem, (2004).

121. Paskind, H.A. (1932). Effects of laughter on muscle tone. *Archives of Neurol. & Psychiatry*, 28, 23-628.

122. Prerost & Ruma (1987).

123. Langorch, W., et al. (1982). Behavior therapy with coronary heart disease patients. *J. of Psychosom. Res.*, 26, 465-484.

124. Blanehard, E., et al. (1982). Sequential comparisons of relaxation training and biofeedback in the treatment of three kinds of chronic headache. *Beh. Res. & Therapy*, 20, 469-481.

125. Leboeuf, A. (1977). The effects of EMG feedback training on state anxiety. *J. of Clin. Psych.*, 33, 251-253.

126. McEwan, B. & Lashley, E.N. (2003). Allostatic load: When protection gives way to damage. *Advances in Mind-Body Med.*, 19, 28-33.

127. Pressman & Cohen (2005).

128. Sapolsky, R.M. (1998). *Why Zebras don't Get Ulcers: An Updated Guide to Stress-related Disease and Coping*. New York: Freeman, p. 7.

129. Linkowski, P. (2003). Neuroendocrine profiles in mood disorders. *Int. J. of Neuropsychopharmacol.*, 6, 191-197.

Miller, A.H. (1998). Neuroendocrine and immune system interactions in stress and depression. *Psychiatric Clinics of North Amer.*, 21, 443-463.

Suarez, E.C., et al. (1998). Neuroendocrine, cardiovascular and emotional responses of hostile men: The role of interpersonal challenge. *Psychosom. Med.*, 60, 78-88.

130. Polk, D.E., et al. (2005). State and trait affect as predictors of salivary cortisol in healthy adults. *Psychoneuroendocrinol.*, 30, 261-272.

131. Gerra, G., et al. (1996). Neuroendocrine responses to emotional arousal in normal women. *Neuropsychobiol.*, 33, 173-181.

Nejtek, V.A. (2002). High and low emotion events influence emotional stress perceptions and are associated with salivary cortisol response changes in a consecutive stress paradigm. *Psychoneuroendocrinol.*, 27, 3, 337-352.

132. Berk et al. (1989).

Hubert, W. & deJong-Meyer, R. (1989). Emotional stress and saliva cortisol response. *J. of Clin. Chem. & Clin. Biochem.*, 27, 235-237.

Hubert, W. & deJong-Meyer, R. (1992). Salivary cortisol response to sad and humorous film segments. In C. Kirschbaum, et al. (Eds.), *Assessment of Hormones and Drugs in Saliva in Biobehavioral Research*. Seattle: Hogrefe and Huber, pp. 213-217.

Vlachopoulos, C., et al. (2009). Divergent effects of laughter and mental stress on arterial

133. Berk, L.S., et al. (2008). Cortisol and catecholamine stress hormone decrease is associated with the behavior of perceptual anticipation of mirthful laughter. *The FASEB J.*, 22:946, 11.

134. Jemmott, J.B. & Locke, S.E. (1984). Psychosocial factors, immunologic mediation, and human susceptibility to infectious diseases: How much do we know? *Psych. Bull.*, 95, 78-108.

Kiecolt-Glaser, J., et al. (1986). Modulation of cellular immunity in medical students. *J. of Beh. Med.*, 9, 5-21.

135. Pressman & Cohen (2005).

136. Berk & Tan (2009).

137. Ishigami, S., et al. (2005). Effects of mirthful laughter on growth hormone, IGF-1 and substance P in patients with rheumatoid arthritis. *Clin. & Exp. Rheumatol.*, 23(5), 651-657.

138. McMahon, C., et al. (2005). Taking blood pressure—no laughing matter. *Blood Pressure Monitoring*, 10(2), 109-110.

139. Fry, W.F., Jr. & Savin, W.M. (1988). Mirthful laughter and blood pressure. *Humor: Int. J. of Humor Res.*, 1, 49-62.

140. Tan, S.A., et al. (1997). Mirthful laughter: An effective adjunct in cardiac rehabilitation. *Canadian J. of Cardiol.*, 13(supplement B), 190.

141. White, S. & Camarena, P. (1989). Laughter as a stress reducer in small groups. *Humor: Int. J. of Humor Res.*, 2(1), 73-79.

142. Kerkkanen, P, et al. (2004). Sense of humor, physical health and well-being at work: A three-year longitudinal study of Finnish Police Officers. *Humor: Int. J. of Humor Res.*, 17(1/2), 21-35.

143. Lefcourt, H.M., et al. (1997). Humor as a stress moderator in the prediction of blood pressure obtained during five stressful tasks. *J. of Res. in Pers.*, 31, 523-542.

144. Pressman & Cohen (2005).

145. Watson, D. (1988). Intraindividual and interindividual analyses of positive and negative affect: Their relation to health complaints, perceived stress, and daily activities. *J. of Pers. & Soc. Psych.*, 54, 1020-1030.

146. Bardwell, W.A., et al. (1999). Psychological correlates of sleep apnea. *J. of Psychosom. Res.*, 47, 583-596.

147. Cohen, S. (2004). Social relationships and health. *Amer. Psychol.*, 59, 676-684.

148. Diener, E. & Seligman, M.E. (2002). Very happy people. *Psych. Sci.*, 13(1), 81-84.

149. American Heart Association (2003). *Heart Disease and Stroke Statistics—2004 Update.* Dallas, TX: American Heart Assn.

150. Futterman, L.G. & Lemberg, L. (1998). Fifty percent of patients with coronary artery disease do not have any of the conventional risk factors. *Amer. J. of Crit. Care*, 7, 240-244.

151. Krantz, D.S., et al. (1981). Behavior and health: Mechanisms and research issues. *Soc. Sci. Res. Council: ITEMS*, 35, 1-6.

152. Blascovich, J. & Katkin, E.S. (Eds.). (1993). *Cardiovascular Reactivity to Psychological Stress and Disease.* Washington, DC: American Psychological Association.

153. Gallo, L.C., et al. (2004). Emotions and cognitions in coronary heart disease: Risk, resilience and social context. *Cog. Therapy & Res.*, 28(5), 669-694.

154. Goldstein, M.G. & Niaura, R. (1995). Coronary artery disease and sudden death. In A. Stoudemire (Ed.), *Psychological Factors Affecting Medical Conditions.* Washington, D.C.: Amer. Psychiatric Press.
Matthews, K.A. & Haynes, S.G. (1986). Type A behavior pattern and coronary disease risk. *Amer. J. of Epidemiol.*, 30, 489-498.

155. Haynes, S.G., et al. (1978). The relationship of psychosocial factors to coronary heart disease in the Framingham Study. III. Eight-year incidence of coronary heart disease. *Amer. J. of Epidemiol.*, 111, 37-58.

156. Blumenthal, J.A., et al. (1978). Type A behavior pattern and coronary atherosclerosis. *Circulation*, 58, 634-639.

157. Goldstein, J.H., et al. (1988). Humor and the coronary-prone behavior pattern. *Current Psych.: Res. & Reviews*, 7(2), 115-121.

158. Gallow, L.C. & Matthews, K.A. (2003). Understanding the association between socioeconomic status and physical health: Do negative emotions play a role? *Psych. Bull.*, 129, 10-51.
Miller, T.Q., et al. (1996). Meta-analytic review of research on hostility and physical health. *Psych. Bull.*, 119, 322-348.

Smith, T.W. & Ruiz, J.M. (2002). Psychosocial influences on the development and course of coronary heart disease: Current status and implications for research and practice. *J. of Consulting & Clin. Psych.*, 70, 548-568.

159. Trieber, F.A., et al. (2003). Cardiovascular reactivity and development of preclinical and clinical disease states. *Psychosom. Med.*, 65, 46-62.

160. Iribarren, C., et al. (2000). Association of hostility with coronary artery calcification in young adults: The CARDIA study. *J. of the Amer. Med. Assn.*, 283, 2546-2551.

161. Mittleman, M.A., et al. (1995). Triggering of acute myocardial infarction onset by episodes of anger. *Circulation*, 92, 1720-1725.

162. Das, S. & O'Keefe, J.H. (2006). Behavioral cardiology: recognizing and addressing the profound impact of psychosocial stress on cardiovascular health. *Current Atherosclerosis Rep.*, 8(2), 111-118. (Quote on p. 111.)

163. Kark, J.D., et al. (1995). Iraqi missile attacks on Israel: The association of mortality with a life threatening stressor. *J. of the Amer. Med. Assn.*, 273, 1208-1210.

164. Leor, J., et al. (1996). Sudden cardiac death triggered by an earthquake. *New England J. of Med.*, 334, 413-419.

165. Everson, S.A., et al. (1997). Hopelessness and 4-year progression of carotid atherosclerosis. *Arteriosclerosis, Thrombosis & Vasc. Biol.*, 17, 1490-1495.

166. Ferketich, A.K., et al. (2000). Depression as an antecedent to heart disease among women and men in the NHANES I study. *Arch. of Internal Med.*, 160, 1261-1268.

167. Murberg, T.A., et al. (1999). Depressed mood and subjective health symptoms as predictors of mortality in patients with congestive heart failure: A two-year follow-up study. *Int. J. of Psychiatry in Med.*, 29(3), 311-326.

168. Neunteufl, T., et al. (1997). Systemic endothelial dysfunction is related to the extent and severity of coronary artery disease. *Atherosclerosis*, 129, 111-118.

169. Schachinger, V., et al. (2000). Prognostic impact of coronary vasodilator dysfunction on adverse long-term outcome of coronary heart disease. *Circulation*, 101, 1899-1906.

170. Faulx, M.D., et al. (2003). Detection of endothelial dysfunction with brachial artery ultrasound scanning. *Amer. Heart J.*, 145(6), 943-951.

171. Ghiadoni, L., et al. (2000). Mental stress induces transient endothelial dysfunction in humans. *Circulation*, 102, 2473-2478.

Gottdiener, J.S., et al. (2003). Effects of mental stress on flow-mediated brachial artery dilation and influence of behavioral factors and hypercholesterolemia in subjects without cardiovascular disease. *Amer. J. of Cardiol.*, 92, 687-691.

172. Harris, K.F., et al. (2003). Associations between psychological traits and endothelial function in postmenopausal women. *Psychosom. Med.*, 65, 402-409.

173. Hemingway, H., et al. (2003). Social and psychosocial influences on inflammatory markers and vascular function in civil servants (the Whitehall II study). *Amer. J. of Cardiol.*, 92, 984-987.

174. Schachinger, et al. (2000).

175. Carver, C.S. & Scheier, M.F. (2002). The hopeful optimist. *Psych. Inquiry*, 13, 288-290.

176. Kubzansky, L.D., et al. (2001). Is the glass half empty or half full? A prospective study of optimism and coronary heart disease in the normative aging study. *Psychosom. Med.. Special Issue: Outerspace Res.*, 63, 910-916.

177. Scheier, M.F., et al. (1989). Dispositional optimism and recovery from coronary artery bypass surgery: The beneficial effects on physical and psychological well-being. *J. of Pers. & Soc. Psych.*, 57, 1024-1040.

178. Scheier, M.F., et al. (1999). Optimism and rehospitalization after coronary artery bypass graft surgery. *Archives of Internal Med.*, 159, 36-49.

179. Middleton, R.A. & Byrd, E.K. (1996). Psychosocial factors and hospital readmission status of older persons with cardiovascular disease. *J. of Applied Rehab. Counseling*, 27, 3-10.

180. Clark, A., et al. (2001). Inverse association between sense of humor and coronary heart disease. *Int. J. of Cardiol.*, 80, 87-88.

181. Berk, et al. (2008).

182. Tan, et al. (1997).

183. Blascovich, J.J. & Katkin, E.S. (1993). *Cardiovascular Reactivity to Psychological Stress and Disease*. Washington, D. C. American Psychological Association.

184. Tugade, M.M. & Fredrickson, B.L. (2004). Resilient individuals use positive emotions to bounce back from negative emotional experiences. *J. of Pers. & Soc. Psych.*, 86, 320-333.

185. Blascovich & Katkin (1993).

186. Fredrickson, B.L. & Levinson, R.W. (1998). Positive emotions speed recovery from the cardiovascular sequelae of negative emotions. *Cog. & Emot.*, 12, 191-220.

Fredrickson, B.L., et al. (2000). The undoing effect of positive emotions. *Mot. & Emot.*, 24, 237-258.

187. Fredrickson, et al. (2000).

188. Quote taken from press release by the University of Maryland Medical News, Nov. 15, 2000.

189. Miller, M., et al. (2006). Impact of cinematic viewing on endothelial function. *Heart*, 92(2), 261-262.

190. Rywik, T.M., et al. (1999). Enhanced endothelial vasoreactivity in endurance trained older men. *J. of Applied. Physiol.*, 87, 2136-2142.

191. Korkmaz, H. & Onalan, O. (2008). Evaluation of endothelial sysfunction: flow-mediated dilation. *Endothelium*, 15, 157-163.

192. Miller, M. & Fry, W. F. (2009). The effect of mirthful laughter on the human cardiovascular system. *Med. Hypotheses*, in press [doi:10.1016/j.mehy.2009.02.044].

193. Vlachopoulos, C., et al. (2009). Divergent effects of laughter and mental stress on arterial stiffness and central hemodynamics. *Psychosom. Med.*, 71(4), 446-453.

194. Berk, et al. (2008).

195. Berk, L.S. & Tan, S. (2009).

196. Matsuzaki, T., et al. (2006). Mirthful laughter differentially affects serum pro-and anti-inflammatory cytokine levels depending on the level of disease activity in patients with rheumatoid arthritis. *Rheumatol.*, 45(2), 182-186.

197. Berk, L.S. & Tan, S. (2009).

198. Svebak, S., et al. (2007). Sense of humor and mortality: A seven-year prospective study of an unselected county population and a sub-population diagnosed with cancer. *Psychosom. Med.*, 69, A-64.

199. Bennett, M.P. & Lengacher, C.A. (1999). Use of complementary therapies in a rural cancer population. *Oncol. Nursing Forum*, 26, 1287-1294.

200. Lengacher, C.A., et al. (2002). Frequency of use of complementary/ alternative medicine (CAM) in women with breast cancer. *Oncol. Nursing Forum*, 29, 1445-1452.

201. Benjamin, H.B. (1987). *From Victim to Victor*. New York: Dell, p. 132-133.

202. Fry, W.F., Jr. (1986). Humor, physiology, and the aging process. In L. Nahemow, et al. (Eds.), *Humor and Aging*. San Diego: Academic Press, pp. 81-98.

203. Fry, W.F. (1994). The biology of humor. *Humor: Int. J. of Humor Res.*, 7(2), 111-126.

204. Personal conversation with Dr. Jonathan Raskin, May 26, 2005.

205. Filippelli M., et al. 2001. Respiratory dynamics during laughter. *J. Appl. Physiol.*, 90, 1441-1446.

206. Brutsche, M.H., et al. (2008). The impact of laughter on air trapping in severe chronic obstructive lung disease. *Int. J. of Chronic Obstructive Pulmonary Dis.*, 3(1), 185-192.

207. American Lung Assn. *Diseases A to Z. Trends in asthma morbidity and mortality.* Available at www.lungusa.org. Assessed March 7, 2000.

208. Miller, B.D. & Wood, B.L. (1997). Influences of specific emotional states on autonomic reactivity and pulmonary function in asthmatic children. *J. of the Amer. Acad. of Child & Adol. Psychiatry*, 36, 669-677.
Ritz, T. (2004). Probing the psychophysiology of the airways: Physical activity, experienced emotion and facially expressed emotion. *Psychophysiol.*, 41, 809-821.
Wright, R.J., et al. (1998). Review of psychosocial stress and asthma: An integrated biopsychosocial approach. *Thorax*, 53, 1066-1974.

209. Kimata, H. (2004). Effect of viewing a humorous vs. nonhumorous film on bronchial responsiveness in patients with bronchial asthma. *Physiol. & Beh.*, 81, 681-684.

210. Liangas, G., et al. (2003). Mirth-triggered asthma: Is laughter really the best medicine? *Ped. Pulmonology*, 36, 107-112.

211. Garay, S. (2007). Paper presented at meeting of the American Thoracic Society (International Conference), San Diego

212. Liangas, et al. (2003).

213. Miller & Wood (1997).

214. Ritz (2004).

215. Pressman & Cohen (2005).

Ritz, (2004).

216. Lask, B. (1991). Psychological treatments of asthma. *Clin. & Exp. Allergy*, 21, 625-626.

217. Richter, R. & Dahme, B. (1982). Bronchial asthma in adults: There is no evidence for the effectiveness of behavioral therapy and relaxation. *J. of Psychosom. Res.*, 26, 533-540.

218. Ritz (2004). P. 818.

219. Liangas, et al. (2003).

220. Rees, W.L. (1980). Etiological factors in asthma. *Psychiatric J. of the Univ. of Ottowa*, 5, 250-254, p. 252.

221. Choy, E.H. & Panayi, G.S. (2001). Cytokine pathways and joint inflammation in rheumatoid arthritis. *New England J. of Med.*, 344, 907-916.

Goldring, S.R. (2003). Pathogenesis of bone and cartilage destruction in rheumatoid arthritis. *Rheumatol.*, 42(supplement 2), ii11-ii16.

222. Matsuzaki, T., et al. (2006). Mirthful laughter differentially affects serum pro- and anti-inflammatory cytokine levels depending on the level of disease activity in patients with rheumatoid arthritis. *Rheumatol.*, 45, 182-186.

Nakajima, A., et al. (1999). Reassessment of mirthful laughter in rheumatoid arthritis. *J. Rheumatol.*, 26, 512-513.

Yoshino, S., et al. (1996). Effects of mirthful laughter on neuroendocrine and immune systems in patients with rheumatoid arthritis. *J. Rheumatol.*, 23, 793-794.

223. Matsuzaki, et al. (2006).

224. Cutolo, M., et al. (1999). Is stress a factor in the pathogenesis of autoimmune rheumatic diseases? *Clin. & Exp. Rheumatol.*, 17, 515-518.

225. Ishigami, S., et al. (2005). Effect of mirthful laughter on growth hormone, IGF-1 and substance P in patients with rheumatoid arthritis. *Clin. & Exp. Rheumatol.*, 23(5), 651-657.

226. Kimata, H. (2003). Enhancement of allergic skin wheal responses and in vitro allergin-specific IgE production by computer-induced stress in patients with atopic dermatitis. *Brain Beh. Immunity*, 17, 134-138.

227. Kimata, H. (2001). Effect of humor on allergen-induced wheal response. *J. of the Amer. Med. Assn.*, 285, 738.

Kimata, H. (2004a). Laughter counteracts enhancement of plasma neurotropin levels and allergic skin wheal responses by mobile phone-mediated stress. *Beh. Med.*, 29(4), 149-152.

228. Kimata, H. (2004b). Differential effects of laughter on allergen-specific immunoglobulin and neurotropin levels in tears. *Perceptual & Motor Skills*, 98(3), 901-908.

Kimata, H. (2004c). Reduction of allergen-specific IgE production by laughter. *European J. of Clin. Investig.*, 34, 76-77.

229. Kimata, H. (2006). Emotion with tears decreases allergic responses to latex in atopic eczema patients with latex allergy. *J. of Psychosom. Res.*, 61, 67-69.

230. Guzik, T.J., et al. (2005). Persistent skin colonization with *Staphylococcus aureus* in atopic dermatitis: relationship to clinical and immunological parameters, *Clin. & Exp. Allergy*, 35, 448-455.

231. Rieg, S., et al. (2005). Deficiency of dermcidin-derived antimicrobial peptides in sweat of patients atopic dermatitis correlates with an impaired innate defense of human skin in vivo. *J. of Immunology*, 174, 8003-8010.

232. Kimata, H. (2007a). Increase in dermcidin-derived peptides in sweat of patients with atopic eczema caused by a humorous video. *J. of Psychosom. Res.*, 62, 57-59.

233. Kimata, H. (2007b). Viewing humorous film improves night-time wakening in children with atopic dermatitis. *Indian Pediatr.*, 44(4), 281-285.

234. Kimata, H. (2007c). Laughter elevates the levels of breast-milk melatonin. *J. of Psychosom. Res.*, 62, 699-702.

235. Hayashi, T., et al. (2003). Laughter lowered the increase in postprandial blood glucose. *Diabetes Care*, 26(5), 1651-1652.

236. Hayashi, T., et al. (2006). Laughter regulates gene expression in patients with type 2 diabetes. *Psychother. & Psychosomatics*, 75, 62-65. Hayashi, et al. (2007a).

Hayashi, T. & Murakami, K. (2009). The effects of laughter on post-prandial glucose levels and gene expression in type 2 diabetic patients. *Life Sci.*, May 19. [Epub ahead of print, *PubMed*.]

237. Surwit, R.S. & Schneider, M.S. (1993). Role of stress in the etiology and treatment of diabetes mellitus. *Psychosom. Med.*, 55, 380-393.

238. Hayashi, T., et al. (2007b). Laughter modulates prorenin receptor gene expression in patients with type 2 diabetes. *J. of Psychosom. Res.*, 62, 703-706.

239. Peach, M.J. (1977). Renin angiotensin system: biochemistry and mechanism of action. *Physiol. Rev.*, 57, 313-370.

240. Miller, J.A., et al. (1996). Effect of hyperglycemia on arterial pressure, plasma rennin activity and renal function in early diabetes. *Clin. Sci.*, (90), 189-195.

Vidotti, D.B., et al. (2004). High glucose concentration stimulates intracellular renin activity and angiotensin II generation in rat mesangial cells. *Amer. J. of Physiol.*, 286, F1039-F1045.

241. Luestscher, J.A., et al. (1985). Increased plasma inactive rennin in diabetes mellitus. A marker of microvascular complications. *New England J. of Med.*, 312, 1412-1417.

242. Nasir, U.M., et al., (2005). Laughter therapy modulates the parameters of renin-angiotensin system in patients with type 2 diabetes. *Int. J. of Molecular Med.*, 16(6), 1077-1081 (quote on p. 1080).

243. Kurtz, M. (1990). Adherence to diabetes regimens: Empirical status and clinical applications. *Diabetes Educ.*, 16, 50-56.

244. Helme, D.W. & Harrington, N.G. (2004). Patient accounts for noncompliance with self-care regimens and physician compliance-gaining response. *Patient Educ. & Counseling*, 55, 281-292.

245. Murakami, K. & Hayashi, T. (2002). Interaction between mind-heart and gene. *J. of Int. Soc. of Life Info. Sci.*, 20(1), 122-126.

246. Hayashi, et al. (2007b). p. 705.

247. Hayashi, et al. (2007b). p. 705.

248. Ichihara, A., et al. (2004). Inhibition of diabetic nephropathy by a decoy peptide corresponding to the "handle" region for nonproteolytic activation of prorenin. *J. of Clin. Investigation*, 114, 1128-1135.

249. Hayashi & Murakami (2009).

250. Hayashi, et al. (2007a).

251. Elinav, E., et al. (2006). Adoptive transfer of regulatory NKT lymphocytes ameliorates non-alcoholic steatohepatitis and glucose intolerance in ob/ob mice and is associated with intrahepatic CD8 trapping. *J. Pathology*, 209, 121-128.

252. Buchowski, M.S., et al. (2007). Energy expenditure during laughter. *Int. J. of Obesity*, 31, 131-137.

253. Callow, K.A. (1985). Effect of specific humoral immunity and some non-specific factors on resistance of volunteers to respiratory coronavirus infection. *J. of Hygiene*, 95, 173-189.

Jemmott, J.B. III & McClelland, D.C. (1989). Secretary IgA as a measure of resistance to infectious disease: Comments on Stone, Cox, Valdimirsdottir and Neale. *Beh. Med.*, 15, 63-71.

254. Smith, D.J. & Taubman, M.A. (1990). Effect of local deposition of antigen on salivary immune responses and reaccumulation of mutans streptococci. *J. of Clin. Immunology*, 10, 273-281.

255. McClelland & Cheriff (1997).

256. Dillon, K.M. & Totten, M.C. (1989). Psychological factors, immunocompetence, and health of breast feeding mothers and their infants. *J. of Gen. Psych.*, 150, 155-162.

257. Annie, C.L. & Groer, M. (1991). Childbirth stress: An immunologic study. *JOGN Nursing*, 20, 391-397.

258. Dowling, J.S., et al. (2003). Sense of humor, childhood cancer stressors and outcomes of psychological adjustment, immune function, and infection. *J. of Ped. Oncol. Nursing*, 20(6), 271-292.

259. Boyle, G. & Joss-Reid, J.M. (2004). Relationship of humour to health: A psychometric investigation. *Brit. J. of Health Psych.*, 9(1), 51-66.

Carroll, J. & Schmidt, S. (1992). Correlation between humorous coping style and health. *Psych. Rep.*, 70, 402.

Ruch, W., et al. (1998). Assessing the humorous temperament: Construction of the facet and standard trait forms of the State-Trait Cheerfulness Inventory. *Humor: Int. J. of Humor Res.*, 9(3/4), 303-339.

Svebak, S., et al. (2008). Some health effects of implementing school nursing in a Norwegian high school: A controlled study. *J. of School Nursing*, 24(1), 49-54.

260. Hehl, F. J. (1990). Beziehungen zwischenkorperlichen Beschwerden und Humor. *Zeitschrift fur Klinische Psychologie, Psychopathologie und Psychotherapie*, 38, 362-368.

261. Hehl, F.J. & Ruch, W. (1988). The location of sense of humor within comprehensive personality spaces: An exploratory study. *Pers. & Indiv. Diff.,* 6, 703-715.

262. Schmitt (1990).

263. Carroll, J. (1990). The relationship between humor appreciation and perceived physical health. *Psych.: The J. of Human Beh.,* 27, 34-37.

Carroll, J. & Shmidt, J. (1992). Correlation between humorous coping style and health. *Psych. Rep.,* 70, 402.

264. Simon, J. (1990). Humor and its relationship to perceived health, life satisfaction and morale in older adults. *Issues in Mental Health Nursing,* 11, 17-31.

265. Labbott, S.M. & Martin, R.B. (1990). Emotional coping, age and physical disorder. *Beh. Med.,* 16, 53-61.

Porterfield, A.L. (1987). Does sense of humor moderate the impact of life stress on psychological and physical well-being? *J. of Res. in Pers.,* 21, 306-317.

Svebak, S., et al. (2004). The significance of sense of humor, life regard and stressors for bodily complaints among high school students. *Humor: Int. J. of Humor Res.,* 17(1/2), 67-83.

Svebak, S., et al. (2004). The prevalence of sense of humor in a large, unselected county population in Norway: Relations with age, sex and some health indicators. *Int. J. of Humor Res.,* 17(1/2), 121-134.

266. Kerkkanen, et al. (2004).

267. Kuiper, N.A. & Nicholl, S. (2004). Thoughts of feeling better? Sense of humor and physical health. *Humor: Int. J. of Humor Res.,* 17(1/2), 37-66.

268. Dowling, J.S. (2001). Sense of humor, childhood cancer stressors and outcomes of psychosocial adjustment, Immune function and infection. *Dissert. Abstr. Int. Section B: The Sci. & Engineering,* Vol. 61 (70B), Feb., 3505.

269. Friedman, M. & Rosenman, R.H. (1974). *Type A Behavior and Your Heart.* New York: Knopf, p. 298.

270. Goldstein, J.H., et al. (1988). Humor and the coronary-prone behavior pattern. *Current Psych. Res. Rev.,* 7, 115-121.

271. Svebak, et al. (2007).

272. Svebak, S., et al. (2006). Sense of humor and survival among a county cohort of patients with end-stage renal failure: A two-year prospective study. *Int. J. of Psychiatry in Med.,* 36(3), 269-281.

273. Friedman, H., et al. (1993). Does childhood personality predict longevity? *J. of Pers. & Soc. Psych.,* 65, 176-185.

274. Martin, L., et al. (2002). A life course perspective on childhood cheerfulness and its relation to mortality risk. *Pers. & Soc. Psych. Bull.,* 28, 1155-1165.

275. Scholl, J.C. (2007). The use of humor to promote patient-centered care. *J. of Applied Communic. Res.,* 35(2), 156-176.

276. Sala, F., et al. (2002). Satisfaction and the use of humor by physicians and patients. *Psych. & Health,* 17(3), 269-280.

277. Bricher, G. (2000). Children in the hospital: Issues of power and vulnerability. *Ped. Nursing,* 26, 277-282.

278. Lindeke, L., et al. (2006). Capturing children's voices for quality improvement. *Amer. J. of Mat./Child Nursing*, 31, 290-295.

279. Schmitt, (1990).

280. Schmidt, C., et al. (2007). Hospitalized children's perceptions of nurses and nurse behaviors. *Amer. J. of Maternal/Child Nursing*, 32(6), 336-342.

281. Penson, R.T., et al. (2005). Laughter: The best medicine? *The Oncologist*, 10, 651-660.

282. Lotzkar, M. & Bottorf, J.L. (2001). An observational study of the development of a nurse-patient relationship. *Clin. Nursing Res.*, 10(3), 275-294.

283. Scholl, J.C. & Ragan, S.L. (2003). The use of humor in promoting positive provider-patient interactions in a hospital rehabilitation unit. *Health Communic.*, 15(3), 319-330.

284. Penson, et al. (2005). p. 653.

285. Penson, et al. (2005). p. 653.

286. Oliffe, J. & Thorne, S. (2007). Men, masculinities and prostate cancer: Australian and Canadian patient perspectives of communication with male physicians. *Qual. Health Res.*, 17(2), 149-161.

287. Chapple, A. & Ziebland, S. (2004). The role of humor for men with testicular cancer. *Qual. Health Res.*, 14(8), 1123-1139.

288. Adamie, K., et al. (2007). Comparing teaching practices about humor among nursing faculty: An international collaborative study. *Int. J. of Nursing Educ. Scholarship*, 4(1).

289. Dean, R.A.K. & Major, J.E. (2008). From critical care to comfort care: The sustaining value of humour. *J. of Clin. Nursing*, 17(8), 1088-1095.

290. Koller, D. & Gryski, C. (2008). The life threatened child and the life enhancing clown: Towards a model of therapeutic clowning. *Evidence-Based Complem. & Alt. Med.*, 5(1), 17-25.

Spitzer, P. (2001). The clown doctors. *Austria Family Physician*, 30, 12-16.

291. Darrach, B. (1990). Send in the clowns. *Life Mag.*, 13(10), 76-85.

292. Wollin, S.R., et al. (2003). Predictors of preoperative anxiety in children. *Anaesthesia Intensive Care*, 31, 69-74.

293. Golan, G., et al. (2006). Clowns for the prevention of preoperative anxiety in children: a randomized controlled trial. *Ped. Anaesthesia*, 16(10), 1019-1027.

Smerling, A.J., et al. (1999). Perioperative clown therapy for pediatric patients. *Anesth. Analg.*, 88, 243-256.

Vagnoli, L., et al. (2005). Clown doctors as a treatment for preoperative anxiety in children: a randomized, prospective study. *Pediatrics*, 116. 563-567.

294. Canto, M.A., et al. (2008). Evaluation of the effect of hospital clown's performance about anxiety in children subjected to surgical intervention. *Cir. Pediatr.*, 21(4), 195-198. (Article in Spanish.)

295. Vagnoli, et al. (2005).

296. Scholl, J.C. & Ragan, S.L. (2003). The use of humor in promoting positive provider-patient interactions in a hospital rehabilitation unit. *Health Communic.*, 15(3), 319-330.

297. Scholl & Ragan (2003). p. 328.

298. Scholl (2007). P. 170.

299. Melnechuk, T. (1988). Emotions, brain, immunity and health: A review. In M. Clynes & J. Panksepp (Eds.), *Emotions and Psychopathology*. New York: Plenum, 181-247.

300. Holden-Lund, C. (1988). Effects of relaxation with guided imagery on surgical stress and wound healing. *Res. in Nursing & Health*, 11, 235-244.

301. Rotton, J. & Shats, M. (1996). Effects of state humor, expectancies and choice on post-surgical mood and self-medication: A field experiment. *J. of Applied Soc. Psych.*, 26, 1775-1794.

302. Adams, E.R. & McGuire, F.A. (1986). Is laughter the best medicine? A study of the effects of humor on perceived pain and affect. *Activities, Adaptation, & Aging*, 8, 157-175.

303. Turner, de S. & Stokes, L. (2006). Hope promoting strategies of Registered Nurses. *J. of Advanced Nursing*, 56(4), 363-372.

304. Dreher, D. (1988). Mind-body interventions for surgery: Evidence and exigency. *Advances in Mind-Body Med.*, 14, 207-222.

305. Mumford, E., et al. (1982). The effects of psychological intervention on recovery from surgery and heart attacks: An analysis of the literature. *Amer. J. of Public Health*, 72, 141-151.

306. Devine, E.C. (1992). Effect of psychoeducational care for adult surgical patients: A meta-analysis of 191 studies. *Patient Educ. & Counseling*, 19, 129-142.

307. Devine, E.C. & Cook, T.D. (1986). Clinical and cost-savings effects of psychoeducational interventions with surgical patients: A meta-analysis. *Res. in Nursing & Health*, 9, 89-105.

308. Dreher (1998).

309. Bennett, M.P. & Lengacher, C. (2006). Humor and laughter may influence health: II. Complementary therapies and humor in a clinical population. *Complem. & Alt. Med.*, 3(2), 187-190.

310. Bennett & Lengacher (1999).

311. Lengacher, et al. (2002).

Chapter 3

1. Alvord, L.A. & Van Pelt, E.C. (2000). *The Scalpel and the Silver Bear*. New York: Bantam Books.

2. Bookheimer, S. (2002). Functional MRI of language: New approaches to understanding the cortical organization of semantic processing. *Annual Rev. of Neurosci.*, 25, 151-188.

3. Suls, J.M. (1972). A two-stage model for the appreciation of jokes and cartoons. In J.H. Goldstein & P.E. McGhee (Eds.), *The Psychology of Humor*. New York: Academic Press.

4. Blumstein, S.E. (1994). Impairment of speech production and speech perception in aphasia. *Philosophical Transactions of the Royal Society of London. Series B: Biol. Sci.*, 346(1315), 29-36.

Damasio, A.R. (1992). Aphasia. *New England J. of Med.*, 326(8), 531-539.

5. Van Lancker, D. & Kempler, D. (1987). Comprehension of familiar phrases by left- but not right-hemisphere damage patients. *Brain & Lang.*, 32(2), 265-277.

6. Wapner, W., et al. (1981). The role of the right hemisphere in the apprehension of complex linguistic materials. *Brain & Lang.*, 14, 15-33.

7. Bihrle, A.M., et al. (1986). Comprehension of humorous and nonhumorous materials by left and right brain-damaged patients. *Brain & Cog.*, 5(4), 399-412.

Gardner, H., et al. (1983). Missing the point: The role of the right hemisphere in the processing of complex linguistic materials. In E. Perecman (Ed.), *Cognitive Processes in the Right Hemisphere*. New York: Academic Press.

8. Bihrle, A.M., et al. (1988). Humor and the right hemisphere: A narrative perspective. In H.A. Whitaker (Ed.), *Contemp. Reviews in Neuropsych.*, New York: Springer-Verlag, pp. 109-126.

9. Brownell, H.H., et al. (1983). Surprise, but not coherence: Sensitivity to verbal humor in right-hemisphere patients. *Brain & Lang.*, 18, 20-27.

10. Bihrle, et al. (1986).

11. Gainotti, A. (1972). Emotional behavior and hemispheric side of lesion. *Cortex*, 8, 41-55.

12. Stuss, D.T., et al. (2001). The frontal lobes are necessary for theory of mind. *Brain*, 124, 279-286.

Winner, E., et al. (1998). Distinguishing lies from jokes: Theory of mind deficit and discourse interpretation in right hemisphere damage patients. *Brain & Lang.*, 62, 89-106.

13. Cheang & Pell (2006).

14. Brownell, H.H., et al. (1990). Appreciation of metaphoric alternative word meanings by left and right brain-damaged patients. *Neuropsychologia*, 28, 375-383.

Martin, I. & McDonald, S. (2006). That can't be right! What causes pragmatic language impairment following right hemisphere damage? *Brain Impairment*, 7(3), 202-211.

15. Giora, R., et al. (2000). Differential effects of right- and left-hemisphere damage on understanding sarcasm and metaphor. *Metaphor & Symbol*, 15, 63-83.

Shamay, S.G., et al. (2002). Deficit in understanding sarcasm in patients with prefrontal lesion is related to impaired empathic ability. *Brain & Cog.*, 48(2-3), 558-563.

Shamay-Tsoory, S.G., et al. (2005). The neuroanatomical basis of understanding sarcasm and its relationship to social cognition. *Neuropsych.*, 19(3), 288-300.

16. Heilman, K.M., et al. (1975). Auditory affective agnosia: Disturbed comprehension of affective speech. *J. of Neurol., Neurosurgery & Psychiatry*, 38, 69-72.

17. Stemmer, B., et al. (1994). Production and evaluation of requests by right hemisphere brain-damaged individuals. *Brain & Lang.*, 47(1), 1-31.

Weylman, S.T., et al. (1989). Appreciation of indirect requests by left- and right-brain-damaged patients: The effects of verbal context and conventionality of wording. *Brain & Lang.*, 36, 580-591.

18. Foldi, N. (1987). Appreciation of pragmatic interpretation of indirect commands: comparison of right and left hemisphere brain-damaged patients. *Brain & Lang.*, 31. 88-108.

19. Brownell, H. (1988). Appreciation of metaphoric and connotative meaning by brain damaged patients. In C. Chiarello (Ed.), *Right Hemisphere Contributions to Lexical Semantics*. New York: Springer-Verlag, pp. 19-31.

MacKenzie, C., et al. (1997). The effects on verbal communication skills of right hemisphere stroke in middle age. *Aphasiology*, 11, 929-945.

Winner, E. & Gardner, H. (1977). The comprehension of metaphor in brain-damaged patients. *Brain*, 100, 717-729.

20. Van Lancker, D.R. & Kempler, D. (1987). Comprehension of familiar phrases by left- but not right-hemisphere damaged patients. *Brain & Lang.*, 32(2), 265-277.

Papagno, C. & Carporali, A. (2007). Testing idiom comprehension in aphasic patients. *Brain & Lang.*, 100, 208-220.

21. Brownell, H.H., et al. (1986). Inference deficits in right brain-damaged patients. *Brain & Lang.*, 27, 310-321.

Lehman-Blake, M.T. & Tompkins, C.A. (2001). Predictive inferencing in adults with right hemisphere brain damage. *J. of Speech, Lang. & Hearing Res.*, 44(3), 639-654.

Winner, et al. (1998).

22. Gardner, H., et al. (1983). Missing the point: The role of the right hemisphere in the processing of complex linguistic materials. In E. Perecman (Ed.), *Cognitive Processing in the Right Hemisphere*. New York: Academic Press.

23. Caplan, R. & Dapretto, M. (2001). Making sense during conversation: An fMRI study. *NeuroRep.*, 12, 3625-3632.

Rehak, A., et al. (1992). Sensitivity to conversational deviance in right-hemisphere-damaged patients. *Brain & Lang.*, 42, 203-217.

24. Zaidel, E., et al. (2002). Effects of right and left hemisphere damage on performance of the "right hemisphere communication battery." *Brain & Lang.*, 80, 510-535.

25. Faust, M. & Chiarello, C. (1998a). Sentence context and lexical ambiguity resolution by the two hemispheres. *Neuropsychologia*, 36(9), 827-835.

Faust, M. & Chiarello, C. (1998b). Constraints on sentence priming in the cerebral hemispheres: Effects of intervening words in sentences and lists. *Brain & Lang.*, 63, 219-236.

26. Burgess, C. & Simpson, G. (1988). Cerebral hemispheric mechanism in the retrieval of ambiguous word meanings. *Brain & Lang.*, 33, 86-103.

27. Coney, J. & Evans, K.D. (2000). Hemispheric asymmetries in the resolution of lexical ambiguity. *Neuropsychologia*, 38, 272-282.

28. Coney & Evans (2000). Quote on p. 280-281.

29. Faust & Chiarello (1998a). Quote on p. 832.

30. Peterson, S., et al. (1989). Positron emission tomographic studies of the processing of single words. *J. of Cog. Neurosci.*, 1, 153-170.

31. McCarthy, G. (1993). Echoplanar magnetic resonance imaging studies of frontal cortex activation during word generation in humans. *Proceedings of the Nat. Acad. of Sci. USA*, 90, 4952-4956.

32. Nakagawa, A. (1991). Role of anterior and posterior attention networks in hemispheric asymmetries during lexical decisions. *J. of Cog. Neurosci.*, 3, 313-321.

33. Posner, M. & Raichle, M. (1994). *Images of the Mind*. New York: Scientific American Library.

34. Burgess & Simpson (1988).
Titone, D. (1998). Hemispheric differences in context sensitivity during lexical ambiguity resolution. *Brain & Lang.*, 65, 361-394.

35. Meyer, M., et al. (2000). Neurocognition of auditory sentence comprehension: event related fMRI reveals sensitivity to syntactic violations and task demands. *Cog. Brain Res.*, 9, 19-33.

36. Bottinni, G., et al. (1994). The role of the right hemisphere in the interpretation of figurative aspects of language. A positron emission tomography activation study. *Brain*, 117, 1241-1253.

37. Rapp, A.M., et al. (2004). Neural correlates of metaphor processing. *Cog. Brain Res.*, 20, 395-402.

38. Giora (2000).
Schmidt, G.L., et al. (2007). Right hemisphere metaphor processing? Characterizing the lateralization process of semantic processes. *Brain & Lang.*, 100, 127-141.

39. Giora, R. (2007). Editorial: Is metaphor special? *Brain & Lang.*, 100, 111-114.

40. Coulson, S. & Van Petten, C. (2002). Conceptual integration and metaphor: an ERP study. *Memory & Cog.*, 30, 958-968.
Gagnon, L., et al. (2003). Processing of metaphoric and non-metaphoric alternative meanings of words after right- and left-hemispheric lesion. *Brain & Lang.*, 87(2), 217-226.
Kirchner, T.T. (2001). Engagement of right temporal cortex during processing of linguistic context. *Neuropsychologia*, 39, 798-809.

41. Duncan, J. & Owen, A. (2000). Common regions of the human frontal lobe recruited by diverse cognitive demands. *Trends in Neurosci.*, 23, 475-483.

42. Xu, J., et al. (2005). Language in context: emergent features of word, sentence, and narrative comprehension. *NeuroImage*, 25, 1002-1015 (quote on p. 1010).

43. Fletcher, P.C., et al. (1995). Brain systems for encoding and retrieval of auditory-verbal memory. An in vivo study in humans. *Brain*, 118, 401-416.

44. Ferstl, E.C., et al. (2005). Emotional and temporal aspects of situation model processing during text comprehension: An evenet-related fMRI study. *J. Cog. Neurosci.*, 17, 724-739.

45. Berns, G., et al. (1997). Brain regions responsive to novelty in the absence of awareness. *Sci.*, 276, 1272-1273.

46. Goldberg, E. & Costa, L.D. (1981). Hemispheric differences in the acquisition and use of descriptive systems. *Brain & Lang.*, 14, 144-173.

47. Fink, G.R., et al. (1999). The neural consequences of conflict between intention and the senses. *Brain*, 122, 497-512.

48. Zeki, S. & Marini, L. (1998). Three cortical stages of colour processing in the human brain. *Brain*, 121, 1669-1685.

49. Ross, E.D. (1984). Right hemisphere's role in language, affective behavior and emotion. *Trends in Neurosci.*, 7, 342-345.

50. Beeman, M., et al. (2000). Right and left hemisphere cooperation for drawing predictive and coherence inferences during normal story comprehension. *Brain & Lang.*, 71, 310-336.

Virtue, S., et al. (2006). Neural activity of inferences during story comprehension. *Brain Res.*, 1084, 104-114.

51. Thoma, P. & Daum, I. (2006). Neurocognitive mechanisms of figurative language processing—Evidence from clinical dysfunctions. *Neurosci. & Biobehav. Rev.*, 30, 1182-1205. Quote on p. 1189.

52. Thoma & Daum (2006). Quote in p. 1190.

53. Ozawa, F., et al. (2000). The effects of listening comprehension of various genres of literature on response in the linguistic area: an fMRI study. *Neurorep.*, 11, 1141-1143.

54. Goel, V. & Dolan, R.J. (2001). The functional anatomy of humor: segregating cognitive and affective components. *Nature Neurosci.*, 4, 237-238.

55. Coulson, S. & Severens, E. (2007). Hemispheric asymmetry and pun comprehension: When cowboys have sore calves. *Brain & Lang.*, 100, 172-187.

56. Coulson, S. & Williams, R.F. (2005). Hemispheric asymmetries and joke comprehension. *Neuropsychologica*, 43, 128-141.

Coulson, S. & Wu, Y.C. (2005). Right hemisphere activation of joke-related information: An event-related potential study. *J. of Cog. Neurosci.*, 17(3), 494-506.

57. Rodden, F.A., et al. (2001). Humour, laughter and exhilaration with functional magnetic resonance imaging (fMRI). *Neuroimage*, 13(6), 466.

58. Shibata, D. & Zhong, J. (2001). Humor and laughter: localization with fMRI. *Neuroimage*, 13(6), 476.

59. Bartolo, A., et al. (2006). Humor comprehension and appreciation: An fMRI study. *J. of Cog. Neurosci.*, 18(11), 1789-1798.

60. Watson, K.K., et al. (2007). Brain activation during sight gags and language-dependent humor. *Cerebral Cortex*, 17, 314-324.

61. Wild, B., et al. (2006). Humor and smiling: cortical regions selective for cognitive, affective, and volitional components. *Neurology*, 66, 887-893.

62. Mobbs, D., et al. (2003). Humor modulates the mesolimbic reward centers. *Neuron*, 40, 1041-1048.

63. Samson, A.C., et al. (2008). Cognitive humor processing: Different logical mechanisms in nonverbal cartoons—an fMRI study. *Soc. Neurosci.*, 3(2), 125-140.

64. Samson, et al. (2008). P. 132.

65. Samson, et al. (2008). Pp. 136-137.

66. Samson, A.C., et al., (2009). Neural substrates of incongruity-resolution and nonsense humor. *Neuropsychologia*, 47, 1023-1033.

67. Just, M., et al. (1996). Brain activation modulated by sentence comprehension. *Sci*, 383, 114-116.

68. von Economo, C. & Koskinas, G.N. (1929). *The Cytoarchitectonics of the Human Cerebral Cortex*. London: Exford University Press.

69. Allman, J., et al. (2002). Two phylogenetic specializations in the human brain. *Neuroscientist*, 8, 335-346.

Nimchinsky, E.A., et al. (1999). A neuronal morphologic type unique to humans and great apes. *Proceedings of the Nat. Acad. of Sci.*, 96, 5268-5273.

70. Watson, et al. (2007).

71. McGhee, P.E. (1976). Children's appreciation of humor: A test of the cognitive congruency principle. *Child Dev.*, 47, 420-426.

72. Brown, W.S., et al. (2005). Comprehension of humor in primary agenesis of the corpus callosum. *Neuropsychologia*, 43, 906-916.

Dennis, M. (1981). Language in a congenitally acallosal brain. *Brain & Lang.*, 12, 33-53.

Jeeves, J.A. & Temple, C.M. (1987). A further study of language function in callosal agenesis. *Brain & Lang.*, 32, 325-335.

Paul, L.K., et al. (2003). Communicative deficits in individuals with agenesis of the corpus callosum: Nonliteral language and affective prosody. *Brain & Lang.*, 85, 313-324.

Schieffer, B.M., et al. (1998). Deficits in complex problem solving in agenesis of the corpus callosum. *J. of the Int. Neuropsych. Society*, 4, 20.

73. Brown, et al. (2005).

74. Brown, et al. (2005). Quote on p. 914.

75. Fletcher, P.C., et al. (1995). Other minds in the brain: A functional imaging study of 'theory of mind' in story comprehension. *Cog.*, 57, 109-128.

Huettner, M.I.S. (1989). Regional cerebral blood flow (rCBF) in normal readers: Bilateral activation with narrative text. *Archives of Clin. Neuropsych.*, 4, 71-78.

Lechevalier, B., et al. (1989). Regional cerebral blood flow during comprehension and speech (in cerebrally healthy subjects). *Brain*, 37, 1-11.

St. George, M., et al. (1999). Semantic integration in reading: engagement of the right hemisphere during discourse processing. *Brain*, 122, 1317-1325.

76. Jung-Beeman, M. (2005). Bilateral brain processes for comprehending natural language. *Trends in Cog. Sci.*, 9(11), 512-518.

77. St. George, et al. (1999). Quote on p. 1322-1323.

78. Stephan, K.E., et al. (2003). Lateralized cognitive processes and lateralized task control in the human brain. *Sci.*, 301, 384-386.

79. Xu, et al. (2005). Quote on p. 1002.

80. Xu, et al. (2005).

81. Mason, R.A. & Just, M.A. (2007). Lexical ambiguity in sentence comprehension. *Brain Res.*, 1146, 115-127.

82. McGhee, P.E. Brain lateralization and humor: Will the funny hemisphere please light up? Journal article submitted for publication.

83. McGhee, P.E. (2002). *Understanding and Promoting the Development of Young Children's Humor.* Dubuque, IA: Kendall/Hunt.

McGhee, P.E. (2004). *Small Medium at Large.* Bloomington, IN: Author House.

84. McGhee, P.E. (1983). The role of arousal and hemispheric lateralization in humor. In P.E. McGhee & J.H. Goldstein (Eds.), *Handbook of Humor Research.* Vol. I. *Basic Issues.* New York: Springer-Verlag, pp. 13-37.

85. Wapner, et al. (1981).

86. Springer, S.P. & Deutsch, G. (1993). *Left Brain/Right Brain.* (Eds.), New York: W. H. Freeman (4th edition).

87. Bever, T.G. (1980). Broca and Lashley were right: Cerebral dominance is an accident of growth. In D. Caplan (Ed.), *Biological Studies of Mental Processes.* Cambridge, MA: MIT Press.

88. Fry, W.F., Jr. (2002). Humor and the brain: A selective review. *Humor: Int. J. of Humor Res.*, 15 (3), 305-333.

89. Alexander, M.P., et al. (1989). Frontal lobes and language. *Brain & Lang.*, 37, 656-691.

90. Baddeley, A.D. (1986). *Working Memory.* Oxford: Clarendon Press.

Goldman-Radic, P.S. & Friedman, H.R. (1991). The circuitry of working memory revealed by anatomy and metabolic imaging. In H.S. Levin, et al. (Eds.), *Frontal Lobe Function and Dysfunction.* New York: Oxford University Press, pp. 72-91.

91. Tulving, E., et al. (1994). Hemispheric encoding/retrieval asymmetry in episodic memory: positron emission tomography findings. *Proceedings of the Nat. Acad. of Sci..* 91, 2016-2020.

92. Stuss, D.T., et al. (1999). Consciousness, self-awareness and the frontal lobes. In S. Salloway, et al. (Eds.), *The Frontal Lobes and Neuropsychiatric Illness.* Washington, D.C.: American Psychiatric Press.

Wheeler, M.A., et al. (1997). Toward a theory of episodic memory: the frontal lobes and autonoetic consciousness. *Psych. Bull.*, 121, 331-354.

93. Goldberg & Costa (1981).

Goldberg, E. (2001). *The Executive Brain.* New York: Oxford University Press.

94. Grossberg, S. (1988). *Neural Networks and Natural Intelligence.* Cambridge: MIT Press.

95. Bever, T.G. & Chiarello, R.J. (1974). Cerebral dominance in musicians and nonmusicians. *Sci.*, 185 (150), 537-539.

96. Marzi, C.A. & Berlucchi, G. (1977). Right visual field superiority for accuracy of recognition of famous faces in normals. *Neuropsychologia*, 15 (6) 751-756.

97. Bever (1980).

Das, J.P., et al. (1979). *Simultaneous and Successive Cognitive Processes*. New York: Academic Press.

98. Iaccino, J.F. (1993). *Left Brain-Right Brain Differences*. Hillsdale, NJ: Lawrence Erlbaum Associates, quote on p. 31.

99. Anderson, B., et al., (1999). Anatomic asymmetries of the posterior superior temporal lobes: a postmortem study. *Neuropsychiat, Neuropsychol., & Behav. Neurol.*, 12, 247-254.

Gur, R.C., et al. (1980). Differences in distribution of gray and white matter in human cerebral hemispheres. *Sci.*, 207(4436), 1226-1228.

Watkins, K.E., et al. (2001). Structural asymmetries in the human brain: A voxel-based statistical analysis of 142 MRI scans. *Cereb. Cortex*, 11, 868-877.

100. Anderson, et al. (1999).

Gur, et al. (1980).

Sa, M.J., et al. (2007). Dentritic right/left asymmetries in the neurons of the human hippocampal formation: a quantitative Golgi study. *Archivos de Neuro-Psiquiatria*, 65(4), 1105-1113.

101. Hayes, T.L., & Lewis, D.A. (1995). Anatomical specialization of the anterior motor speech area: hemispheric differences in magnopyramidal neurons. *Brain & Lang.*, 49, 289-308.

102. Galuske, R.A.W. (2000). Interhemispheric asymmetries of the modular structure in human temporal cortex. *Sci.*, 289, 1946-1949.

103. Buxhoeveden, D.P., et al. (2001). Lateralization of minicolumns in human planum temporale is absent in nonhuman primate cortex. *Brain & Behav. Evol.*, 57, 349-358.

Seldon, H.L. (1982). Structure of human auditory cortex. III. Statistical analysis of dentritic trees. *Brain Res.*, 249, 211-221.

104. Galluske, R.A.W., et al. (1998). Patterns of long range intrinsic connectivity in different language related areas of the human cerebral cortex. *Soc. Neurosci. Abstr.*, 24, 15.

105. Galaburda, A. (1995). Anatomical basis of cerebral dominance. In R. Davidson & K. Hugdal (Eds.), *Brain Asymmetry*. Cambridge, MA: MIT Press.

106. Hutsler, J. & Galuske, R.A.W. (2003). Hemispheric asymmetries in cerebral cortical networks. *Trends in Neurosci.*, 26(8), 429-435.

107. Keller, S.S., et al. (2009). Broca's area: Nomenclature, anatomy, typology and asymmetry. *Brain & Lang.*, 109, 29-48. Quote on p. 45.

108. Azim, E., et al. (2005). Sex differences in brain activation elicited by humor. *Proceedings of the Nat. Acad. of Sci.*, 45, 16496-16501.

Bartolo, et al. (2006).

Mobbs, et al. (2003).

Shibata & Zhong (2001).

Watson, et al. (2007).

109. Shultz, W. (2002). Getting formal with dopamine and reward. *Neuron*, 36, 241-263.

110. Okun, M.S., et al. (2004). What's in a "smile?" Intra-operative observations of contralateral smiles induced by deep brain stimulation. *Neurocase*, 10, 271-279.

111. Mobbs, et al. (2003).

112. Bartolo, et al. (2006).

113. Clynes, M. (1978). *Sentics: The Touch of Emotions*. Garden City, NY: Doubleday.

114. Panksepp, J. & Gordon, N. (2003). The instinctual basis of human affect: affective imaging of laughter and crying. *Consciousness & Emot.*, 4, 197-205.

115. Burgdorf, J., et al. (2007). Neurobiology of 50-kHz ultrasonic vocalizations in rats: electronic mapping lesion and pharmacological studies. *Behav. Brain Res.*, 182(2), 274-283.

Burgdorf, J. & Panksepp, J. (2006). The neurobiology of positive emotions. *Neurosci. Biobehav. Rev.*, 30, 173-187.

116. Hernandez, L. & Hoebel, B.G. (1988). Food reward and cocaine increase extracellular dopamine in the nucleus accumbens as measured by microanalysis. *Life Sci.*, 42(18), 1705-1712.

Smith, G. (1995). Dopamine and food reward. In S. Fluharty, et al. (Eds.), *Progress in Psychobiol. & Physiol. Psych.* (vol. 16), New York: Academic Press, pp. 83-144.

117. Melis, M.R. & Argiolas, A. (1995). Dopamine and sexual behavior. *Neurosci. & Biobeh. Rev.*, 19(1), 19-38.

Pfaus, J.G., et al. (1995). Sexual activity increases dopamine transmission in the nucleus accumbens and striatum of female rats. *Brain Res.*, 693(1-2), 181-191.

118. Fibiger, H.C., et al. (1992). The neurobiology of cocaine-induced reinforcement. *Ciba Foundation Symp.*, 166, 96-111 [discussion on pp. 111-124]. Hernandez & Hoebel (1988).

119. Knutson, B., et al. (2001). Dissociation of reward anticipation and outcome with event-related fMRI. *Neurorep.*, 12(17), 3683-3687.

120. Hansen, S., et al. (1993). Interaction with pups enhances dopamine release in the ventral striatum of maternal rats: a microdialysis study. *Pharmacol. & Biochem. of Beh.*, 45(3), 673-676.

121. Blood, A.J. & Zatorre, R.J. (2001). Intensely pleasurable responses to music correlate with activity in brain regions implicated in reward and emotion. *Proceedings of the Nat. Acad. of Sci.*, 98(20), 11818-11823.

122. Vanderschuren, L.S., et al. (1997). The neurobiology of social play behavior in rats. *Neurosci. & Biobeh. Rev.*, 21(3), 309-326.

123. Azim, et al. (2005).

Breinigsville, PA USA
29 January 2010
231587BV00002B/1/P